Mechanisms of Tumor Immunity

BASIC AND CLINICAL IMMUNOLOGY

SERIES EDITORS: Stanley Cohen, University of Connecticut Health Center, Farmington. Robert T. McCluskey, Massachusetts General Hospital, Harvard Medical School

Mechanisms of Cell-Mediated Immunity

ROBERT T. MCCLUSKEY AND STANLEY COHEN, *Editors*

Mechanisms of Tumor Immunity

IRA GREEN, STANLEY COHEN, AND ROBERT T. MCCLUSKEY, *Editors*

Mechanisms of Tumor Immunity

EDITED BY

IRA GREEN

National Institute of Allergy and Infectious Diseases, National Institutes of Health

STANLEY COHEN

University of Connecticut Health Center, Farmington

ROBERT T. McCLUSKEY

Massachusetts General Hospital and Harvard Medical School

A WILEY MEDICAL PUBLICATION

JOHN WILEY & SONS   New York ● London ● Sydney ● Toronto

Library of Congress Cataloging in Publication Data:

Main entry under title:

Mechanisms of tumor immunity.

(Basic and clinical immunology)
Includes bibliographical references.
1. Cancer—Immunological aspects. 2. Cellular immunity. I. Green, Ira. II. Cohen, Stanley, 1937- II. McCluskey, Robert T. [DNLM: 1. Neoplasms—Immunology. QA200 M486]
RC268.3.M4   616.9′92′079   76-48047
ISBN 0-471-32481-7

Printed in the United States of America

10 9 8 7 6 5 4 3 2 1

Contributors

Atul K. Bhan, M.D.
Department of Pathology
Massachusetts General Hospital and
Harvard Medical School
Boston, Massachusetts 02114

Stanley Cohen, M.D.
Department of Pathology
University of Connecticut Health
Center
Farmington, Connecticut 06032

Ronald M. Ferguson, M.D.
Department of Surgery
University of Minnesota School of
Medicine
Minneapolis, Minnesota 55455

Ira Green, M.D.
Laboratory of Immunology
National Institute of Allergy and
Infectious Disease
National Institutes of Health
Bethesda, Maryland 20014

Karl Erik Hellström, M.D.
Ingegerd Hellström, M.D.
Department of Pathology
University of Washington Medical
School
Seattle, Washington 98195

Christopher S. Henney, Ph.D.
Department of Medicine
Johns Hopkins University
School of Medicine
Baltimore, Maryland 21205

Ronald B. Herberman, M.D.
Laboratory of Immunodiagnosis
National Cancer Institute
Bethesda, Maryland 20014

Martin S. Hirsch, M.D.
Department of Medicine
Massachusetts General Hospital and
Harvard Medical School
Boston, Massachusetts 02114

Elaine S. Jaffe, M.D.
Hematopathology Section
Laboratory of Pathology
National Cancer Institute
National Institutes of Health
Bethesda, Maryland 20014

Geraldine S. Konior, M.D.
Pediatric Oncology Branch
National Cancer Institute
National Institutes of Health
Bethesda, Maryland 20014

Brigid G. Leventhal, M.D.
Pediatric Oncology Branch
National Cancer Institute
National Institutes of Health
Bethesda, Maryland 20014

Robert T. McCluskey, M.D.
Department of Pathology
Massachusetts General Hospital and
Harvard Medical School
Boston, Massachusetts 02114

Charles F. McKhann, M.D.
Department of Surgery
University of Minnesota School of
Medicine
Minneapolis, Minnesota 55455

Sandra Ristow, Ph.D.
Department of Microbiology
University of Minnesota School of
Medicine
Minneapolis, Minnesota 55455

Jon R. Schmidtke, Ph.D.
Department of Surgery
University of Minnesota School of
Medicine
Minneapolis, Minnesota 55455

Richard L. Simmons, M.D.
Department of Surgery
University of Minnesota School of
Medicine
Minneapolis, Minnesota 55455

Osias Stutman, M.D.
Memorial Sloan-Kettering Cancer
Center
1275 York Avenue
New York, New York 10021

Peter A. Ward, M.D.
Department of Pathology
University of Connecticut Health
Center
Farmington, Connecticut 06032

Takeshi Yoshida, M.D.
Department of Pathology
University of Connecticut Health
Center
Farmington, Connecticut 06032

Preface

For many years it has been suspected that the immune system may be involved in host defense against neoplastic disease. This notion was based in part on early speculations as to the role of immunologic reactions in maintaining cellular homeostasis, in part on the rare but documented phenomenon of spontaneous regression of tumors, and in part on analogies with situations involving the response to infectious agents or organ transplants. It received support from the discovery of a wide variety of tumor-specific antigens and the development of a number of animal models in which immunization against such antigens modified the behavior of transplanted, induced, or spontaneous neoplasms. A large amount of clinical data has accumulated as well. It has become apparent in these studies that although all the known forms of immunologic reactivity may play a role, cell-mediated immunity seems to be of central importance in many cases, especially those involving solid tumors.

Thus, there is a wealth of evidence that the immune system can play a protective role in neoplastic disease. Nevertheless, in the natural state, tumors frequently grow in an unrelenting, lethal manner, often in the face of a demonstrable immune response against the tumor. This has had three major consequences, all potentially beneficial. First, it has prompted a reexploration and critical reevaluation of the concept of immune surveillance itself. Second, it has led to the investigation of a multiplicity of factors which serve to modify, limit, or regulate the immune response in tumor-bearing animals and man. Third, it has led to various procedures for increasing immunologic reactivity, either by specific immunization or by nonspecific methods of augmentation. Although these clinical approaches have had limited success to date, they provide a framework upon which our increasing knowledge of basic immunologic mechanisms can be applied in the future. Also, they have provided data which have given new insight into fundamental processes.

Although the above subjects have been discussed in reviews and workshops, no single comprehensive text has covered all these major advances. The present volume has been designed to provide such a treatise. It begins with a general overview of cell-mediated immunity and a critical discussion of the evidence for and against immune surveillance. Next, various mechanisms by which the immune system can destroy tumors are described. Following is a review of immunologic enhancement as a category of reactions that may limit the in vivo effectiveness of tumor immunity. With this as background, the evidence for the existence of tumor immunity in man is presented, followed by definitive reviews of the current status of immunotherapy, both in experimental models and in human disease. Subsequent chapters deal with the known neoplasms of the immune system and with the interactions of lymphocytes with oncogenic viruses. The final chapter reemphasizes the links between the immune and inflammatory systems and discusses in a speculative manner possible ways by which such interactions might be spontaneously inhibited in tumor-bearing subjects. Experimental circumvention of such inhibitory mechanisms might lead to new kinds of therapeutic approaches.

A certain amount of repetition has accompanied the attempt for broad coverage. This is unavoidable and in fact desirable. Although the available information in the literature is vast, it is finite. Each author has dipped into the same pool of published data, and it is not surprising that the cited references often overlap. Each has organized and interpreted a subset of these data to focus on his or her assigned topic, and the multiplicity of views that emerge provide a well-balanced summary of our present state of knowledge. We believe that this text should therefore prove of value to immunologists, students, and clinicians who have interest in any of the basic or applied aspects of tumor immunity.

September 1976

IRA GREEN
STANLEY COHEN
ROBERT T. McCLUSKEY

Contents

Mechanisms of Tumor Immunity

Chapter One

Cell-Mediated Reactions in vivo

ROBERT T. MCCLUSKEY AND ATUL K. BHAN

Department of Pathology, Massachusetts General Hospital and Harvard Medical School, Boston, Massachusetts

The acquisition of solid knowledge concerning tumor immunity began about two decades ago, when it was shown that inbred strains of mice were capable of rejecting syngeneic or autologous neoplasms against which they had previously been immunized (1). These and subsequent experiments led to the widely held concept that effective tumor immunity usually depends upon recognition of tumor-associated antigens on the surface of neoplastic cells and that tumor destruction is effected by mechanisms similar to those responsible for the destruction of solid tissue allografts—that is, primarily through cell-mediated mechanisms. Indeed, Thomas proposed that the "purpose" of the allograft rejection mechanism is to recognize and destroy autochthonous neoplasms at an early stage (2). However, the validity of this concept has been seriously challenged in recent years (3), and the possibility that the mechanisms of cell-mediated destruction observed in tumor models are of little relevance to most spontaneously arising tumors cannot be dismissed at present (see Chapter 2).

Although the first definitive studies on tumor immunity were carried out in vivo, in the past decade most investigations concerning cell-mediated destruction of neoplastic cells have been performed in vitro, which has resulted in the delineation of several distinct mechanisms (see Chapters 3 and 4). However, as noted by numerous authors, the relevance of many of these observations remains to be established.

This chapter will review the salient cellular events occurring in several forms of cell-mediated reactions (delayed hypersensitivity, cutaneous basophil hypersensitivity reactions (CBH), allograft reactions, and certain autoimmune diseases) and attempt to relate these findings to observations made in tumor immunity.

Cell-mediated reactions in vivo are by no means homogeneous in terms of the nature of the infiltrating cells, a fact that has not been sufficiently appreciated until recently. The most important factors known to influence the character of the reaction are: the species studied; the route and method of immunization (espe-

1

cially the use and type of adjuvant); the physical properties of the antigen; the site of challenge; the presence or absence of humoral antibodies; and the capacity of the host to mount an appropriate inflammatory response, in large part by virtue of possessing sufficient circulating leukocytes and by having the capacity to produce or release adequate mediator substances. (For more extensive discussion of these factors see refs. 4,5,6.)

The first form of cell-mediated reaction to be studied was delayed hypersensitivity response to bacterial antigens, in particular the tuberculin reaction (7). In the 1920s Dienes showed that similar reactions could be produced by purified proteins, such as ovalbumin (8). The criteria for defining these prototype delayed hypersensitivity reactions are relatively precise and well known. They are immunologically specific responses that develop in appropriately sensitized hosts following local (usually intradermal) challenge with antigen. Typical reactions occur in animals without demonstrable antibodies. The reactions appear several hours after challenge and then exhibit gradually increasing erythema and induration. Histologically a predominantly mononuclear infiltrate is seen. Reactivity can be transferred with lymphoid cells, but not with serum. The antigens used for elicitation of delayed reactions generally must possess carrier specificity, in contrast with most antibody-mediated reactions, which can be elicited with hapten-specific antigens (9). Lymphocytes from animals with delayed sensitivity can be stimulated by antigen in vitro to produce a variety of mediator substances (lymphokines). The carrier specificity requirements for such stimulation parallel those required for in vivo elicitation of delayed reactions (10).

Within the past two decades the concept of delayed hypersensitivity (or cell-mediated immune reactivity) has expanded to include responses to a variety of antigens other than bacterial products and purified proteins, including simple reactive chemicals (contact sensitivity), viruses, allografts, autologous antigens (in certain autoimmune diseases), and tumor-associated antigens (11). In most of these instances it has been possible to obtain convincing evidence for cell-mediated mechanisms. Nevertheless, it is not always possible to be certain that a given inflammatory reaction is cell mediated, especially when all criteria cannot be examined (as is true of studies in man). The histologic features, although characteristic, are not pathognomonic. Indeed, even certain lesions that are mediated by humoral antibodies can be characterized by an almost exclusively mononuclear cell infiltrate (12). Further, certain reactions with no known immunologic mechanisms can show mononuclear infiltrates. Perhaps the most conclusive evidence for a cell-mediated mechanism is the demonstration that typical reactivity can be transferred with lymphocytes but not with serum. Obviously, this type of evidence can be obtained only in experimental animals. The demonstration of in vitro correlates of cell-mediated immunity, employing the host's lymphocytes and the antigen in question, indicates that the host possesses cell-mediated reactivity against that antigen but does not prove that this accounts for reactions observed in vivo. Clearly, new methods are needed for the recognition of cell-mediated reactions in vivo.

CELLULAR EVENTS IN PATHOGENESIS OF CELL-MEDIATED REACTIONS

The principal cellular events occurring in experimental animals developing cell-mediated reactions of a variety of types can be summarized as follows. The immunizing antigen, administered in the form of a local injection (usually with adjuvant), or as a graft, stimulates the proliferation of T lymphocytes, including some with specificity against the immunizing antigen, especially in the draining lymph nodes. Many of these newly formed T lymphocytes enter the circulation, which provides them with the opportunity to come in contact with the immunizing antigen at the site of challenging injection of antigen, tumor, or graft implantation or in an organ containing a tissue-specific antigen. Contact between a few specifically sensitized cells and antigen causes these cells to produce and release a group of lymphokines. These mediators bring about an inflammatory reaction, in which most of the leukocytes exhibit no specificity toward the responsible antigen.

Published descriptions of the kinds of cells present in cell-mediated reactions vary widely; this appears to stem not only from the heterogeneity of these reactions but also differences in terminology, differences in emphasis and bias of the authors, variations in techniques used to study the cells, and the growth of knowledge (which is still far from complete) on the nature and identifying characteristics of subpopulations of mononuclear cells.

Knowledge concerning important aspects of cell-mediated reactions—changes in draining lymph nodes, effector mechanisms, and the nature and immunologic specificity of the mononuclear cells in infiltrates—are best considered in the light of experiments carried out with several types of reactions. These topics will be discussed separately after brief descriptions of the major morphologic features of the individual types of reactions.

DELAYED HYPERSENSITIVITY REACTIONS

Delayed hypersensitivity reactions have been most thoroughly studied in human beings, guinea pigs, and rats. In experimental animals immunization usually involves local injections of microgram amounts of antigen (often modified in some way so as to reduce antigenicity) (9) in complete Freund's adjuvant. The reactions are generally elicited by intradermal injection, although they can be evoked in other sites. The rate of development varies in different species; it is fastest in guinea pigs and slowest in man. The most consistent microscopic feature, as seen at 24–48 hours, is perivascular accumulation of mononuclear cells, some of which extend into the dermis as a more diffuse infiltrate. Dermal lymphatics are often dilated and packed with mononuclear cells. Mononuclear cells can also be seen invading the epidermis, a feature which is much more conspicuous in contact reactions than in reactions elicited by intracutaneous injections. In severe reactions necrosis may be found. Two additional features have recently been recognized as characteristic of delayed reactions: one, the accumulation of substantial amounts of fibrin in the interstitial tissue, which accounts for the induration typical of these reactions (13); two, changes in the microvasculature, characterized by endothelial cell damage with lumenal narrowing and later by irregular basement membrane thickening (14).

Identification of many of the mononuclear cells is not possible on morphologic grounds. In particular, large lymphocytes cannot always be distinguished from monocytes. Small lymphocytes have been estimated to account for about 20–25% of the cells in the guinea pig and rat (15). The remaining mononuclear cells have been considered to be mostly either mononuclear phagocytes (monocytes and macrophages), especially in the rat, or large ("activated") lymphoctyes (15). However, in man only a small percentage of the mononuclear cells in tuberculin or contact reactions can be identified on morphologic grounds as mononuclear phagocytes (16). Additional information concerning the nature of the infiltrating cells in experimental animals has been obtained in transfer studies; as will be discussed, these findings indicate that a large proportion of the cells are mononuclear phagocytes.

It is worth noting that delayed reactions elicited by ordinary protein antigens do not usually exhibit features generally considered to be characteristic of granulomatous reactions—i.e., lesions with nodular accumulation of epitheloid cells and giant cells—although such changes have been described in late tuberculin reactions (17). However, it has recently been shown that delayed sensitivity to purified proteins *can* express itself to some extent in the form of a granulomatous response, if the antigen is coupled to sepharose beads prior to challenging injection (18,19), probably because the antigen is rendered nondiffusible and nondegradable. In addition, granulomas can be induced by poorly understood immunologic mechanisms, even in situations where no immunologic factors appear to be operating.

Neutrophils are present to some degree in most delayed reactions. Although generally seen only in small numbers, they are sometimes quite numerous, especially in the rat and the mouse. Their presence can sometimes be attributed to irritating properties of the challenging material, to a response to necrosis, or to an antibody-mediated component of reaction. Nonetheless, they cannot all be explained away in this fashion, and they must be considered an intrinsic part of some reactions.

Eosinophils are sparse or lacking in most delayed reactions but in some instances are quite numerous, especially after several days. Moreover, eosinophils often appear in abundance in reactions elicited by repeated injections of antigen in the same skin site in guinea pigs with delayed sensitivity (retest reaction) (20). One mechanism that could account for eosinophil accumulation involves a combined effect of cell-mediated and humoral immunity. Thus, it has been shown that lymphocytes from sensitized guinea pigs can be stimulated by antigen to produce a substance that interacts with immune complexes of the same specificity to generate a potent eosinophil chemotactic factor (21). Production of eosinophil chemotactic factors may also be mediated by mechanisms related to anaphylaxis (22).

Basophils are found in only small numbers or are lacking in "classical" delayed hypersensitivity reactions in guinea pigs but are quite numerous in so-called cutaneous basophil hypersensitivity reactions (CBH). The participation of basophils and mast cells in cell-mediated reactions is discussed below.

A few plasma cells may be seen after several days in tuberculin reactions, or in delayed reactions elicited by purified proteins, obviously reflecting the stimulation of antibody production. However, plasma cells are never numerous, as they are in the later stages of active Arthus reactions (23).

Thus, all kinds of leukocytes participate in delayed hypersensitivity reactions. The percentage of cell types varies in different reactions and can be modified by several factors, including the concomitant presence of antibodies.

CUTANEOUS BASOPHIL HYPERSENSITIVITY IN THE GUINEA PIG

In the past several years Dvorak and his associates have recognized and analyzed the important participation of basophils in cell-mediated reactions to a variety of antigens and have coined the term cutaneous basophil hypersensitivity (CBH)* to describe basophil-rich reactivity seen in guinea pigs (24).

CBH can be reproducibly induced in guinea pigs by immunization with a variety of soluble proteins administered locally in microgram amounts in saline or in *incomplete* Freund's adjuvant. Reactivity is maximal at 6 or 7 days, before the appearance of detectable antibody. The reactions begin several hours after challenge, with perivascular accumulations of mononuclear cells. However, basophils soon appear in considerable numbers, and at 24–48 hours generally comprise 20–60% of the infiltrating cells. It is important to realize that basophils cannot be reliably identified in ordinary histologic preparations; their recognition in CBH reactions depended upon improved morphologic techniques, involving fixation and embedding of the type used in electron microscopy (25).

The possibility that appreciable numbers of basophils in the infiltrate exhibit specificity toward the eliciting antigen, which might occur as the result of coating by homocytotrophic γ_1 antibody, has been excluded (26).

Some of the basophils in the infiltrate exhibit degranulation. Using tracers that can be followed by electron microscopy, Dvorak et al. (27) demonstrated that basophils can release their granule contents by means of a previously unrecognized vesicular transport mechanism, which permits prolonged release of mediators over a span of hours or days, rather than in the explosive fashion seen with anaphylactic reactions.

CBH reactions lack the deposits of fibrin in the intervascular dermis that are characteristic of delayed reactions and for this reason do not exhibit induration (13).

Basophil-rich reactivity can be induced in guinea pigs not only against soluble protein antigens but also against a variety of antigens of greater biologic importance, such as contact allergens, vaccinia virus, allogeneic tumor cells, schistosomes, and skin allografts (28). Indeed, in guinea pigs the usual type of cell-mediated reactivity against these agents appears to be basophil-rich reactivity, rather then the classical type of delayed sensitivity. Moreover, in contrast to the reactivity induced against soluble protein antigens, which is evanescent and typically wanes when humoral antibodies appear, basophil-rich reactivity persists indefinitely following immunization with contact-sensitizing antigens and allogeneic tumors (28).

Basophil-rich hypersensitivity is considered to be a form of cell-mediated immunity, since reactivity can be transferred with lymph node cells (29). However, the exact nature of the responsible lymphocytes and their relation to those that mediate "classical" delayed hypersensitivity have not been established.

Moreover, several reports of transfer of reactivity with serum have appeared (30,31,32). Although further confirmation of these reports would be desirable,

---

*This was perhaps an unfortunate choice, since similar reactions can be elicited in sites other than the skin.

they are sufficiently provocative to suggest that mechanisms other than direct initiation of CBH reactions by sensitized cells is possible. The claim that 7s γ_1 antibody is responsible awaits confirmation (32).

BASOPHIL-RICH CELL-MEDIATED REACTIONS IN MAN

The distinction between CBH and delayed hypersensitivity reactivity in man is not as clear-cut as in the guinea pig. Thus, although a variety of cell-mediated reactions in man show appreciable numbers of basophils (16), their numbers are quite variable, even in similar types of reactions. Moreover, they are never seen in such large numbers as may be found in guinea pigs. Nearly all contact reactions studied in man have been found to contain abundant basophils. They are seen in smaller numbers in many tuberculin reactions. Basophils have also been seen in early renal allografts (34).

Mast cells appear to play an active role in cell-mediated reactions in man. In early reactions degranulated cells are often found. In later stages hyperplasia may occur (14,16). It has been postulated that basophils and mast cells are supplementary cells with similar or identical functions and that participation of these cells in delayed reactions is governed by their relative frequency in a given species and by the duration of the reaction, with mast cells assuming a greater role late in the reaction (35).

ALLOGRAFT REACTIONS

Rejection of first-set allografts of solid tissues or organs is believed to result from cell-mediated mechanisms. The composition of the infiltrate varies, depending on such factors as the nature of the graft, the species studied, the state of sensitization of the recipient, and the time of examination of the graft. The infiltrate is best studied in experimental animals, where the reactions need not be modified by immunosuppressive agents.

The most extensive studies of the infiltrating cells have been carried out in skin, kidney, and cardiac allografts. Interpretation of skin grafts is complicated to some extent because of the nonspecific inflammatory component that occurs during vascularization. However, the cells invading the graft itself and especially the epidermis can be considered to be the result of the rejection process. The majority of these cells have been described as lymphocytes, or as cells intermediate in morphology between lymphocytes and monocytes (36). Early first-set renal allografts are characterized by infiltration of the interstitium, tubules, and blood vessel walls by mononuclear cells, the great majority of which appear to be small or large lymphocytes, as judged in histologic sections or by electron microscopy (37). In this respect the infiltrates differ from those of cutaneous delayed reactions, where other leukocytes, especially mononuclear phagocytes, are often prominent. However, some macrophages are seen in early renal allografts, as well as appreciable numbers of basophils in some instances. In older grafts increasing numbers of plasma cells and mast cells may be found. With the onset of necrosis, the number of macrophages increases and numerous neutrophils appear.

Tilney et al. (38,39) have performed careful and revealing studies on the cells infiltrating recently transplanted cardiac heterotopic allografts in rats. On the basis of examination of histologic preparations and of cells isolated from 4- to 5-day-old grafts they estimated that about 75% were lymphocytes, 15–20% macrophages, and the rest neutrophils. The time of appearance and distribution of macrophages were studied after intravenous injections of India ink. Lymphocytes appeared early, followed by increasing numbers of carbon-bearing macrophages. At day 4, many of the macrophages were seen in groups in areas of frank necrosis, although scattered isolated cells were also seen. With complete rejection, which occurred at 6 to 7 days, macrophages and neutrophils appeared in very large numbers.

AUTOIMMUNE LESIONS

Certain tissue-specific autoimmune diseases (adrenalitis, thyroiditis, encephalitis) are characterized by a predominantly mononuclear cell infiltrate. Since in some instances these diseases can be transferred with lymph node cells but not with serum, the lesions are presumed to result from cell-mediated mechanisms. However, it also appears that at least in some cases humoral antibody is responsible for such lesions, since they can be transferred with serum, if it is collected at the appropriate time after immunization or after removal of the target organ (40,41). Furthermore, in certain tissue-specific autoimmune lesions, plasma cells and germinal centers are conspicuous, especially in the later stages (42), providing evidence for an antibody-mediated component. Moreover, eosinophils are numerous in some lesions and probably result from a combined effect of cell-mediated immunity and humoral antibodies (43). Accordingly, the conclusion that a given tissue-specific autoimmune lesion results principally or entirely from cell-mediated mechanisms can be considered fairly secure only if transfer can be accomplished with cells and not with serum. These criteria are met in certain models, including autoimmune encephalitis and adrenalitis induced in rats by immunization with tissue-specific antigen in Freund's adjuvant plus pertussis (44). The infiltrates in these lesions typically contain very high percentages (up to 80%) of lymphocytes, as judged morphologically, and thus resemble early allografts but differ from cutaneous delayed reactions.

Basophils have apparently not been described in autoimmune lesions, but it is not known whether they have been looked for by appropriate techniques.

NATURE AND SPECIFICITY OF THE MONONUCLEAR CELLS
IN CELL-MEDIATED REACTIONS

Because of the limitations of morphologic criteria applied to tissue sections, other methods have been used to investigate the nature of the cells in infiltrates. Autoradiographic tracer studies have been of value, especially in transfer studies, and in experiments in which populations of lymphoid cells were labeled in situ (45,46). As described in Chapter 11, techniques are available that permit identification of mononuclear phagocytes and B lymphocytes in tissue sections.

Although these techniques have been used to study a variety of infiltrates (including those in and around neoplasms), they apparently have not been systematically used to study the prototype delayed hypersensitivity reactions.

Another method is to prepare suspensions of cells present in the infiltrate and to study their properties in vitro. This offers the advantage of permitting identification of certain surface markers that cannot be detected in tissue sections and makes it possible to study certain functional properties of the cells in vitro. There is at present no way of identifying various subpopulations of T or B cells in inflammatory infiltrates except by isolating cells from the lesions and studying their functional properties.

This type of investigation presents several problems, however. For one thing, with scanty infiltrates and small lesions it may not be possible to obtain sufficient cells. Furthermore, it is possible that the recovered cells are selected populations, rather than representative of all the infiltrating cells. In addition, some of the recovered cells may be circulating cells or cells from lymphoid tissue normally present in the region (as in the alimentary tract), rather than cells that have emigrated. In addition, treatment with enzymes, which are often used in the preparations of cell suspensions, may modify surface markers. Moreover, topographic relationships between cells are destroyed.

It has been clearly shown in autoradiographic studies that the majority of mononuclear cells in delayed reactions are not specifically sensitized to the eliciting antigen. Thus, when delayed sensitivity is transferred from immunized to normal guinea pigs with labeled lymph node cells, only small numbers of labeled cells are found in reactions in the recipient (47). In contrast, when prospective recipients are given repeated injections of ^{3}H thymidine for several days prior to transfer of unlabeled lymph node cells, the great majority of cells at the test site are labeled.

These findings show that most of the cells are of recipient origin and that they are derived from precursors that are rapidly and continuously dividing in the absence of specific antigenic stimulation. Mononuclear phagocytes are probably the most numerous circulating mononuclear cells with these properites, although a certain percentage of T cells and even of B cells possess these attributes. Studies by Lubaroff and Waksman have provided evidence that the majority of mononuclear cells in tuberculin reactions in rats are derived from bone marrow and are therefore probably monocytes (48,49). It is also possible, however, that some of the bone-marrow-derived cells are B lymphocytes. In a study of cells recovered from acutely rejecting cardiac allografts in rats, Tilney et al. concluded that about 15–25% of cells were macrophages and about 75% were lymphocytes (38,39).

Even among the lymphocytes in cell-mediated reactions, the great majority do not appear to be sensitized to the eliciting antigen. This has been shown in experiments in which labeled lymph node cells (almost all of which are lymphocytes) obtained from donors stimulated with a particular antigen have been traced into reactions elicited by the same antigen and by unrelated antigens. In most such studies no difference in the percentage of labeled cells was found between the two sites (4). However, in some reports more labeled cells were found in the appropriate site, although usually not to an impressive degree. Studies of this sort have been performed in animals with delayed or contact reactions, allografts, and autoimmune lesions (4). This lack of consistent or marked preferential accumulation shows that lymphocytes of many specificities are present in the infiltrates.

It has been found that the lymphocytes which emigrate at sites of cell-mediated reactions, and certain other kinds of inflammatory reactions, are predominantly large, newly formed cells with a limited capacity to recirculate (4,44). Although, as discussed later, both T and B cells may exhibit these properties, probably most such cells are T lymphocytes. Cells of this type have been variously referred to as large lymphocytes, immunoblasts, inflammatory lymphocytes, or large pyroninophilic cells.

There is relatively little direct information concerning the proportions of T and B lymphocytes present in cell-mediated reactions. A priori, one might conclude that most or nearly all of the lymphocytes are T cells, since there is abundant evidence that they initiate the reactions. However, it is possible that a few such cells trigger the influx of other kinds of lymphocytes (as they clearly do for monocytes and basophils). Although the available evidence suggests that T cells do predominate, at least in early stages of reactions, there are certain problems involved in the interpretation of the published data. In a study of early tuberculin reactions in rats Williams and Waksman (50) found that the majority of cells were T cells; however, the cells were teased from the lesions, and it is possible that the recovered population was not representative of the cells in the infiltrate. In a similar study on recently transplanted cardiac allografts in rats, Tilney et al. reported finding that Ig-bearing mononuclear cells, thought to be B lymphocytes, made up 35 to 47% of the mononuclear cells collected (38,39). The rest of the lymphocytes were presumed to be T cells. In an immunofluorescence study employing a specific anti-T lymphocyte Balch et al. (51) concluded that the majority of cells in early rat renal allografts are T cells. However, it is questionable whether cell surface markers can be reliably detected on individual cells in tissue sections by immunofluorescence. Electron-microscopic examination of early renal allografts and skin grafts has also provided evidence for a great preponderance of T cells, since in early allografts cells with free ribosomes are described, and only at later stages are there frequent cells with conspicuous endoplasmic reticulum, characteristic of differentiating and mature plasma cells (37,52).

Using another approach, the capacity of purified populations of lymphocytes to emigrate into recently applied skin allografts in mice has been studied (53). Spleen cells were separated on immunoabsorbent columns into highly purified populations of T and B cells, labeled in vitro with ^{3}H uridine and injected intravenously into mice with 7-day-old skin iso- and allografts. The animals were sacrificed 24 hours later and studied by autoradiography. Following transfer of either whole spleen cells or T cells, large numbers of labeled cells were found in the cellular infiltrate of allografts, whereas extremely few were seen in the isografts. In contrast, following transfusion of B cells, almost no labeled cells were detected in either the allografts or the isografts. B cells did, however, home to lymphoid tissue, indicating that their capacity to migrate in vivo had not been abolished by the isolation procedures.

These findings show that T cells emigrate in appreciable numbers in recent skin grafts and thus possess the characteristic of the inflammatory lymphocytes described above. However, they do not exclude the possibility that "null" cells (which may include immature B cells and other mononuclear cells) also accumulate in the graft in large numbers. If this is so, maturation of some of these cells into antibody-secreting cells could account for the presence of Ig-bearing lymphocytes and plasma cells, which are often found in allografts in large numbers. Findings made in chickens with spontaneous autoimmune thyroiditis clearly show that bursal cells can behave as inflammatory lymphocytes (54). This model is of particular interest, since it represents a tissue-specific autoimmune disease in which B cells are mainly responsible for the tissue damage (55,56). It has not been shown that all inflammatory lymphocytes (whether T or B) have been recently stimulated to proliferate by antigens; some may be virgin cells.

EFFECTOR MECHANISMS IN CELL-MEDIATED REACTIONS

Relatively little direct evidence has been obtained from in vivo experiments concerning final effector pathways in most forms of cell-mediated reactions. In the case of destruction of a graft or neoplasm, or the elimination of invading microorganisms, the end point is fairly definite. However, when dealing with delayed or contact reactions, or autoimmune disease, whose "purpose" is not clear, we usually judge the operation of effector mechanisms by whether or not the reactions reach their full expression.

Several approaches have been used to investigate effector mechanisms operating in vivo. Many of these are extensions of methods used to identify the nature of the infiltrating cells. One way to obtain useful information is through morphologic analysis of the cells in the infiltrate. Obviously, if one cell is present in overwhelming numbers, it becomes a prime candidate to be the main effector cell, especially if in vitro studies support the postulated role (for example, of tumor or allogeneic cell destruction). Morphologic studies also permit analysis of the topographic relationship of cells in the reaction; frequent association between a possible effector cell and its target supports an in vivo role of such a cell.

Another approach to the analysis of effector mechanisms operating in vivo is to prepare suspensions of cells present in the infiltrate and to study their functional capabilities in vitro. The advantages and disadvantages of this method have been discussed above.

In vivo cell functions can also be investigated in transfer experiments. It was, of course, through transfer of tuberculin sensitivity by cells that Landsteiner and Chase (57) first directly revealed the basic nature of cell-mediated immunity. The development in recent years of methods for the preparations of purified populations of mononuclear cells has increased the usefulness of this approach. In transfer studies a clear distinction should be made between cells that *initiate* the reaction and those that function as final effector cells. There is little doubt that cell-mediated reactions are initiated by T lymphocytes, following contact with antigen. (This, in fact, has essentially become the definition of cell-mediated reactions.) A wealth of indirect evidence supports this view, chiefly observations indicating that animals or human beings lacking T lymphocytes fail to display normal delayed reactivity. Recently more direct evidence has been obtained by the demonstration that purified populations of T lymphocytes can initiate delayed-type hypersensitivity reactions in inbred guinea pigs following intradermal injection in the presence of antigen (local transfer reaction) (58). Under similar circumstances purified populations of B lymphocytes fail to produce significant reactions (59).

To some extent the role of individual cell types can be further delineated by transfer of purified populations of cells into irradiated recipients, since such animals cannot contribute appreciable numbers of circulating leukocytes to the reaction. In particular, the relative importance of lymphocytes and mononuclear phagocytes has been explored in this fashion.

Transfer of cell-mediated reactivity can be attempted either systemically or locally. Systemic transfer offers the advantage of providing the recipient with circulating cells capable of reacting with allografts, tumor cells, or other antigens in much the same fashion as host circulating cells. On the other hand, very large numbers of donor cells are often required and the results are generally not quantifiable. The local transfer of cells and antigens or tumor cells (60) requires far fewer cells and can be more easily used to obtain quantitative data. However, even though carried out in vivo, certain local conditions can be created that are very unlikely to occur under ordinary conditions, as for example through the use of very high ratios of effector to target cells.

The source of the donor cells used in local transfer experiments (and in in vitro studies of cell-mediated immunity) is of importance. The use of lymph node and spleen cells can be objected to on the grounds that many of the cells would not normally enter the circulation and therefore could not ordinarily participate in inflammatory reactions. Moreover, spleen and lymph nodes from different locations contain varying proportions of subpopulations of lymphocytes (suppressor cells, etc). Thoracic duct lymph provides a source of cells en route to the circulation, which can therefore legitimately be expected to participate in inflammatory reactions. Populations of peritoneal exudate cells contain a high proportion of inflammatory lymphocytes but also frequently contain activated macrophages, which may influence local reactions.

One area about which considerable information *has* been obtained in vivo concerns the mechanisms by which animals defend themselves against bacteria that can survive and grow within cells. Much of this knowledge has been obtained in studies on mice or rats infected with Listeria monocytogenes (61). In brief, after appropriate immunizing procedures the animals develop resistance to infection by virtue of acquisition of macrophages with increased antibacterial mechanisms. These "activated" macrophages can destroy with increased efficiency not only Listeria but other intracellular organisms as well. The production of these macrophages in turn depends upon interaction between specifically sensitized T lymphocytes and Listeria organisms, which results in the secretion of mediators capable of activating macrophages (61).

There is reason to believe that this type of interaction between sensitized lymphocytes and macrophages occurs locally in sites of infection. As noted earlier, the newly formed large lymphocytes that develop in large numbers during immunization are the kind of lymphocytes with the propensity to emigrate in areas of inflammation (inflammatory lymphocytes); in fact, such cells have been recovered in substantial numbers from the peritoneal cavities of animals infected with Listeria (61).

Macrophages also appear to be required for the full development of classical cutaneous delayed hypersensitivity reactions. Lubaroff and Waksman found that irradiated recipient rats do not exhibit delayed reactivity following transfer of lymph node cells unless they are also given a source of bone marrow, presumably because this supplies a source of monocytes (48,49). Similar results have been obtained in experiments dealing with the transfer of autoimmune encephalitis and adrenalitis in rats (44).

In contrast, there is evidence that at least in some cases allograft destruction does not require macrophages but can be accomplished directly by lymphocytes. Lubaroff (62) has reported that renal allografts in irradiated thymectomized rats are rejected following transfusions of lymph node cells, even though the animals are not supplied with bone marrow cells. The conclusion that lymphocytes alone can destroy renal allografts is given further support by the morphologic features; as noted above, early allografts show a very high percentage of lymphocytes, and these cells are seen invading blood vessels and renal tubules. Further, lymphocytes capable of exerting a cytopathic effect on cells of donor origin have been isolated in substantial numbers from renal (63) and cardiac allografts (38). These findings provide impressive evidence for a crucial in vivo role of target cell destruction by T lymphocytes. However, even if this mechanism is primary, damage to blood vessels leading to ischemic necrosis probably accounts for the final destruction of much of the graft. Furthermore, certain experiments in mice suggest that lymphocytes alone are unable to reject skin allografts and presumably require the cooperation of macrophages (64).

As noted above, in all types of cell-mediated reactions numerous lymphocytes are found with specificities directed against antigens not present in the reactions; the function of these cells is unknown.

The role of the basophils in cell-mediated reactions has not been clarified, but it seems likely that release of mediators through the process of slow degranulation referred to above may be important. Neutrophils in cell-mediated reactions presumably perform their usual well-known functions. The role of eosinophils remains obscure.

This discussion of effector mechanisms has been mainly concerned with the relatively simple question as to which types of cells are effector cells. Definition of how the cells exert their effects, in biochemical terms, will probably have to come principally from in vitro studies (see Chapter 3).

ALTERATIONS IN DRAINING LYMPH NODES IN THE IMMUNE RESPONSE

There is considerable interest in the possible relationship between changes in draining lymph nodes and the prognosis in certain forms of human cancer, especially breast cancer. Accordingly, the major changes occurring in lymph nodes during immune responses will be considered.

With antigens that stimulate primarily or exclusively a cell-mediated response (skin allografts, certain tissue-specific antigens, contact sensitization), the principal change is a dramatic increase in lymphocytes in paracortical areas (thymus-dependent areas). This increase results from two processes: lymphocyte trapping (i.e., arrest of circulating lymphocytes within the node and prevention of egress of cells from the node) and proliferation of cells within the node. The former process accounts for most of the increase in the size of the node during the first 2 days (65). At least with several nonliving antigens that have been studied, trapping has been found to be a transient phenomenon.

From a teleological point of view, trapping is desirable, since it brings to the node a large population of cells of differing specificities, thus facilitating the selection of a minor population of antigen specific reactive lymphocytes. However, by arresting cells in the node it may prevent them from participating in inflammatory responses elsewhere.

After day 2, marked proliferation of lymphocytes in paracortical areas begins, resulting in the appearance of large dividing cells. These cells (large lymphocytes, large pyroninophilic cells, immunoblasts) are characterized ultrastructurally by free ribosomes but no endoplasmic reticulum. It seems highly unlikely that most of these cells are specifically reactive with the immunizing antigens, although there appear to be no data directly bearing on this point. The fate of the large dividing cells has been studied by autoradiography following labeling with ^{3}H thymidine, either by systemic or local administration (46). The labeled cells within the node become progressively smaller, until after several days they assume the appearance of small lymphocytes. However, many of the large labeled cells leave the node via the efferent lymphatics to enter the circulation. As described earlier, these are the inflammatory lymphocytes that emigrate at sites of cell-mediated (and certain other) inflammatory reactions, whether elicited by the immunizing antigen or by an unrelated antigen.

Immunization with antigens that exclusively stimulate antibody production, such as pneumococcal polysaccharides, leads to the formation of germinal centers and the appearance of numerous plasma cells in the medullary cords. Obviously, most immunizing procedures result in the stimulation of both cell-mediated and humoral immunity, so that a combination of changes is seen. Eosinophils often appear in large numbers in nodes draining a site of antigen injection in guinea pigs (65); their accumulation may depend upon combined effects of humoral and cell-mediated immunity (21). Mast cells may be also seen in large numbers in stimulated nodes.

A feature that has been described in human lymph nodes draining tumor-bearing areas consists of accumulation of numerous macrophages in the sinuses (sinus histiocytosis); this does not appear to be a direct manifestation of the immune response and probably results from presentation to the node of large amounts of highly phagocytosable material, such as intact cells or nondegradable material, which could be either immunogenic or nonimmunogenic. Similarly, the development of granulomas in lymph nodes is not necessarily a direct reflection of cell-mediated immunity, although, as noted earlier, with certain nondegradable and nondiffusible antigens a cell-mediated response may take on a granulomatous appearance. Complete Freund's adjuvant may result in granulomas in draining nodes and distant sites.

CELL-MEDIATED TUMOR IMMUNITY IN EXPERIMENTAL ANIMALS

The evidence favoring the conclusion that immunologically mediated destruction of solid autochthonous or syngeneic transplantable neoplasms generally depends on cell-mediated mechanisms is substantial, including the fairly convincing demonstration in several systems that it ultimately depends on T cells (67). However, it appears that the responses to tumors are as heterogeneous as other forms of cell-mediated reactions, indicating that the mechanisms responsible for tumor destruction are diverse. Much of the current thinking about mechanisms of cell-mediated tumor destruction are understandably based on in vitro studies. It has become commonplace to say that the in vitro observations need not reflect what occurs in vivo; yet this problem can hardly be exaggerated. For one thing, the demonstration in vitro that a single component of a system involved in tumor destruction is intact may be irrelevant to what happens in vivo, if other essential components are defective. Lymphocytes from guinea pigs bearing large tumor masses may be responsive to stimulation by tuberculin (PPD) in vitro (68), even though such animals are unable to develop a delayed reaction following cutaneous challenge with PPD. Moreover, such animals do not develop effective tumor immunity following transfer of lymphocytes from appropriately sensitized donors. Presumably the animals are deficient in certain immunologically nonspecific factors that are required for the full expression of the delayed inflammatory response and for the destruction of at least some types of neoplasms.

Another example of an in vitro finding that may be irrelevant in some instances is the demonstration that lymphocytes from a tumor-bearing host are stimulated by preparations of tumor tissue; if the responsible antigens are intracellular antigens, whose release from areas of tumor necrosis provided the immunogenic stimulus, this could not be the basis for tumor cell destruction (Chapter 7). In addition, lymph node cells or circulating leukocytes with the capacity to destroy neoplastic cells, as shown in vitro, could not be expected to have much effect on the fate of neoplasms in vivo unless these cells actually infiltrate the tumor (although perhaps some effects could be mediated by lymphokines produced elsewhere; see Chapter 4).

The remainder of this chapter will examine certain patterns of cellular reactions to experimental and human neoplasms, as they relate to the types of cell-mediated reactions reviewed above.

RELATION OF TUMOR IMMUNITY AND ALLOGRAFT IMMUNITY

Cell-mediated tumor destruction is often equated with allograft rejection. Although this interpretation may be basically correct, certain differences between the two situations are obvious. First, there is a major difference in the "efficiency" of the two reactions; thus, whereas grafts of normal allogeneic tissue are almost invariably destroyed, unless special pains are taken to preserve them, most established neoplasms exhibit progressive growth, even in situations where it can be shown that the host has developed cell-mediated immunity against tumor-associated antigens. Similarly, whereas adoptive transfer of lymphocytes from immune donors leads to destruction of established allografts (in tolerant animals), this rarely succeeds in the case of established neoplasms, although when immune lymphocytes are incubated with tumor cells, or administered to animals shortly before or after challenge with a small number of tumor cells, tumor growth is often prevented (69,70). The most frequently offered explanations for these differences are that tumor-associated antigens are "weaker" than transplantation antigens, that tumors present an increasing and sometimes tolerizing antigenic load, and that blocking factors are formed that prevent cell-mediated mechanisms from achieving their goal. Further, as noted by Gershon, the blood vessels in tumor tissue do not possess tumor-associated antigens and thus fail to provide a stimulus to the lymphocytes circulating through the tumor (71). Whether any or all of these explanations fully account for the differences between allograft rejection and tumor destruction remains to be seen.

It should also be remembered that not all allografts are destroyed by cell-mediated mechanisms. Humoral antibodies can account for destruction of isolated cells (leukocytes, erythrocytes) and under special circumstances for rejection of organs (hyperacute rejection of the kidney). Similarly, it seems that humoral antibodies may account for destruction of isolated tumor cells (leukemia, ascites tumors). It is generally agreed that humoral antibodies either do not affect solid tumors or actually protect them from cell-mediated destruction. However, it is possible that isolated tumor cells that break off from solid neoplasms to enter the circulation may be destroyed by humoral antibodies; this could be an important mechanism in the prevention of metastases (72), although even in the case of such isolated cells, blocking by antibodies or complexes might promote their growth. (For a discussion of the possible role of thymus-independent immune mechanisms in surveillance, see Chapter 2.)

In instances where cell-mediated mechanisms are responsible for tumor destruction, the relative importance of macrophages, lymphocytes, or other leukocytes may vary widely from one tumor or allograft to another.

NATURE AND FUNCTIONAL PROPERTIES OF THE INFILTRATING MONONUCLEAR CELLS IN EXPERIMENTAL TUMORS

It has long been recognized that tumors frequently evoke a mononuclear cell infiltrate. However, many of the reported descriptions are concerned with allogeneic-tumor transplants, whose relevance to autochthonous or syngeneic transplantable tumors is questionable at best. In some such tumors lymphocytes are considered to be the predominant cell, whereas in others macrophages or plasma cells are most numerous (73,74). Spontaneously arising tumors in animals (and in man) often show no mononuclear infiltrate.

There appear to be relatively few detailed descriptions on the nature of the mononuclear cells infiltrating autochthonous or syngeneic transplantable tumors. Moreover, the type of autoradiographic tracer studies that have revealed information about the origin and nature of cells in various cell-mediated reactions have apparently not been performed with tumors.

One group of syngeneic transplantable tumors that have been extensively studied from the point of view of reacting cells are hepatomas induced in inbred strain-2 guinea pigs by the carcinogen diethylnitrosamine. These tumors can be grown either in solid form or as ascites tumors. Several antigenically distinct tumor lines are available, and systemic tumor resistance is readily induced by immunization with tumor cells alone or in combination with mycobacteria. Immunity appears to be cell mediated.

The nature of the inflammatory reaction to hepatoma cells injected into the skin of sensitized and control animals has been the subject of a careful morphologic study (75). In nonimmunized animals a mild reaction developed, characterized by lymphocytes, macrophages, neutrophils, and rare basophils; the tumor cells remained viable. In contrast, injections of tumor cells into immunized animals resulted in a delayed-type inflammatory reaction, associated with tumor cell necrosis, and a more intense inflammatory infiltrate, which included substantial numbers of basophils.

In order to gain information about the mechanisms of tumor cell destruction, anatomic relationships between tumor cells and inflammatory cells were studied. In control reactions close associations between tumor cells and inflammatory cells were rarely seen. In contrast, in specifically sensitized animals, where the ratio of inflammatory cells to tumor cells was much higher, such associations were frequent. A large percentage of the tumor cells in sensitized animals were damaged or dead by morphologic criteria, and such cells were commonly surrounded by apparently viable neutrophils and macrophages containing phagocytosed material. In some instances individual lymphocytes were found in relation to apparently viable or damaged tumor cells, but this was quite uncommon. A striking feature of reactions in sensitized animals was the frequency of intimate associations between basophils and tumor cells, both viable and necrotic. Some of the basophils had disintegrated and others exhibited degranulation.

The findings in this study fail to provide evidence for an appreciable role of direct tumor cell killing by lymphocytes in vivo, although because of the limitations of static studies this mechanism cannot be entirely discounted. Moreover, the observations suggest a role of basophils in tumor destruction. However, no in vitro model of tumor cell destruction by basophils has been described.

In a different kind of morphologic study, Russell and Cochrane (76) investigated the relationship between the progressive or regressive behavior of a murine (Moloney) tumor and the extent and nature of the inflammatory infiltrate. Tumors were induced in adult and neonatal mice by intramuscular injections of a cultured Moloney sarcoma line. In neonates, injection of either 10^4 or 10^6 cells resulted in progressively growing neoplasms, whereas in adult mice only the larger inoculum resulted in progressive tumor growth; in adults given the smaller dose the tumors generally underwent regression, beginning at 12–14 days. At 2–3 days all tumors were infiltrated with neutrophils. By 12–14 days tumors in adult mice showed a mononuclear infiltrate, which was at first localized to the periphery of the tumors. In tumors that regressed, the infiltrates extended throughout the neoplastic tissue, whereas in progressive tumors the mononuclear infiltrate remained confined to peripheral portions of the tumor and later disappeared. In either progressing or regressing tumors, neoplastic cells in close association with mononuclear cells often showed evidence of damage. Tumors in neonates, which almost always progressed, never developed an appreciable mononuclear infiltrate. The findings provide impressive evidence for a direct role of infiltrating mononuclear cells in the destruction of the neoplasm. In a later study these authors presented evidence that macrophages were the principal effector cells in the tumor destruction (77).

Another approach to the identification of the cells infiltrating neoplasms is to analyze the cells present in cell suspensions prepared from the tumor, obtained through either mechanical disruption or enzymatic digestion. The advantages and drawbacks of this method have been discussed above. Even the limited studies of this type that have been carried out indicate that different effector mechanisms may operate in different tumors.

Particularly revealing studies have been performed by Haskill et al. on the nature of the cells infiltrating a murine mammary adenocarcinoma (78), a rat fibrosarcoma (79), and a tumor induced by murine sarcoma virus (80). The mouse adenocarcinoma, which originated as a spontaneous tumor in DBA/2 mice and is carried in tissue culture (T1699 line), was found to grow progressively (in about 80% of hosts) when injected subcutaneously at 10^5 cells in the shoulder fat pad area, but to regress spontaneously when similarly injected into the abdominal area. Histologic examination of tumors undergoing regression at day 7 showed numerous inflammatory cells in the region of the tumors, most of which appeared to be lymphocytes and eosinophils. Studies on enzymatically dispersed cells revealed the inflammatory cells to consist of T lymphocytes, Fc receptor-bearing cells, and eosinophils. The functional capacity of the cells was investigated by the colony inhibition assay. Cells recovered from 14-day-old tumors exhibited cytotoxic effects that were specific for the T1699 tumor cells. The majority of the effector cells had the appearance of small lymphocytes and carried Fc receptors but did not have detectable T or B cell markers. The population of T lymphocytes recovered from the tumor displayed no cytotoxic effects in colony inhibition tests.

In contrast, in methylcholanthrene-induced sarcomas in rats (79), macrophages were found to be the predominant cell, and these cells were capable of inhibiting tumor growth in vitro. Similar studies on tumors induced by murine sarcoma virus in C57Bl/6 mice indicated that at least two types of effector cells are found in the infiltrate, specific cytotoxic T cells and macrophages (80).

A number of studies have also been performed on the tumoricidal properties of lymph node cells, circulating cells, or peritoneal exudate cells at various stages in tumor-bearing animals (81). Obviously, unless such cells can be shown to be actually present at the tumor site, it cannot be concluded that they have any role in elimination of the neoplasm. Nevertheless, such studies may reveal potential effector mechanisms and when employed in the local transfer system, as developed by Winn (60), may provide some information about how effective these mechanisms can be in vivo.

Simes et al. (82) have used the local transfer system to investigate the cellular basis for immunity against a syngeneic transplantable methylcholanthrene induced sarcoma in CBA/J mice. Peritoneal exudate cells from tumor-bearing mice had a marked tumor-suppressive effect. If adherent cells were removed, the resulting lymphocyte-enriched population still exhibited a marked tumor-suppressive effect in normal recipients but was effective in irradiated recipients only with very high lymphocyte-tumor cell ratios. However, when whole peritoneal exudate cells were added back to the lymphocyte-enriched population, the mixture was effective in suppressing tumor growth in irradiated recipients, even at low ratios. These results indicate that lymphocytes alone can destroy the tumor cells but are much more effective if they can initiate an amplifying mechanism involving macrophages.

Howell et al. (67) employed the local transfer technique to study the cells involved in the destruction of a syngeneic transplantable Simian virus 40-induced murine tumor. It was found that T cells were the only kind of donor cells required to bring about tumor rejection. The data also indicated that the transferred donor T cells were by themselves not capable of tumor destruction but required help from recipient cells, probably either macrophages or B cells.

Aside from evidence that cell-mediated reactivity directed against tumor-associated antigens can bring about destruction of neoplasms bearing these antigens, certain observations indicate that delayed hypersensitivity reactions elicited by unrelated antigens can exert deleterious effects on tumor cells present at the inflammatory site. This has been shown in studies on guinea pigs injected with different non-cross-reacting hepatoma cell lines (83). All of the following observations were made in animals sensitized to line 1 cells: the injection of line 1 cells intracutaneously resulted in a delayed-type hypersensitivity response, in which the tumor cells were killed; injection of line 7 cells alone did not elicit an appreciable inflammatory reaction, and the tumor exhibited progressive growth; injection of line 1 and line 7 cells together resulted in a delayed-type reaction in which *both* types of cells were destroyed. Possibly analogous observations have been made in man by Klein (84), who has shown that elicitation of contact reactions to DNCB and other sensitizing agents often results in destruction of epidermal neoplasms, using concentrations that produce no apparent injurious effect on normal skin. Immunologically nonspecific mechanisms capable of tumor destruction also can be brought into play by BCG or *C. parvum*.

LYMPH NODE CHANGES IN TUMOR-BEARING ANIMALS

There appear to be relatively few descriptions of alterations occurring in lymph node draining sites bearing autochthonous or syngeneic tumors. Russell and Cochrane (76) studied popliteal and lumbar nodes draining a transplanted syngeneic Moloney sarcoma. Within 2 weeks the nodes became several times larger than the contralateral nodes. They gradually diminished in size following regression of sarcomas but remained enlarged in mice with progressive tumors until the onset of severe cachexia. Histologically, proliferation of both T and B cells elements was evident, with enlargement of paracortical areas, germinal center formation, and appearance of numerous plasma cells in medullary cords. Similar changes have been observed in nodes draining a syngeneic transplantable sarcoma in rats (72).

In studies on the allogeneic transplantable lymphoma in hamsters, Gershon et al. (85) noted massive proliferation of macrophages (sinus histiocytosis) in the draining nodes of animals' nonmetastasizing tumors; this did not occur in hamsters with metastasizing tumors. The sinus histiocytosis apparently resulted from ingestion of tumor cells reaching the node. Although the changes occurred in response to an allogeneic tumor, the findings may be relevant to those sometimes found in nodes draining autochtonous neoplasms, as in human breast cancer.

LYMPHOCYTE TRAPPING IN LYMPH NODES OF TUMOR-BEARING ANIMALS

The implantation of irradiated syngeneic sarcoma cells in the hindquarter region of rats has been shown to result in the appearance of numerous large lymphocytes (immunoblasts) in the thoracic duct lymph (TDL), reflecting the production and release of these cells from draining lymph nodes (86). When viable tumor cells were used, the number of TDL immunoblasts increased initially but soon fell to normal levels (72). If the tumor was excised, a sudden increase in the TDL immunoblasts was seen.

It was concluded that the tumor mass interfered with the release of immunoblasts from the node, preventing these cells from traveling to tumor sites where they might have engaged in tumor cell destruction. This hypothesis may provide an explanation for the observation (87) that rats with primary, chemically induced sarcomas are not able to reject an autograft of their own tumor given subcutaneously as long as some of the primary tumor remains in situ. If, however, the entire primary tumor is removed, the autograft is rejected.

As an illustration of the complexity of immunologic reactions to tumors, it is of interest to compare the findings just described with certain observations made by Gershon et al. (85) in studies on an allogeneic transplantable lymphoma. This tumor arose spontaneously in a random-bred hamster and has been maintained by serial transfer. The tumor elicits a classical state of "concomitant" immunity: tumor-bearing animals can reject considerably larger numbers of tumor cells than normal animals. Immunity can be transferred with lymphoid cells, but not with serum, to normal syngeneic hamsters. The surprising finding has been made that if the primary tumor is resected, the host's immunity sometimes disappears rapidly and is associated with the appearance of distant metastases. This has been shown to result from an effect of specific suppressor cells.

MONONUCLEAR CELL INFILTRATION OF HUMAN NEOPLASMS

That human cancers are often associated with a mononuclear cell reaction has been recognized for over a century. However, the presence, intensity, and nature of the infiltrate is quite variable from one neoplasm to another, and many neoplasms evoke no reaction. Although interest in this subject has heightened in the past few years with the development of knowledge of tumor immunity, there have been surprisingly few systematic studies on the nature of reacting cells, employing the best techniques available for the identification of mononuclear cells.

When a tumor exhibits an inflammatory reaction, we can ask whether this simply reflects a response to infection, especially in ulcerated tumors, or is secondary to necrosis. However, in many instances these explanations do not appear to apply, and the infiltrate may be considered to represent a response to viable tumor cells.

The possible prognostic implications of mononuclear cell infiltration of human tumors has recently been reviewed by Underwood (88). In most of the published reports a correlation between the presence of an infiltrate and prolonged survival has been claimed, especially in breast cancer. In contrast, in an international study of breast cancer, no clear evidence of a correlation between mononuclear cell reaction and prognosis was found (89). This is perhaps not surprising, in view of the fact that the nature of the infiltrate was not carefully analyzed, and even its distribution with respect to the tumor was not studied. One report claimed that diffuse (rather than peripheral) mononuclear cell infiltration or the presence of perivenous infiltrates showed a good correlation with survival (90). In certain types of neoplasms, in particular germinal cell tumors (seminoma and dysgerminomas) and medullary cell carcinomas of the breast, extensive infiltration of the tumor by mononuclear cells is often seen. These malignant tumors in general have a relatively good prognosis, and the claim has been made that among these tumors those showing the most intense infiltrate are associated with the longest survival. In contrast, undifferentiated carcinomas of the nasopharynx (lymphoepitheliomas) evoke an intense mononuclear response and yet behave as highly malignant tumors.

Primary malignant melanomas often show intense mononuclear cell infiltration. This is of particular interest in view of the demonstration that peripheral lymphocytes from some patients with melanoma can destroy autologous or allogeneic melanoma cells in vitro (9) and because of the wide variations in prognosis among melanomas. However, there are conflicting reports as to whether the presence or intensity of infiltrates in or around primary melanomas indicates a relatively favorable prognosis (88). Nevertheless, it has been claimed that spontaneous regression of malignant melanoma is associated with pronounced mononuclear cell infiltration (92). Mononuclear infiltrates are reportedly less conspicuous around metastatic melanomas, suggesting a diminished host response (93). Halo nevi, which are spontaneously regressing pigmented moles, are typically accompanied by a dense inflammatory infiltrate (94,95).

Nature of Inflammatory Cells Infiltrating Human Tumors

There have been relatively few investigations on the nature of the inflammatory cells seen in association with human neoplasms. Even careful morphologic studies are scarce. In most tumors lymphocytes have been considered to be the predominant type of cell, as judged histologically. Plasma cells or macrophages are conspicuous in some tumors. Eosinophils have been observed in certain neoplasms, notably in some cases of Hodgkin's disease and in instances of gastric or colonic carcinoma, and in the latter two neoplasms it has been claimed to indicate a better-than-average prognosis (96). Basophils have not often been noted, but there does not appear to have been any systemic search for these cells, using appropriate techniques. However, in a study of the response to frozen sections of breast cancer, using the skin-window technique of Rebuck, basophils were sometimes found to accumulate in considerable numbers, and this was said to correlate with limited disease, with "lymphoreticular" infiltration of the tumor, and with sinus histiocytosis of draining nodes (97).

Reports have recently begun to appear on the characterization of mononuclear cells through identification of surface markers, either in tissue section or in suspension (see Chapter 11). Edelson et al. (98) reported that most of the mononuclear cells infiltrating cells in six primary melanomas and three halo nevi lacked surface characteristics of B cells or mononuclear phagocytes, as studied in frozen sections, suggesting the cells were T lymphocytes. Direct demonstration of T cells through sheep cell rosetting was accomplished in two melanomas, where sufficient tissue allowed the preparation of cell suspensions from the tumor. In contrast, the majority of cells infiltrating melanoma metastases in four patients were identified as histiocytes (mononuclear phagocytes) by their IgG receptors and ultrastructural appearance. In another study on the surface characteristics of suspensions of cells from cutaneous neoplasms Claudy et al. found a higher percentage of B cells than T cells in primary melanomas; in the same study T cells were found to predominate in basal and squamous cell carcinomas (99). In a report in which cells in suspension were examined for surface Ig, as a B cell marker, wide variations in the percentage of Ig positive cells were found in colon cancer (8–64%) and in malignant melanomas (14–47%) (100). When cell suspensions are prepared from sites that normally contain lymphoid tissue, such as the gastrointestinal tract, care must be taken to avoid contamination by these cells.

There have been very few attempts to assess the functional capabilities of the mononuclear cells infiltrating human tumors. In one study, cells obtained from malignant melanoma and colonic carcinoma showed no in vitro response against cultured tumor cells (100). However, in more than half of these patients the circulating lymphocytes did show cytotoxic activity. Negative lymphocytoxicity to autologous cancer cells was said to be associated with diffuse stromal infiltrates of lymphocytes, while positive cytotoxicity was associated with perivascular aggregation of small lymphocytes.

ALTERATIONS IN LYMPH NODES DRAINING HUMAN NEOPLASMS

There have been numerous studies of changes in lymph nodes draining human tumors, and attempts have been made to relate the findings to prognosis. Several factors might result in stimulation of such nodes aside from tumor-associated antigens, namely intact tumor cells reaching the nodes, material released from necrotic foci, including intracellular antigens capable of stimulating an autoimmune response, and infectious agents, especially in ulcerated tumors.

Attempts have been made to relate the morphologic findings in the lymph nodes to the nature of antigen reaching the lymph node; it has been suggested that sinus histiocytosis is due to intact tumor cells, and germinal center formation to necrosis (101).

Several studies have been concerned with changes in the axillary lymph nodes in patients with carcinoma of the breast. A variety of patterns have been described; no consistent correlation has been found between the changes and prognosis. Sinus histocytosis has been considered by some to be a favorable prognostic sign (90); others have failed to find such a correlation (102,103). It has been claimed that germinal center formation is associated with a poor prognosis, even when sinus histocytosis is present (101). Black and his co-workers (90) have also claimed that there is a good correlation between the extent of sinus histocytosis and the intensity of the inflammatory response to autologous breast cancer tissue, as judged by the skin-window technique (97).

Recently Tsakralides et al. (104) attempted to correlate survival with nodal morphologic features other than sinus histocytosis in 227 patients with breast cancer. A lymphocytic-predominant pattern was interpreted as evidence of response by the cells in the predominantly thymus-dependent cortex and was associated with high survival rates, whereas lymphocytic depletion was associated with poor prognosis. Germinal center predominance and unstimulated lymph nodes were seen in those with intermediate survival. However, Fisher et al. in a similar study found no such correlation (105).

CONCLUDING REMARKS

In the present chapter we have attempted to highlight the complexity and heterogeneity of the cellular events occurring in cell-mediated reactions in vivo, including reactions that develop in association with neoplasms. It should be clear that generalizations about effector mechanisms in various forms of reactions are unwarranted. Although much of the recent progress in cell-mediated immunity has come from in vitro studies, it is obvious that much more information is needed about their relevance to in vivo situations. Moreover, even though a large amount of information has been gathered lately about various aspects of tumor immunity, relatively little attention has been devoted to the inflammatory cells directly participating in reactions that develop in and around neoplasms. Studies are beginning to appear on the nature and functional properties of such cells; it is reasonable to hope that these investigations will help elucidate further the ways in which the immune system can bring about the destruction of neoplasms.

REFERENCES

1. Foley, E. J., *Cancer Res.* **13,** 835 (1953).
2. Thomas, L., in *Cellular and Humoral Aspects of the Hypersensitive State* (H. Sherwood Larence, ed.), Hoebner-Harper, New York, 1959, p. 529.
3. Moller, G., and Moller, E., *J. Nat. Cancer Inst.* **55,** 755 (1975).
4. McCluskey, R. T., and Leber, P. D., in *Mechanisms of Cell-Mediated Immunity* (R. T. McCluskey and S. Cohen, eds.), John Wiley & Sons, New York, 1974, p. 1.
5. Vassalli, P., and McCluskey, R. T., in *Inflammation, Immunity and Hypersensitivity* (H. Z. Movat, ed.) Harper & Row, New York, 1971, p. 179.
6. Dvorak, H. F., in *The Inflammatory Process* (B. W. Zweifach, L. Grant, and R. T. McCluskey, eds.), Academic Press, New York, 1974, p. 291.
7. Zinser, H., *J. Exp. Med.* **34,** 495 (1921).
8. Dienes, L., *J. Immunol.* **17,** 531 (1929).
9. Gell, P. G. H., and Benacerraf, B., *Adv. Immunol.* **1,** 319 (1961).
10. David, J. R., Lawrence, H. S., and Thomas, L., *J. Immunol.* **93,** 279 (1964).
11. Waksman, B. H., in *Ciba Foundation Symposium on Cellular Aspects of Immunity*, Churchill, London, 1960, p. 280.
12. Van Zwieten, M., Bhan, A. K., McCluskey, R. T., and Collins, A. B., *Am. J. Pathol.* **83:**531 (1976).
13. Colvin, R. B., Johnson, R. A., Mihm, M. C., Jr., and Dvorak, H. F., *J. Exp. Med.* **138,** 686 (1973).
14. Dvorak, A. M., Mihm, M. C., Jr., Dvorak, H. F., *Lab. Invest.* **34,** 179 (1976).
15. Kosunen, T. U., Waksman, B. H., Flax, M. H., and Tihen, W. S., *Immunology* **6,** 276 (1963).
16. Dvorak, H. F., Mihm, M. C., Jr., Dvorak, A. M., Johnson, R. A., Manseau, E. J., Morgan, E., and Colvin, R. B., *Lab. Invest.* **31,** 111 (1974).
17. Turk, J. L., *Delayed Hypersensitivity*, 2nd ed., North Holland American Elsevier, Amsterdam-Oxford-New York, 1975.
18. Unanue, E., and Benacerraf, B., *Am. J. Pathol.* **71,** 349 (1973).
19. Kasdon, E. J., and Schlossman, S. F., *Am. J. Pathol.* **71,** 365 (1973).
20. Arnason, B. G., and Waksman, R. H., *Lab. Invest.* **12,** 737 (1963).
21. Cohen, S., and Ward, P. A., *J. Exp. Med.* **133,** 133 (1971).
22. Kay, A. B., Stechschulte, D. J., and Austen, K. F., *J. Exp. Med.* **133,** 602 (1971).

23. Gell, P. G. H., and Hinde, I. T., *Int. Arch. Allergy Appl. Immunol.* **5,** 23 (1954).

24. Richerson, H. B., Dvorak, H. F., and Leskowitz, S. J., *Exp. Med.* **132,** 546 (1970).

25. Dvorak, H. F., Dvorak, A. M., Simpson, B. A., Richerson, H. B., Leskowitz, S., and Karnovsky, M. J., *J. Exp. Med.* **132,** 558 (1970).

26. Dvorak, H. F., and Dvorak, A. M., *Clin. in Hematol.* **4,** 651 (1975).

27. Dvorak, A. M., Mihm, M. C., and Dvorak, H. F., *J. Immunol.* **116,** 687 (1976).

28. Dvorak, H. F., and Dvorak, A. M., in *Progress in Immunology* II, Vol. 3 (L. Brent and E. J. Holborous, eds.), Amsterdam, 1974, p. 171.

29. Dvorak, H. F., Simpson, B. A., Bast, R. C., Jr., and Leskowitz, S., *J. Immunol.* **107,** 138 (1971).

30. Askenase, P. W., *J. Exp. Med.* **138,** 1144 (1973).

31. Askenase, P. W., Haynes, J. D., Tauben, D., and Debernardo, R., *Nature* **256,** 52 (1975).

32. Haynes, J. D., Kantor, F. S., and Askenase, P. W., *Fed. Proc.* **34,** 1039 (1975). (Abstract)

33. Dvorak, H. F. and Mihm, M. C., Jr. *J. Exp. Med.* **135:**235, (1972).

34. Colvin, R. B., and Dvorak, H. F., *Lancet* **1,** 212 (1974).

35. Dvorak, H. F., and Dvorak, A. M., *Human Pathol.* **3,** 454 (1972).

36. Weiner, J., Spiro, D., and Russell, P. S., *Am. J. Pathol.* **44,** 319 (1964).

37. Porter, K. A., in *Pathology of the Kidney,* 2nd ed. (R. H. Heptinstall, ed.) Little, Brown and Co., Boston, 1974, p. 977.

38. Tilney, N. L., Strom, T. B., MacPherson, S. G., and Carpenter, C. B., *Transplantation* **20,** 323 (1975).

39. Tilney, N. L., Strom, T. B., MacPherson, S. G., and Carpenter, C. B., *Surgery* **79,** 209 (1976).

40. Rose, N. R., and Kite, J. H., in *First International Convocation on Immunology* (N. R. Rose and F. Milgrom, eds.), S. Karger, Basel, 1969, p. 247.

41. Vladutui, A., and Rose, N. R., *Science* **174,** 1137 (1971).

42. Flax, M. H., in *Cellular Interactions in the Immune Response* (S. Cohen, G. Cudkowicz, and R. T. McCluskey, eds.), S. Karger, Basel, 1970.

43. Cohen, S., Ward, P. A., and Bigazzi, P. E., in *Mechanisms of Cell-Mediated Immunity* (R. T. McCluskey, S. Cohen, eds.), John Wiley & Sons, New York, 1974.

44. Werdelin, O., and McCluskey, R. T., *J. Exp. Med.* **133,** 1242 (1971).

45. Werdelin, O., McCluskey, R. T., and Witebsky, E., *Lab. Invest.* **23,** 144 (1970).

46. Werdelin, O., Wick, G., and McCluskey, R. T., *Lab. Invest.* **25,** 279 (1971).

47. McCluskey, R. T., Benacerraf, B., and McCluskey, J. W., *J. Immunol.* **90,** 466 (1963).

48. Lubaroff, D. M., and Waksman, B. H., *J. Exp. Med.* **128,** 1425 (1968).

49. Lubaroff, D. M., and Waksman, B. H., *J. Exp. Med.* **128,** 1437 (1968).

50. Williams, R. M., and Waksman, B. H., *J. Immunol.* **103,** 1435 (1969).

51. Balch, C. M., Wilson, C. B., Lee, S., Feldman, J. D., *J. Exp. Med.* **138,** 1584 (1973).

52. Andre-Schwartz, J., *Blood* **24,** 113 (1964).

53. Bhan, A. K., Reinisch, C. L., Levey, R. H., McCluskey, R. T., and Schlossman, S. F., *J. Exp. Med.* **141,** 1210 (1975).

54. Moorhead, J. W., Kite, J. H., McCluskey, R. T., Werdelin, O., and Wick, G., *Clin. Immunol. and Immunopath.* **2,** 160 (1974).

55. Wick, G., Kite, J. H., Cole, R. K., and Witebsky, E., *J. Immunol.* **104,** 45 (1970).

56. Wick, G., Kite, J. H., Cole, R. K., and Witebsky, E., *J. Immunol.* **104,** 54 (1970).

57. Landsteiner, K., and Chase, M. W., *Proc. Soc. Exp. Biol. Med.* **49,** 688 (1942).

58. Jaffer, A. M., Jones, G., Kasdon, E. J., Schlossman, S. F., *J. Immunol.* **111,** 1268 (1973).

59. Stashenko, P. P., Bhan, A. K. Schlossman, S. F., and McCluskey, R. T. (in preparation).

60. Winn, H. J., *J. Immunol.* **86,** 228 (1961).

61. North, R. J., in *Mechanisms of Cell-Mediated Immunity* (R. T. McCluskey and S. Cohen, eds.), John Wiley & Sons, New York, 1974, p. 185.

62. Lubaroff, D. M., *J. Exp. Med.* **138,** 331 (1973).

63. Strom, T. B., Tilney, N. L., Carpenter, C. B., and Busch, G. J., *N. Eng. J. Med.* **292,** 1257 (1975).

64. Giroud, J. P., Spector, W. G., and Willoughby, D. A., *Immunology* **19,** 857 (1970).

65. Werdelin, O., Foley, P. S., Rose, N. R., and McCluskey, R. T., *Immunology* **21,** 1059 (1971).

66. Cohen, S., Vassalli, P., Benacerraf, B., and McCluskey, R. T., *Lab. Invest.* **15,** 1143 (1966).

67. Howell, S. B., Dean, J. H., Esber, E. C., and Law, L. W., *Int. J. Cancer* **14,** 662 (1974).

68. Bernstein, I. D., and Rapp, H. J., *Fed. Proc.* **30,** 245 (1971).

69. Alexander, P., *Prog. Exp. Tumor Res.* **10,** 22 (1968).

70. Katz, D. H., Ellman, L., Paul, W. E., Green, I., and Benacerraf, B., *Cancer Res.* **32,** 133 (1972).

71. Gershon, R. K., in *Immunologic Parameters of Host- Tumor Relationships* (D. W. Weiss, ed.), Vol. 3, Academic Press, New York, 1975, p. 198.

72. Alexander, P., and Hall, J. G., *Adv. Cancer Res.* **13,** 1 (1970).

73. Gorer, P. A., *Adv. in Immunol.* **1,** 345 (1961).

74. Diamandopolous, G. T., *Arch. für die gesamte Viruss forschung.* **22,** 108 (1967).

75. Dvorak, H. F., Dvorak, A. M., and Churchill, W. H., *J. Exp. Med.* **137,** 751 (1973).

76. Russell, S. W., and Cochrane, C. G., *Int. J. Cancer* **13,** 54 (1974).

77. Russell, S. W., Doe, W. F., and Cochrane, C. G., *J. Immunol.* **116,** 164 (1976).

78. Haskill, J. S., Yamamura, Y., and Radov. L., *Int. J. Cancer* **16,** 798 (1975).

79. Haskill, J.. S., Proctor, J. W., and Yamamura, Y., *J. Nat. Cancer Inst.* **54,** 387 (1975).

80. Holden H. T., Haskill, J. S., Kirchner, H., and Herbermann, R. B. *J. Immunol.* **117,** 440 (1976).

81. Lamon, E. W., Wigzell, H., Klein, E., Anderson, B., and Skurzak, H. M., *J. Exp. Med.* **137,** 1472 (1973).

82. Simes, R. J., Kearney, R., and Nelson, D. S. *Immunol.* **29,** 343 (1975).

83. Rapp, H. J., in *Immunological Parameters of Host-Tumor Relationships,* Vol. II (D. W. Weiss, ed.), Academic Press, New York, 1973, p. 162.

84. Klein, E., *Cancer Res.* **29,** 235 (1969).

85. Gershon, R. K., Carter, R. L., Lane, N. J., *Am. J. Path.* **51,** 1111 (1967).

86. Delorme, E. J., Hall, J. G., Hadgett, J., and Alexander, P., *Proc. Roy. Soc.* **B 174,** 229 (1969).

87. Mikulsha, Z. B., Smith, C., and Alexander, P., *J. Natl. Cancer Inst.* **36,** 29 (1966).

88. Underwood, J. C. E., *Brit. J. Cancer* **30,** 538 (1974).

89. Morrison, A. S., Black. M. M., Lowe, C. R., MacMahon, B., and Yuasa, S., *Int. J. Cancer* **11,** 261 (1973).

90. Black, M. M., in *Immunological Parameters of Host-Tumor Relationships,* Vol. II (D. W. Weiss, ed.), Academic Press, New York, 1973, p. 80.

91. Mavlight, G., Gutterman, J. U., McBride, C., and Hersh, E. M., *Progr. Exp. Tumor Res.* **19,** 222 (1974).

92. Lloyd, O. C., *Proc. Roy. Soc. Med.* **62,** 543 (1969).

93. Payan, H. M., Gilbert, E. F., and Jacobs, W. H., *South. Med. J.* **63,** 1350 (1970).

94. Wayte, D. M., and Helwig, E. B., *Cancer* **22,** 69 (1968).

95. Jacobs, J. B., Edelstein, L. M., Snyder, L. M., and Fortier, N., *Cancer Res.* **35,** 352 (1975).

96. Yoon, I. L., *Am. J. Surg.* **97,** 195 (1959).

97. Black, M. M., and Leis, H. P., Cancer **28,** 263 (1971).

98. Edelson, R. L., Hearing, V. J., Dellon, A. L., Frank, M., Edelson, E. K., and Green, I., *Clin. Immunol. and Immunopath.* **4,** 557 (1975).

99. Caludy, A. L., Schmitt, D., Viac, J., Alario, A., Staquet, M. J., and Thivolet, J., *Clin. Exp. Immunol.* **23,** 61 (1976).

100. Nind, A. P. P., Nairn, R. C., Rolland, J. M., Gulli, E. P. C., and Hughes, E. S. R., *Brit. J. Cancer* **28,** 108 (1973).

101. Hunter, R. L., Ferguson, D. J., and Coppleson, L. W., *Cancer* **36,** 528 (1975).

102. Berg, J. W., *Cancer* **9,** 935 (1956).

103. Kister, S. J., Sommers, S. C., Haagensen, C. D., Friedell, G. H., Cooley, E., and Varma, A., *Cancer* **23,** 570 (1969).

104. Tsakralides, V., Olson, P., Kersey, J. H., and Good, R. A., *Cancer* **34,** 1259 (1974).

105. Fisher, E. R., Gregorio, R., Redmond, C., Dekker, A., and Fisher, B., *Am. J. Clin. Path.* **65,** 21 (1976).

Chapter Two

Immunodeficiency and Cancer

OSIAS STUTMAN

Memorial Sloan-Kettering Cancer Center, New York, New York

The idea that immune responses are the principal defense mechanisms against neoplasia has deeply influenced cancer research during the past decade. This idea, although suggested by Paul Ehrlich in 1909 (1), lay dormant until it was reformulated in 1959 (2) and crystallized as a general theory of "immunologic surveillance" by Burnet (3–5). On the whole, the present chapter is included in a volume dedicated to cancer immunology as a result of such persistent influence. This is especially true since the association of immunologic deficiency with increased risk for tumor development has represented the main source of experimental support (3–7), as well as the main prediction (3–5), derived from the immune surveillance theory. However, the analysis of available information concerning this relationship has shown the association to be a very special and restricted one, instead of the general phenomenon predicted by the theory (8–12). Although the immune surveillance concept is commonly accepted as established fact, a small chorus of critics has developed during the past 5 years (8,10–18, of which refs. 10 to 12 are extensive reviews of the problem).

In its current formulation the immune surveillance theory is proposed as a teleological justification for the efficiency of cell-mediated immunity against transplanted tissues (2). In a strict neo-Darwinian stance, Thomas suggested that, because of the "universal requirement of multicellular organisms to preserve uniformity of cell type ... homograft rejection will turn out to represent a primary mechanism for natural defense against neoplasia" (2). Another interpretation for the unusual vigor with which surgical artifacts such as transplants are rejected was that "the homograft reaction may be regarded as the price paid for an efficient system of defense against bacterial and viral invasion" (19). Our present knowledge of immune defenses against a wide variety of bacterial, viral,

Generation of the experimental data mentioned in this review was supported by U.S. Public Health Grants CA-08748, CA-15988, and CA-16599.

protozoan, and fungal parasites (usually intracellular) supports this view, since cell-mediated immunity is the main defense mechanism against such infectious threats (20–23). Indeed, it was indicated that "the ability to reject foreign transplants is so consistent in phylogeny that it must represent an important survival advantage to the species endowed with it, an advantage that has no relation to modern organ transplantation" (24).

The biological paradox, pointed out by Thomas (25), of the apparent drive to maintain absolute biological self-identity (through immunologic and other mechanisms) versus the opposing force capable of generating successful symbiosis, may explain the multiple "escape" mechanisms by which "invaders" avoid the immunologic defense mechanisms. For example, compare the persistence of adult schistosoma worms in the presence of a powerful host immunity against reinfection with cercariae (26) with any of the many experiments showing concomitant immunity to tumors in experimental animals (e.g., 27). Luckily for the tumor biologist, cancer cells probably do not exhibit the unique capacity to generate new antigenic variants or to acquire human antigens to the degree that protozoans and other pathogens do (7,21,28).

The main contention of the theory of immunologic surveillance is that immune functions have evolved, in part, as a mechanism to prevent the emergence of cancer cells that arise through somatic mutation (3–5,29). The purported role of immune surveillance is not to mediate the regression of established tumors, but rather to seek and destroy clinically unrecognized in situ tumors (3–5,29). Thus, we are not going to discuss the response that a host produces against its own growing tumor, a post factum event that is the main subject of this book. In a way, the established tumor (as well as the ongoing immune response to it, when detectable) would represent the actual failure of the immune surveillance mechanism (3–5). This chapter will discuss mainly the experimental and clinical evidence that has been used to support the immune surveillance theory. It is quite difficult to be comprehensive within a relatively few pages. Much of the documentation to support some of our criticism for the generality of immune surveillance has been presented in a more extensive review (12), which, although comprising more than one thousand references and most of the pertinent literature, still proved to be incomplete. As Charles Darwin suggested: ". . . the only object in writing (a book) is a proof of earnestness, and that you do not form your opinions without undergoing labor of some kind" (30). As its title indicates, this chapter will address itself mainly to an area that has been considered the strongest support of the immune surveillance theory: the association of spontaneous or induced immune deficiencies with increased incidence of tumors in both experimental animals and man (3–7,29,31–40).

GENERAL ASPECTS OF IMMUNE SURVEILLANCE

In a review on cancer biology Burnet stated: "It is by no means inconceivable that small accumulations of tumor cells may develop and because of their possession of new antigenic potentialities provoke an effective immunologic reaction with regression of the tumor and no clinical hint of its existence" (41). This "foreshadowing" (5) of the theory has remained almost unchanged in essence, albeit clothed in new terminology (3–5). For example: "The thesis is that when aberrant cells with proliferative potential arise in the body, they will carry new antigenic determinants. . . . When a significant amount of new antigen has developed, a thymus-dependent immunologic response will be initiated which eventually eliminates the aberrant cells in essentially the same way as a homograft is destroyed." (3). This definition also contains axioms that have become integral parts of the theory (3–5,29,42): 1) tumor cells have distinct antigens, and 2) such antigenic differences can "under appropriate conditions be recognized as foreign and provoke an immune response, based on thymus-dependent immunocytes" (5). These two axioms are assumed to be ". . . now acceptable to all" (5).

Immune surveillance has been repeatedly equated to homograft reactions (2,5,29,42), and the thymus-dependent immune system has been declared to be "almost solely responsible for surveillance" (4, p. 161). At the clinical level the predictions of the theory are (3–5): 1) the age incidence of tumors should reflect higher emergence of tumors "initiated at ages of relative immunologic inefficiency" (5), i.e., the ante- and perinatal period as well as old age; and 2) "conditions associated with depression of the thymus-dependent system, whether genetic, induced by drugs, or of other origin, should increase the likelihood of cancer" (5). These two predictions pertain directly to the subject of this chapter. Two other predictions are (3–5) that spontaneous tumor regressions may be immunologic in nature and that histologic studies of common sites of cancer show a higher proportion of premalignant or small cancerous lesions than those expected to emerge clinically. These two last points have been previously considered only as "indirect" evidence for immune surveillance in humans (42). At the experimental level the prediction is that immunodepressive procedures (such as thymectomy) should facilitate the appearance of spontaneous as well as experimentally induced tumors (3–5,29,42). Additional support is given by the observation that carcinogens are immunodepressive by themselves (3) and may serve as a permissive factor to bypass surveillance (a theory proposed in 1964 by Prehn for chemical carcinogenesis, see 43). We will briefly discuss some of these axioms before addressing the main subject of the chapter.

As indicated in a previous review (12), many of the experimental data on immunodepression and tumor development, generated during both the pre- and postsurveillance days, do not support the generality of the theory. Thus, a remark such as ". . . there is now an extremely large body of experimental work on immunological aspects of malignant diseases in laboratory animals and one must be rather highly selective in choosing investigations which are directly relevant to the concept of immunological surveillance" (3), although it may economize effort, may also generate dogmatic stances and confusion. For example, such a selective procedure has induced even severe critics of the immune surveillance theory to state that the experimental support of the theory ". . . in aggregate constitute(s) a quite compelling case" (44). Conversely, some other critics assume, after reviewing some of the available literature, that most aspects of immune surveillance cannot be tested experimentally (16). Perhaps we should keep in mind that "surveillance, if it exists, is a negative factor in the natural history of (human) cancer" (4, p. 161) and that "malignant disease is initiated by factors intrinsic to individual cells and its emergence will depend on a variety of factors in the microenvironment. . . . immunological effects will be superimposed upon others. . . ." (4, pp. 161–162)—which shows that in book form authors tend to be more cautious than in shorter presentations of the same facts and theories.

The problems of tumor antigenicity and of the efficiency of the immune system to act as a true surveillance mechanism have been the main sources of Prehn's criticism of the theory (13,14). Some of his conclusions can be summarized in one quotation: "There is an immune defense mechanism in cancer biology. However, in most systems it is ineffective and late-acting rather than a surveillance mechanism against incipient tumors. . . . There is evidence for surveillance in some chemically induced and some viral tumor systems, in both of which these tumors are unusually immunogenic. These systems may be laboratory artifacts that have little to say about the naturally occurring disease" (14). Prehn adds: "The evidence overall seems to suggest that immunological surveillance of nascent tumors, as originally conceived, may not exist in most tumor systems. On the other hand, there is a late-acting and inefficient immunological defense mechanism. Hopefully, this mechanism may be subject to augmentation for purposes of immunotherapy" (14).

Tumor antigenicity in many experimental systems may be difficult to demonstrate, and it is accepted that not all tumors (spontaneous or induced) show detectable antigenicity when measured in vivo (8,45–47), albeit some may show antigenicity in in vitro testing (as seems to be the case with mouse lung adenomas, 48). Burnet addressed this point (5,49), as supportive of the theory; i.e., the emerging tumors had been immunoselected for low antigenicity (5), albeit he conceded that "there is no evolutionary need for tumors to be antigenic" (49). However, tumors with low or no detectable antigenicity can appear regardless of the immunologic status of the host (46) and can even be detected in mice with lifelong profound immunodepression (8,12). Similarly, in many instances tumors generated in environments sheltered from the immune response show low or no detectable antigenicity (i.e., tumors produced in vitro, 50, or produced within cell-impermeable diffusion chambers, which are impermeable to cell-mediated immunity, 51–53). The theory would have predicted the emergence of tumors with high antigenic strength in the absence of immunologic influences (5,43,44).

As a matter of fact, the presence or absence of antigens in sarcomas produced by chemical carcinogens within diffusion chambers seems related to cell cycle stage: nonimmunogenic sarcomas are induced by treatment of replicating cell populations with methylcholanthrene, while immunogenic tumors arise when cells are treated during the resting phase of growth (54). On the other hand, proliferating cells are more susceptible to chemically induced transformation than their resting counterparts (55–57). These two observations may explain the fact that even in the chemically induced tumor systems, antigenicity is not the general rule (8,45–47). In addition, the rare spontaneous tumors appearing in mice that have no clear viral etiology are usually weakly antigenic or do not show detectable antigenicity (44,45). One report indicates that antigenicity of sarcomas induced in mice by methylcholanthrene was proportional to the carcinogen dose; lower doses produced tumors with low antigenicity (58). Prehn's suggestion concerning these results is that low levels of environmental oncogens will tend to produce sporadic tumors of low antigenicity (58). Using a single suboptimal dose of methylcholanthrene injected subcutaneously, we observed that antigenicity seems not to correlate with carcinogen dose: the incidence of nonantigenic as well as antigenic tumors was comparable in mice receiving a carcinogen dose that would produce 100% tumor incidence and those receiving a dose that would produce 20% tumor incidence (12). It is apparent that further research in this area is required, especially studies determining the effects of cumulative low doses of chemical carcinogens.

Experiments designed to demonstrate that immune responses are capable of dealing efficiently with incipient in situ tumors gave negative results both with early mammary tumor lesions in mice (59) and with chemically induced skin tumors (60–62). The skin tumor experiments clearly showed that in the intact normal host there is no immunologic recognition of the in situ tumor, unless traumatic nonphysiological procedures are used, such as transplantation of the tumor-containing skin (62). Andrews (62) observed that when skin treated with methylcholanthrene was autografted (i.e., removed and placed back in the same animal), no tumors developed in the autografted sites in normal hosts. Conversely, normal mice with their skin left unmolested or groups of grafted or nongrafted immunodepressed hosts had significant local tumor development. These experiments indeed support Prehn's contention that early immunologic recognition of incipient tumors seems to be a rare event (14). Andrews concludes that "in a natural situation where most tumors are small and weakly antigenic, immunosurveillance is ineffective because the weak antigenicity of the tumors is not detectable and undisturbed tumors are not recognized by host immunity" (62).

The concept of immune surveillance would have also suggested that "immunologically privileged sites" should have a naturally high incidence of tumors or that it would be relatively easy to induce tumors in such sites. However, although these experiments seem "directly relevant to the concept of immunological surveillance" (3), they were never discussed, probably because they did not support the theory (12). We will briefly comment on tumors in the hamster cheek pouch and in the brain (see 12 for extensive review). Immunologically privileged sites have been defined as sites where "the physiological pathways necessary for either evocation or the putting into effect of an immunological response are incomplete in some respect" (63). The exact mechanism by which some of these sites have unique properties that permit even transplantation of xenogeneic tissues is still undetermined, but peculiarities of lymphatic drainage seem the most probable reason (63).

Although hamster cheek pouches have been extensively used in tumor research (64–66), spontaneous tumors are indeed rare, and only two slow-growing mesenchymal tumors have been reported (67 and W. G. Banfield, quoted in 68). This compares with approximately 7% incidence of spontaneous epithelial and mesenchymal tumors at other sites (64–66,68) and probably many thousands of animals under study. However, direct application of chemical carcinogens can induce tumors in the cheek pouch at a rate usually lower than that produced by the same dosages applied to skin (64–66). In some instances treatment with steroids increased tumor incidence after application of chemical carcinogens in the cheek pouch (69–70); similarly, treatment with antilymphocyte serum produced an increase in tumor incidence and some decrease in latency periods for tumor development (71,72). Several studies with exteriorized cheek pouch autografts implanted in the skin (73–76) have yielded variable results. In general, the exposed cheek pouch was less susceptible to tumor induction by polycyclic hy-drocarbons than either the surrounding skin or the pouch in situ (the exception being the data presented in ref. 76, showing opposite results). For additional discussion of this subject, see ref. 12.

A very similar picture emerges from the analysis of spontaneous or induced brain tumors in animals (see also 12 for extensive review). Spontaneous brain tumors occur infrequently among laboratory animals (77), and induction of brain tumors by several procedures has proven a complex and difficult task (12). Two examples will be used to indicate that experimental brain tumors do not fit with a strict interpretation of immunologic surveillance. First, with resorptive car-cinogens that have a high selectivity for nervous tissue, the incidence of tumors of the central nervous tissue is usually comparable to or lower than that of tumors appearing in the peripheral nervous tissue (i.e., in the sites that do not behave as immunologically privileged), as demonstrated by several authors (78–80). Second, additional immunodepression had no effect on tumor development, including central nervous tissue (81,82).

In summary, it is apparent that tumor development within immunologically privileged sites (whatever the mechanism for such privileged status) grow and develop either at a reduced rate or at a rate comparable to that of similar tumors in immunologically exposed sites, which does not fit with the predictions of the immune surveillance theory. It is interesting that, although the majority of the literature on cheek pouch or brain was generated during the presurveillance or early surveillance days (see ref. 12 for review), no direct attempts to use these models as a test for the theory were made until recently (76,81,82).

An additional variable complicating many of these studies has been the de-monstration in vivo and in vitro that the incipient immune response may be stimulatory for tumor growth (83,84) and that such effects seem to be mediated both by immune cells (83,84) and antibodies (85). The consequences of "im-munostimulation" on tumor development and growth are quite apparent and in need of further confirmation and additional study.

Lastly, we are still ignorant of the fine details as to which type of immune reponse is the most effective in controlling cancer development and/or cancer spread in animals or man. In addition, the poor characterization of human tumor antigens (86) complicates the comparison between clinical and experimental situations. Thus, it becomes apparent (especially in the experimental models) that it is difficult to evaluate the degree and relevance of the immunodepressive procedure when we still ignore which are the main mechanisms for local or generalized antitumor reactions.

One final example will serve to close this introduction. Mice infected with *Toxoplasma gondii* show a marked and persistent suppression of immune func-tions, especially thymus-dependent responses (measured as blastogenesis after exposure to phytohemagglutinin, etc., 87). Such infected mice also show a reduc-tion in the incidence of spontaneous tumors and are even capable of destroying transplanted tumors, perhaps as a consequence of macrophage activation by the chronic infection (88). This represents a paradox that clearly does not fit present-day immunologic dogma; while "conventional" immune responses are depressed, the overall response to tumors may be highly efficient. It should be noted that the immune parameters depressed in this experimental situation include many of those that are studied in cancer patients for evaluation of their general immune status (89).

EXPERIMENTAL EVIDENCE

The direct action of the oncogenic agent on the immune system of the host has been considered a necessary but not sufficient factor for its carcinogenic action (43), and the "carcinogen as immunosuppressive agent" concept has been incorporated in several enunciations of the immune surveillance theory (3–6,29,42). The basis for testing the immunodepressive effect of a variety of chemical carcinogens (90) was the observation that "Rous sarcoma virus in addition to initiating tumors will also depress antibody levels" (91) and that "x-irradiation, in addition to inhibiting and initiating neoplastic growth, depresses antibody levels in experimental animals" (90). Extensive experimental work has demonstrated that a variety of chemical carcinogens and oncogenic viruses have, indeed, immunodepressive properties (12). We will not dwell upon this subject, since it has been reviewed elsewhere *in extenso* (12,92,93).

For chemical carcinogens, it is our opinion that the association is probably trivial in relation to cancer etiology (12). The main argument bearing on this point is that the immunodepressive effects are observed with carcinogen dosages that are usually 100 to 1000 times the optimal oncogenic dosage (12,94), a sitution rarely occurring in natural environments. On the other hand, by dosage adjustment, the oncogenic effects can be clearly dissociated from the immunodepressive capacities (94): carcinogen doses will still be oncogenic without detectable effects on the immune system of the host, a situation which probably mimics environmental exposure to chemical carcinogens (12). Concerning the immunodepressive effects of oncogenic viruses (12,92,93), it is apparent that such effects are mainly associated with the highly pathogenic "laboratory" viruses and are usually not observed in the animals with endogenous viruses or viruses transmitted vertically—i.e., the "high-tumor" mouse strains (12,93). This last fact weakens the significance of the association of immunodepression and oncogenicity.

The results of different immunodepressive procedures on tumor development after exposure to chemical or viral oncogenic agents show that the issue is not a simple one, since either no detectable effects, inhibition, or facilitation of tumor development have been observed (facilitation expressed as increased tumor incidence and/or decreased latency periods for tumor development), depending on the experimental systems (see refs. 10 and 12 for comprehensive reviews). Some examples will be cited to show the complexities of the experimental evidence available. However, the inescapable conclusion is that if such experiments are supposed to represent the main support of the immune surveillance theory, the theory actually applies to a most restricted set of experimental situations (12). While the experimental data are weak for most oncogenic agents, it is accepted that immunodepression will influence tumor development by some DNA and herpes viruses, supporting the idea of a restricted surveillance directed to "tumor-associated antigen systems that have been regularly encountered by most members of the species, at least during their recent evolution" (7) and not to products of our relatively new socioeconomic environment.

Table 1 shows a distribution of the experimental results concerning the effects of different immunodepressive procedures on systemic and local tumor development after exposure of mice and rats to chemical carcinogens (mostly polycyclic hydrocarbons, urethane, and nitrosamines).

It appears that while some experiments indeed show facilitation of tumor development by immunodepression, the majority of the experiments give results that do not fit with the surveillance interpretation. For example, early thymectomy produces marginal effects (mainly a moderate diminution of latency periods), and even some of the positive experiments, extensively quoted as support for the theory (3–6), showed intrinsic discrepancies (ref. 95 shows no effects of thymectomy on tumor induction by 3,4–9,10-dibenzanthracene while showing a facilitating effect with methylcholanthrene, and such facilitating effect was observed only in female C3H mice and not in males; in ref. 101 the facilitating effect of thymectomy was observed in only one of the three mouse strains studied; in ref. 96 the differences in latency period were observed only at 14 weeks after carcinogen administration, etc.; for review of the effects of thymectomy see refs. 12 and 153). With antilymphocyte serum (ALS) the results also show some interesting discrepancies, which may be related to nonimmunological factors. For example, in at least two reports showing facilitation (107,116) ALS had marked toxicity for the animals, while two of the more extensive studies showing no detectable effects expressly stated that the ALS had no toxicity (111) or that actual tolerance to rabbit immunoglobulins was induced in the recipients (8). On the other hand, one experiment comparing the effect of neonatal thymectomy versus chronic ALS treatment in rats showed no effect in the former and facilitation in the latter (151).

Very few studies tested the effects of immunodepression on different dosages of carcinogen (8,108). The results showed no differences in one study (8), while those in the other showed no effect at the higher dose and some facilitation at the lower dose of carcinogen (108). No significant effects of ALS treatment were observed with a variety of chemical carcinogens and different systems—i.e., subcutaneous sarcoma induction (8,111), skin tumors (112), lung adenomas (115,116), neurological tumors (81,82), mammary tumors (117), liver and colon tumors (121a and b). In experiments using systemic carcinogens, immunodepression had no effect on most of the tumors in different organ sites, with the exception of bladder tumors, which were increased in the ALS-treated rats (81). The degree of immunodepression by the different procedures was measured concomitantly in only a few experiments (8,81,111), and in most of the studies effective immunodepression was only assumed. This also applies to most of the studies using chemical immunodepression.

The observations with nude athymic mice showed surprising unanimity: the results of three different laboratories indicate that the incidence and latency periods for tumor development after exposure to chemical carcinogens are comparable in the immunodepressed nudes and the immunologically normal heterozygote siblings (12,15,104,122–124). This last observation is in clear disagreement with predictions of the immune surveillance dogma.

The effects of chemical immunodepressive agents (see Table 1) cover both systemic and topical carcinogenesis. Azathioprine either inhibited tumor development (125,131) or had only marginal facilitating effects (129). The effect of

Table 1   Summary of References Describing the Effects of Immunodepression on Systemic and Local Tumor Development after Chemical Carcinogens in Mice and Rats

Experimental Procedure	No Effect	Ref. Number Facilitation	Inhibition
Thymectomy (early, plus irradiation)	12, 97, 98, 99 100, 101, 102, 104, 151	95, 96, 101, 103	—
Antilymphocyte serum (ALS)	8, 108, 109, 110, 111, 112, 81, 82, 115, 116, 117, 120, 121a and b	105, 106, 107, 114, 118, 119, 151	113, 152
Nude athymic mice	12, 15, 104, 122, 123, 124	—	—
Chemical immunosuppression[a]	87, 125, 126, 127, 128	129, 130	118, 120, 131, 132
Steroids	133, 134, 135	136, 137, 138, 139, 140	134, 141, 142, 143, 144, 145
Whole-body irradiation	—	114	146, 147, 148, 149, 150

[a] Including 6-mercaptopurine, azathioprine, iododeoxyuridine, fluorodeoxyuridine, methotrexate, cyclophosphamide.

steroids are of interest, since, as with ALS, comparable experiments produced quite different results, especially on skin carcinogenesis, where both facilitation (138–140) and inhibition of papilloma development have been reported. Reference 145 shows an even more interesting result: no effect on skin carcinogenesis and inhibition of lung tumor formation in mice after methylcholanthrene administration. Whole-body irradiation at different dosages also has paradoxical effects: it prevents skin papilloma regression (114) as predicted by the immune surveillance theory, while it inhibits development of subcutaneous sarcomas (146) and lung adenomas (147–150). The lung adenoma issue is important, because it has been considered a positive example of immune surveillance even by critics of the theory (14); however, the experimental data with the effects of thymectomy of ALS on lung adenoma formation show extensive variation even within experimental groups, which makes the actual evaluation somewhat difficult (see ref. 12 for extensive analysis of this problem); also, lung adenoma formation is most susceptible to environmental factors and/or infections, which may enhance or inhibit lung tumor development (154). It should be noted that the incidence of lung adenomas after methylcholanthrene or urethane administration in nude mice was comparable to the incidence observed in the immunologically normal heterozygote siblings (15,122,123).

In summary, the analysis of almost all the available literature dealing with the effect of different immunodepressive procedures or situations on the development of local or systemic tumors in mice and rats after exposure to chemical carcinogens clearly supports our contention at the beginning of this section. It appears that the number of exceptions to the predictions of the immune surveillance theory is too high to assure us of its generality. As a matter of fact, it is not easy to predict the effects of a given drug or immunodepressive procedure on tumor development (10–12), and in many instances it is impossible to conclude that the observed effects of these agents or procedures on carcinogenesis are indeed due to their immunodepressive properties (8,10,12).

In the epilogue to his book on immune surveillance Burnet indicates that the "important" experiment would be to maintain a large number of thymectomized and sham-operated animals "throughout their life span" and determine tumor incidences (4, p. 236). And he adds: "I am reasonably certain that Medawar would agree that it is a good experiment" (4).

Several experiments have been done concerning this question using either early thymectomy (12,97,98,155–164), lifelong administration of antilymphocyte serum (8,167), or athymic nude mice (15,123,124,168). In the majority of these experiments the animals were observed for the duration of their natural life span, and with one exception (168) the observation period ranged from 12 to 30 months. No significant differences were observed between thymectomized and control animals on the incidence of hepatomas, reticular cell tumors, and lung adenomas in C57B1/Ks, (C57B1/Ks × C3H)F₁ (155), C3H/Hef (156), and BALB/C mice (157). No differences were observed in the incidence of postcastrational adrenal tumors in CE and their hybrids (12). Thymectomy had no effect on lung adenoma or hepatoma development in C3H-Avy mice (156), the viable yellow gene (Avy) being a dominant gene that increases tumor incidence in mice (12,169). In one study thymectomized animals showed increased incidence of nonviral mammary tumors (155), while no difference in that type of breast cancer was observed in another study (156). A moderate increase in lymphoma incidence was observed in thymectomized (C57BL × A)F₁ hybrids (158). The spontaneous mammary tumors of mice, which are induced by a virus, consistently showed a decrease in incidence and delay in latency periods in thymectomized mice of different strains (12,97,98,159–163). In his original description Martinez indicated that "the interpretation of these results must remain a matter of conjecture at the present time" (159), and it is apparent that more than 10 years later the situation has not changed substantially. Incidentally, a moderate decrease in incidence of breast cancer has been described in patients thymectomized for myasthenia gravis (165), although in the overall studies there is no evidence that adult thymectomy in humans is followed by an increased risk of neoplastic disease (165–166; see also 12 for review).

Two studies in which lifelong administration of ALS was used showed no increase in spontaneous tumors when compared to the controls in C3Hf, I, and CBA mice (8,167), although in one experiment (167) contamination of the animals with polyoma induced high incidence of tumors in the ALS-treated mice. The polyoma studies will be discussed further in this chapter. Upon the whole, it seems that these immunodepressive procedures do not significantly influence the actual incidence of spontaneous tumors in mice.

The studies using the nude athymic mice have confirmed, in essence, these results (12,15,123,124). In one study the incidence of lung adenomas, hepatomas, and lymphomas was comparable between nude mice in a CBA/H background and their immunologically normal counterparts (12,15,123). These animals were observed for 20 to 30 months and were preserved in pathogen-free environments.

Similarly, the insertion of the dominant gene viable yellow (Avy) showed no difference in tumor incidence between the nudes and controls (15,123). Another study using germ-free nudes in a BALB/C background showed an overall incidence of 8.3% (22 of 265) lymphomas in the nudes, appearing late in life usually after 12 months of age, while the heterozygote controls had only 1.2% (2 of 162) incidence of lymphomas. No significant differences in incidence of other tumors were observed. This observation is of interest. However, the lymphoma incidence observed in the nudes is in accord with the published data on lymphoma incidence in normal BALB/C mice (which ranges from 1 to 20%, see refs. 157,170–174) and actually cannot be considered as a true increase in lymphoma incidence. Lymphoma incidence in normal germ-free BALB/C mice was 8%, with a mean appearance time of 23 months (174). Similarly "lymphoid hyperplasia" (171,172) and spontaneous amyloidosis are common in older BALB/C males (173), both situations capable of producing enlarged spleens and possible diagnostic problems. Amyloidosis was described in carcinogen-treated nude mice (122,123).

All these points are made concerning this observation because already it has been quoted as a "very high incidence of neoplasia in these long-lived, severely immunodeficient animals" (17). Also, the fact that the tumors are mainly of the lymphoreticular tissues was used, on the one hand, to criticize the generality of immune surveillance, and on the other to stress the similarities between the nude model and the tumors appearing in immunodeficient humans (17). Similarly, the observation described in ref. 168 was used in an editorial that stated "nude mice do not develop spontaneous tumors" (18) and "there is no immune surveillance" (18). Neither of those generalizations seems to be correct. The paper by Rygaard and Povlsen indicates that no tumors were observed in 2,900 nude mice," many observed over the whole of their life span (approximately 7 months)" (168). These animals were kept in conventional conditions, and it is apparent that the observation period was too short (most spontaneous tumors in mice appear at 12 or more months of age, depending on strains; see 12). These sweeping generalizations are dangerous and do not help to elucidate any of the problems discussed. If Dr. J. J. Bittner had observed his mice for only 7 months, we could have concluded that the incidence of mammary tumors was less than 5%!

An alternative interpretation of the results in nude mice (12,15) is that antitumor surveillance is exerted by thymus-independent immune pathways. This interpretation is supported by the demonstration of natural cytotoxic cellular reactivity against syngeneic and allogeneic tumor cells in vitro in nude mice (175,176) and by the late appearance of immune resistance against polyoma oncogenesis in nude mice (15,177). Natural antibodies capable of lysis of tumor cells in the presence of complement have been also detected in nude mice (178). Concerning natural resistance, nude mice can express the genes for myxovirus resistance (179) and for resistance to focus formation by Friend virus (15,123). In summary, what the experiments on tumor development in nude mice may actually dispel is mainly the idea that immune surveillance is a thymus-dependent mechanism.

As indicated at the beginning of this section, the possible role of immune functions controlling tumor development induced by DNA and herpes viruses seems to be established on more solid grounds (7,98,156). Thymectomy and other immunodepressive procedures have a marked effect, overcoming age, sex, or strain-dependent resistance to tumor induction by a variety of DNA-oncogenic viruses in mice, rats, and hamsters (see 12 for extensive review, also 7,98,156). We will discuss mainly the studies with polyoma virus, which best exemplify the role of immune functions in oncogenesis by DNA viruses. For information on effects on immunodepression on tumor development after infection with adenoviruses see 180,181, and for data on SV-40 see 102.

Increased susceptibility to polyoma virus oncogenesis after early thymectomy has been observed in rats (182,183), hamsters (95), and mice (97,98,156,184–186). Nude athymic mice also show an increased susceptibility to polyoma tumor induction (15,177,187,188), and treatment with antilymphocyte serum also sensitizes mice and rats to polyoma oncogenesis (189,190). For reviews on immune functions and polyoma oncogenesis see 98,156,191,192. It is apparent that in the polyoma model there is absolute concordance with the results obtained in different laboratories, using different polyoma strains, as well as different species and mouse strains: in every instance an increased susceptibility to tumor development was observed in the immunodepressed animals. Polyoma infection has been detected in wild mice as well as in laboratory colonies, although it may be questioned whether it is an etiologic agent for tumor development in wild mice (193,194). It appears that under natural conditions polyoma does not produce tumors as a consequence of several interacting mechanisms: low probability of infection during the susceptible perinatal period (maternal antibodies?, etc.); low dosages of virus likely to be acquired by inhalation or ingestion; the dominance of genetic resistance and the effectiveness of cell-mediated immunity in the adult mouse (7,98,156,192).

Although polyoma is prevalent in many mouse colonies, it is not pathogenic (tumorigenic) unless inoculated early in life and in high titers (193,194). However, several reports of tumor development in immunodepressed mice after room infection or other forms of accidental infection with polyoma virus (97,102,167,195) clearly support the view that an intact immune system is critical for preventing this form of oncogenesis. Immunodepression could either overcome mouse strain-dependent resistance (184–186), increase susceptibility or overcome age-dependent resistance in susceptible strains (98,177,187), or increase oncogenic potential of polyoma virus strains with low oncogenicity in either susceptible or resistant strains (98,185). Restoration of immune functions by administration of immunologically competent lymphoid cells or different thymus replacements (97,98,156,177,182,183,186,191) indicates that all those procedures could prevent the effects of immunodepression on polyoma oncogenesis and supports the view of the thymus dependency of this resistance mechanism.

However, although these models seem to be one of the paradigms of effective immune surveillance (98,192), two remarks seem pertinent. First, no tumors appear after polyoma infection in the presence of an intact immune system; however, it is still not clear whether this is due to a true surveillance-type mechanism (i.e., elimination of nascent tumors) or to other mechanisms that act before transformation occurs (i.e., control of virus spread, infectivity, etc.). Second, the detection of a late-appearing natural resistance to polyoma oncogenesis in nude athymic mice, which is dependent on non-T cells for its expression and probably mediated by B cells (177), indicates that alternate pathways—i.e., thymus-independent—should be kept in mind. A third point concerns the type of tumors in nude mice: in two reports (177,187) the type of tumors appearing in normal and nude mice were comparable, although in both studies an increase of uterine tumors was observed in the nudes, and in a third study (188) the predominant tumor type was in the skin (these three studies used nude mice with different inbred backgrounds). Could it be that some tumor types are more susceptible to immunologic control than others? This presumption is supported by studies in which immunodepression increased only tumors of one type without affecting the incidence of others (81; see also previous paragraphs on effects of immunodepression on chemical carcinogenesis) and also by the preponderance of certain epithelial tumors in immunodepressed patients (see next section).

The many immunologic concomitants, such as development of successful vaccines or peculiar oncogenicity spectra, support the view that some kind of immunologic surveillance may be effective in controlling lymphotropic herpes viruses in birds and primates (see 7 for extensive review). However, even this issue is not clear. For example, thymectomy either had no effect (196) or increased (197) the incidence of Marek's disease in birds, while bursectomy either showed no effect (198–200), decreased incidence (196,201), or increased incidence of the disease (202,203).

In summary, the association of immunodeficiency and increased risk for tumor development in experimental animals is apparent only in a limited number of systems (i.e., polyoma and other DNA viruses and perhaps herpes), and the number of exceptions to the predictions of the immune surveillance theory is quite high.

I will close this section with two additional remarks concerning the experimental evidence. First, other models in which there is a profound immune deficit, such as the pituitary dwarf mouse (see ref. 204 for review), do not show increase in susceptibility to development of spontaneous or induced tumors (see 12 and 205), even when examined for long periods (205). Second, the effects of immaturity or aging on the immune system are considered important evidence supporting the surveillance concept (see pp. 27–28). However, the experimental data are not strong. Owing to space limitations we will address this question very briefly. It is evident that in most cases, when weight-adjusted dosages of carcinogens were used in newborn animals, susceptibility was comparable to that observed in older animals (12; especially see 206 for review); thus the "increased susceptibility" appears to be more of a dosage artifact than a consistent effect. However, the increase in susceptibility of newborn or weanling animals to oncogenesis by viruses (especially DNA viruses) may have an immunologic basis and may also be related to availability of special target cells for virus replication, etc. (see ref. 12 for discussion). On the other hand, we could not define a true association between age-dependent immunologic decay (or development of autoimmunity) and spontaneous tumor development in mice (see 12 and 207 for extensive review). However, the peculiar age-related incidences of tumors in man require incisive analysis, and generalizations are difficult, since the natural history of the many cancers shows vast complexities and differences (see 12 and 208 for reviews). At least with some industry-associated cancers it appears that "time of exposure" as well as "time at exposure" are critical factors in tumor risk (208).

Finally, the peculiar association of immunodepression plus chronic antigenic stimulation has been considered as one possible factor explaining the appearance of lymphomas in immunodeficient patients. Chronic antigen administration alone (209) or associated with chronic immunodepression with ALS or azathioprine (210,211) produces an increase in development of reticular cell tumors and lymphomas in mice. It should be pointed out that in one experiment the antigenic stimulation was provided by the lactic dehydrogenase elevating virus, which is an endemic contaminant of many mouse colonies, a problem rarely discussed in the experiments using immunodepression in mice (12). The interpretation for these experiments (as well as for the immunodepressed humans) is that lymphomas arise as a consequence of the imbalanced immune response (211,212), especially the imbalance of immunoregulatory mechanisms (212,213), perhaps in association with activation of leukemia (or other) virus as result of those uncontrolled immune reactions (11,17,211–214). In man, one group has proposed that immunodepression plus activation of herpes virus may explain the peculiar array of tumors appearing in immunodepressed transplant patients (214).

This rapid overview of the experimental evidence supporting immune surveillance shows that at the peak of acceptance of the theory, a time during which most of the discussed data were generated, there was an obvious tendency to discuss mainly the experiments that seemed to support the theory. However, although the immune surveillance theory has on occasion been interpreted as strict dogma, especially in the hands of the *exegetae*, it is still a valid and stimulating hypothesis. Perhaps the problems are derived from the proliferation of reviews, which in many cases replace the original texts as source material, plus the fact that "Men who have excessive faith in their theories . . . make very poor observations."*

CLINICAL EVIDENCE

In this section we will discuss briefly two main clinical situations: the association of primary immunologic deficiencies with high incidence of malignancy (6,31–33,38–40) and the increased incidence of tumor development in immunodepressed patients undergoing organ transplantation (34–37). Both clinical observations have been considered as prime support for the immune surveillance concept (5,6,31,32). However, it soon became apparent that even this type of evidence presented problems, mainly that in both situations the increased risk for tumor development was due mostly to an inordinate incidence of lymphomas (9,36–40) and rarely to other types of tumors. As a matter of fact, neither in the pediatric groups, comprising most of the primary immunodeficiency cases (9), nor in the adult cases, comprised mostly of transplanted patients (215), was there any increase in the common tumors appearing in each age group. This made a case for either a very restricted form of immune surveillance or for alternative interpretations (11,12,40,210–214).

An additional factor that complicates both issues (especially the primary immune deficiencies) is that the majority of the material has been collected as case reports (see 33), and the actual size of the population at risk is difficult to assess. The problem with case reports is that they "are known to be subject to a myriad of

---

*Written by Claude Bernard in 1865. See the English translation, *Introduction to the Study of Experimental Medicine* (New York: Dover Publications, Inc., 1957), p. 38.

selective biases and they could hardly be expected to include all the data which future readers might deem useful" (216). The recently developed "Immunodeficiency Cancer Registry" (38) as well as the "Denver Transplant Tumor Registry" (34–37) may help in the collection and analysis of this clinical information.

In the case of the primary immunodeficiencies several problems should be kept in mind. The size of the population at risk for the different diseases is unknown—which helps explain some of the marked discrepancies in the estimation of tumor incidence (e.g., compare 33 with 34–37 or 217,218). With the exception of a recent paper (9) that analyzed the pediatric cases, no age-specific rates for tumor incidence were clearly defined. The combination of diseases with different clinical course and age incidence within a single category of "primary immune deficiencies" also compounds the problems (the severe combined immune deficiencies may bias toward lower tumor incidence, since these patients die early in infancy; the inclusion of the common variable immunodeficiency of late onset may bias toward a normal age-dependent adult type of cancer; relatively well-tolerated deficiencies with good survival may alter overall incidence when the patients are followed up for long periods, etc.; see also 11 and 12 for further discussion of sampling problems). An additional factor is the accuracy of the diagnosis of "lymphoma" in some of these cases, especially since biopsies from patients who have had multiple infections may show hyperplastic and/or granulomatous abnormalities that may be difficult to diagnose (11,12). Marked lymphoid hyperplasia without overt malignancy is common in certain immune deficiencies such as ataxia-telangiectasia and common variable immunodeficiency (see 12 and 129 for review). A good example of this problem is one case of common variable immunodeficiency reported by Douglas et al. (220) that was diagnosed as having a lymphosarcoma at biopsy and 20 years later was "in remission," a most bizarre evolution of lymphosarcoma in an immunodeficient patient. This patient apparently has been included in the "Registry" (38).

However, with all the provisos discussed above, the tentative incidence of 5% (2 to 10% range) for the overall group of primary immunodeficiencies (38–40,221) is far above the expected rate. Moreover, when the age-specific tumor incidence was calculated for tumor mortality in children under 15 years of age with primary immunodeficiencies, compared with unselected children in the United States, the picture showed some important characteristics (9,39,40,221), the only tumor category showing an increased risk in the immunodeficiency group being the lymphoreticular (reticulum cell sarcoma, lymphosarcoma, etc.). While the expected incidence was 8% in the unselected children, it was 67% and 69% respectively for all the collected cases and the cases of the United States only (9,221). All the other common types of pediatric tumors were either lower or absent in the immunodeficient group—for example: leukemias (all types), 48% in the unselected children, 25% in the immunodeficient children, etc. (9,221). This tendency holds for the total group of all ages, and in the series of 145 patients discussed in the first presentation of the Registry data (38), 58% had lymphoreticular tumors, 17% had leukemias of all types, and only 18% had epithelial tumors. This distribution has so far remained unchanged as new cases have been incorporated into the Registry (39,40, and J. H. Kersey, personal communication).

As indicated earlier, the high incidence of the lymphoreticular tumors provides only questionable support for the immune surveillance theory, since there is no clear cause-effect relationship and the tumors are of tissues that are affected by the disease and/or by its consequences. Indeed, a relationship between frequent infections, chronic antigenic stimulation, and the development of lymphoreticular tumors has been proposed for the immunodeficient patients (210–211,222). However, some possible correlations may be derived from the available data, such as the relative high incidence of gastrointestinal tract tumors associated with ataxia-telangiectasia, common variable immune deficiency, and IgA deficiency (38). The validity of this association may be questioned, since numbers are small and the age of tumor appearance quite different (17–21 years in ataxia and 50 years in common variable immune deficiency). In addition, other genetic factors may be operative in ataxia, since there is a high incidence of tumors in first-degree relatives of these patients, relatives who do not show immune deficiency (223,224). Is this another case of possible restricted surveillance to certain tumor types (as discussed in the "Experimental Evidence" section), or is it a special case of genetic susceptibility to tumor development (see 225 for review)? The existence of conditions (mostly with a genetic basis) associated with a high risk for tumor development but with no detectable immunologic alterations is well documented (221,225) and is beyond the scope of this review.

The early appearance of tumors in the severe combined immune deficiencies (i.e., 3 to 45 months of age; see 38) would suggest the possibility of tumor developing in the embryo, related or not to actual transplacental carcinogenic influences. However, the tumors were all lymphoreticular and not of the types that appear early in life (i.e., Wilms' tumor, neuroblastoma, primary carcinoma of the liver or presacral teratoma; see 226).

Some brief remarks concerning leprosy, sarcoidosis, and Hodgkin's disease are in order. Certain forms of leprosy as well as sarcoidosis and Hodgkin show moderate to severe immunologic deficiency, despite which tumor incidence is usually not increased. In leprosy, especially the lepromatous form, there is a severe deficit of cellular immunity, comparable to that observed in the primary immune deficiencies (see 227 for review); however, no differences between observed and expected incidence of leukemia-lymphoma, Hodgkin, or epithelial tumors was found in a large group of patients (217), as well as in necropsy material (228). It was concluded that "the results of this study provide no support for the hypothesis that defects of cellular immunity play an important role in the pathogenesis of human malignancies or that chronic intense stimulation of the lymphoreticular system predisposes that system to malignant transformation" (217). Sarcoidosis produces a moderate immunologic deficit (229), and most of the studies with large numbers of patients do not mention increased tumor incidence (229,230). One study showed some interesting features: in a total of 2,544 patients, 48 developed tumors (expected 33.9); however, the increase was due to lung cancer in males (9 observed versus 2.8 expected) and lymphoma (6 observed versus 0.5 expected), while no significant differences were observed for all the other forms of cancer (231). Again, the immune surveillance predictions are not fulfilled. In patients with Hodgkin's disease there has been a reported increased incidence of second malignancies complicating Hodgkin in remission (6 tumors in 452 patients); however, as indicated by the authors, "The mechanism of oncogenesis may represent a combination of the immunosuppressive effects and cellular effects of . . . treatment" (232). The group with highest tumor incidence in this case was the one that had a combination of chemotherapy and intense radiotherapy (232).

In summary, a reflective analysis of the incidence of tumors in patients with primary (as well as "secondary") immunodeficiencies does not support the generality of immunologic surveillance as an operative mechanism; it suggests a more restricted possibility (which may be explained also by alternative mechanisms) related especially to the development of lymphoreticular tumors. The orthodox theory of surveillance would have predicted higher incidence of tumors of all classes and probably multiple tumors in the same patient (as is the case with polyoma virus oncogenesis in immunodepressed mice, which still remains as the prime example of a surveillance of immunologic nature).

Since the initial descriptions of *de novo* appearance of lymphomas in patients immunodepressed for kidney transplantation (34,233), this peculiar association has been considered as additional supportive evidence for the concept of immunologic surveillance (3–5). For extensive discussion of these cases as they have been accumulating since 1968, also through a "registry," see refs. 34–37 and 233–235. If the latest figure of 256 tumor cases (235) is related to the total number of kidney transplants of the latest "Human Renal Transplant Registry" (236), which includes 16,444 patients, the tumor incidence is 1.5% and 2% if calculated from the 12,389 patients of the 11th Registry of Renal Transplants (237). Thus, the 5–6% risk for tumor development frequently quoted (36,37,233–235) seems too high. Another large epidemiologic study from the Scandia Transplant Program (238) showed a tumor incidence of 1.6% (30 tumors in 1,862 patients). The main types of tumors appearing in the transplanted patients were, for a total of 256 cases: 100 tumors of skin and/or lip (39%); 69 lymphomas (27%), of which 30 (44%) had mainly involvement of the central nervous system; and 19 tumors of the cervix uteri (7%) (see ref. 235). This distribution is fairly similar to those recorded in the earlier reports (34–36,233,234). However, when proper epidemiologic analysis was used in a study based on 6,297 transplant patients at risk (215), it became apparent that while the risk for development of reticulum cell sarcomas was 350 times greater than expected, the risk for development of other tumors was usually comparable to the expected figures. This observation was confirmed in a smaller series of 1,862 patients (238). Both studies noted that none of the common tumors for the adult age group were increased in incidence—i.e., breast, lung, prostate, etc. (215,238). Similarly, none of the reports on renal transplantation in aged patients (55 or older) showed an inordinate increase in tumors of any kind (239–241). Thus, it seems that again, as was the case with the primary immune deficiencies, the tumors appearing in these patients seem to be quite restricted, represented mostly by the solid lymphoma category.

The large differences in tumor incidence and tumor type reported by different centers (see ref. 12 for discussion) may be due to "a reporting artifact in that there would be a tendency to report the more florid and lethal malignancies to the registry" (233). Conversely, it could be argued that the high incidence of skin, lip, and uterine tumors reported from some centers may be due to the meticulous search for such tumors, a search to which few other patients are subjected (see 11,12). It should also be emphasized that, as with the primary immunodeficient patients, the main problem of the transplant immunodepressed patients is the high incidence of recurrent infections and sepsis, which accounts for most of the deaths (236,237). Thus, much of the discussion concerning the possible origin of the lymphoreticular tumors in immunodepressed patients undergoing chronic antigenic stimulation (by infections and the grafted organ) is similar to that concerning the primary immune deficiencies. Another interesting observation is that while the prognosis of the solid lymphomas is poor, the prognosis and survival of the patients with skin, lip, or uterine tumors was quite good after conventional surgical treatment (34–36,233–235).

The role of uremia as an additional immunodepressive factor in these patients cannot be excluded (242), especially since the vast majority of the transplants are for kidney disorders. Uremia produces a profound deficit of cell-mediated immunity (242,243), and one publication has reported a high incidence of primary tumors in uremic patients after the onset of chronic renal failure: 10 tumors appearing in 9 of 646 patients in chronic hemodialysis (244). The most interesting point of this study is that the tumor types were the ones expected in the normal age-matched population (i.e., breast, kidney, lung, etc.) and not of the types observed in the immunodepressed kidney transplants (244). If these trends are confirmed and extended, especially with respect to the differences in tumor types, the immunodepressive effect of chronic uremia may represent a good case for immunologic control of malignant development in man. However, the available information on patients in chronic hemodialysis, albeit incomplete, does not support the report described above (245–248), either in adult (245–246) or pediatric patients (248). Reference 247 concerns a "National Registry of Long-Term Dialysis Patients" with "about 5,000 patients" and records 1% tumors "as cause of death" in these patients, without clear indication of tumor incidence, age of the patients, etc.

Concerning the etiology of the lymphoreticular tumors in the transplant patients, we have mentioned the possible role of immune depression plus chronic antigenic stimulation (209–211), the possible deregulation of the immune system as a consequence of immunodepression (212,213), activation of endogenous viruses (212), and a possible role for herpes viruses (214), to which we could also add cytomegalovirus, since it has a marked prevalence in the immunodepressed transplant patients (249) and both herpes and cytomeglovirus can produce malignant transformation in vitro (250).

The high incidence of central nervous tissue involvement in the patients developing lymphomas, especially the solitary brain localizations, is unprecedented (251,252), reticulum cell sarcomas of the brain being extremely rare (253). As discussed in one review (11), "Why should lymphomas arise preferentially in the brain of an already immunodepressed person? Why do the transplant recipients develop cerebral lymphomas and not gliomas?" A third question is: Why are central nervous system tumors (including lymphomas) rare in the patients with primary immunologic deficiencies? It is apparent that we do not have answers to such questions.

One proposed interpretation of the brain lymphoma problem (11) suggests that they may be related to corticosteroids used in such patients, which may "alter the permeability of the blood-brain barrier to lymphoid cells" (11). However, long-term steroid treatment in experimental animals and in man has not produced such preferential effect on the central nervous system (see 12 for review).

An example: in a group of six patients with lymphoid malignancies immunodepression with antilymphocyte serum (in addition to chemotherapy) was added to treat concomitant autoimmune diseases (254); however, "neither spread nor activation of the tumors" was observed and no preferential brain localization was detected (254).

In summary, the clinical data on transplanted patients, although offering a most intriguing set of questions and problems pertaining to cancer biology, do not fit with the orthodox view on immune surveillance. In addition, the clinical behavior of the more conventional tumors appearing in the immunodepressed transplant patients is quite comparable to that observed in nonimmunodepressed patients (34–37). Concerning the incidence of distant metastasis recorded for the epithelial tumors, although the information is incomplete in the published material, it does not seem inordinately high (9 liver metastases plus one to pancreas in 182 cases analyzed by Penn, 37).

Another revealing group that does not fit with the surveillance theories is that of organ transplant recipients with preexisting tumors—i.e., patients who had cancer 5 years or less before organ transplantation (37). In a report of 76 such cases Penn indicates that in 27% of the patients the cancer was incidental, while in the remaining cases the organ replacement was performed specifically for the treatment of cancers involving kidney or liver (37). Although the group is heterogeneous and the age of the patients is not indicated, Penn remarks that "when all the malignancy was completely eradicated before the time of transplantation, there was little chance of subsequent recurrence" (37). Of the 76 patients discussed, no recurrences were observed in 41 (54%); however, 4 patients (5%) developed unrelated *de novo* malignancies (37); unfortunately, no additional information is provided concerning the second tumor. In relation to the clinical course Penn states: "At present it is not possible to determine what influence the immunosuppressive therapy exerted in patients where the cancer was not completely eradicated. In some recipients this treatment apparently did not alter the natural history of the neoplasms" (37).

Finally, we will discuss briefly the case for chronic immunodepression and tumor development in nontransplanted patients (see 11 and 12 for review). Some of the cautionary remarks concerning case reports, anecdotal collection of cases, clusterings, lack of proper controls for comparison, and inability to determine the actual population at risk, which were discussed at the beginning of this section, are pertinent here. Penn has begun a compilation of some of these cases (36,37) and has data on 49 tumors appearing in immunodepressed patients with nonmalignant disease and on new malignancies in 135 cancer patients treated with chemotherapy. The danger of this approach is one of creating false relationships, the main problem being that of relating the effects of the drugs to immunodepression (and not to other direct mechanisms) (see 11,12 for review)—especially since in the majority of the cases there is no evidence that the treatment was indeed immunodepressive (there are at least two studies in which patients treated with azathioprine alone or with prednisone showed normal immunologic responses, 255,256). Concerning positive versus negative data, Penn included in his series 7 patients with rheumatoid arthritis treated with immunodepressive agents who developed leukemia lymphoma (37). However, in a controlled trial on the effects of azathioprine treatment on rheumatoid arthritis (27 patients received drug and

27 received placebo for 30 months) 3 lymphomas developed in the placebo group (257). The authors observe that "it is interesting to speculate on the conclusions which might be drawn had the tumors occurred in the azathioprine-treated group" (257). Concerning the extensive use of immunodepressive chemotherapy in patients with disorders other than cancer, two extensive reviews show that the risk for tumor development in those conditions is relatively low (258,259). The possibility of direct action of the drugs (or treatments) as oncogenic agents has been discussed for the Hodgkin patients (232) and in reviews (11,12,258,259). Indeed, a recent report suggests direct oncogenicity of the bladder in patients treated with cyclophosphamide, mostly for myeloma (260).

In summary, the association of increased risk for tumor development in immunodepressed patients with diseases other than those requiring organ transplantation is not well established and needs further definition, especially concerning actual tumor incidences and prevalences.

CONCLUDING REMARKS

On the whole, it is apparent that the cause of the increased incidence of certain tumors in immunodepressed hosts is still unexplained. It is also apparent that the orthodox interpretation of immunologic surveillance as a thymus-dependent immune mechanism capable of destroying in situ tumors can be questioned concerning its generality, efficiency, and perhaps even its reality. Under certain special conditions it appears that immune surveillance-like mechanisms may be operative (i.e., polyoma oncogenesis, other DNA viruses). Certain models, notably the nude athymic mice, while not fulfilling many of the predictions of the immune surveillance theory, may represent an excellent model for the study of thymus-independent antitumor immune mechanisms. It is felt that by unbiased study of the multiple exceptions to the theory, a better understanding of tumor host interactions, especially during early tumor development, may evolve.

ACKNOWLEDGMENT

I would like to thank Linda Stevenson for her help in preparing this manuscript.

REFERENCES

1. Ehrlich, P., in *The Collected Papers of Paul Ehrlich*, Vol. II (F. Himmelweit, ed.), London, Pergamon Press, 1957, p. 559.
2. Thomas, L., in *Cellular and Humoral Aspects of the Hypersensitivity States* (H. S. Lawrence, ed.), Hoeber-Harper, New York, 1959, p. 529.
3. Burnet, R. M., *Progr. Exp. Tumor Res.* **13**, 1–27 (1970).
4. Burnet, F. M., *Immunological Surveillance*, Pergamon, London, 1970.
5. Burnet, F. M., *Transplant. Rev.* **7**, 3 (1971).
6. Good, R. A., *Proc. Natl. Acad. Sci.* (U.S.A.) **69**, 1026 (1972).

7. Klein, G., *The Harvey Lectures,* Series 69, Academic Press, New York, 1975, p. 71.

8. Stutman, O., *Natl. Cancer Inst. Monogr.* **35,** 107 (1972).

9. Kersey, J. H., Spector, B. D., Good, R. A., *Pediatrics* **84,** 263 (1974).

10. Kripke, M. L. , Borsos, T., *Israel J. Med. Sci.* **10,** 888 (1974).

11. Melief, C. J. M., Schwartz, M. A., in *Cancer: A Comprehensive Treatise,* Vol. 1. (F. Becker, ed.), Plenum Press, New York, 1975, p. 121.

12. Stutman, O., *Adv. Cancer Res.* **22,** 261 (1975).

13. Prehn, R. T., in *Immune Surveillance* (R. T. Smith and M. Landy, eds.), Academic Press, New York, 1970, p. 451.

14. Prehn, R. T., in *Clinical Immunobiology,* Vol. 2 (F. H. Bach and R. A. Good, eds.), Academic Press, New York, 1974, p. 191.

15. Stutman, O., *Excerpta Medica International Congress Series No. 349,* Vol. 1, *Prox. XI International Cancer Congress,* Excerpta Medica, Amsterdam, 1974, p. 275.

16. Kripke, M. O., Borsos, T., *J. Natl. Cancer Inst.* **52,** 1393, 1974.

17. Schwartz, R. S., *N. Eng. J. Med.* **293,** 181 (1975).

18. Moller, G., Moller, E., *J. Natl. Cancer Inst.* **55,** 755 (1975).

19. Brent, L., *Progr. Allergy* **5,** 271 (1958).

20. MacKaness, G. B., in *Progress in Immunology* (B. Amos, ed.), Academic Press, New York, 1971, p. 413.

21. Brown, K. N., *Nature* **230,** 163 (1971).

22. Targett, G. A., in *Contemporary Topics in Immunobiology,* Vol. 2. (A. J. S. Davies and R. L. Carter, eds.), Plenum Press, New York, 1973, p. 217.

23. Nelson, D. S., *Transplant. Rev.* **19,** 226 (1974).

24. Stutman, O., and Good, R. A., in *Advances in Biology of Skin,* Vol. 11, *Immunology and the Skin* (W. Montagna and R. E. Billingham, eds.), Appleton, New York, 1971, p. 357.

25. Thomas, L., in *The Immune System and Infectious Diseases,* 4th Intl. Convoc. Immunol., Karger, Basel, 1975, p. 2.

26. Smithers, S. R., and Terry, R. J., *Trans. Roy. Soc. Trop. Med. Hyg.* **61,** 517 (1967).

27. Mikulska, Z. B., Smith, C., Alexander, P., *J. Natl. Cancer Inst.* **36,** 29 (1966).

28. Clegg, J. A., Smithers, S. R., Terry, R. J., *Nature* **232,** 653 (1971).

29. Burnet, F. M., *Brit. Med. Bull.* **20,** 154 (1964).

30. C. Darwin, letter to J. M. Herbert, in *The Life and Letters of Charles Darwin* (F. Darwin, ed.), Vol. 1, Murray, London, 1887, p. 334.

31. Good, R. A., and Finstad, J., *Natl. Cancer Inst. Monogr.* **31,** 41 (1969).

32. Good, R. A., in *Immune Surveillance* (R. T. Smith and M. Landy, eds.), Academic Press, New York, 1970, p. 437.

33. Gatti, R. A., and Good, R. A., *Cancer* **28,** 89 (1971).

34. Penn, I., Hammond, W., Brettschneider, L., and Starzl, T., *Transplant. Proc.* **1,** 106 (1969).

35. Penn, I., *Malignant Tumors in Organ Transplant Recipients,* Springer-Verlag, New York, 1970.

36. Penn, I., *Cancer* **34,** 858 (1974).

37. Penn, I., *Cancer* **34,** 1474 (1974).

38. Kersey, J. H., Spector, B. D., Good, R. A., *Int. J. Cancer* **12,** 333 (1973).

39. Kersey, J. H., Spector, B. D., Good, R. A., *Adv. Cancer Res.* **18,** 211 (1973).

40. Kersey, J. H., Spector, B. D., in *Immunodeficiency in Man and Animals, Birth Defects Original Article Series,* The National Foundation, Vol. 9, No. 1 (1975), p. 289.

41. Burnet, F. M., *Brit. Med. J.* **1,** 841 (1957).

42. Burnet, F. M., *Lancet* **1,** 1171 (1967).

43. Prehn, R. T., *J. Natl. Cancer Inst.* **32,** 1 (1964).

44. Prehn, R. T., in *Cellular Antigens* (A. Nowotny, ed.), Srpinger-Verlag, New York, 1972, p. 308.

45. Prehn, R. T., *Ann. N.Y. Acad. Sci.* **164,** 449 (1969).

46. Bartlett, G. L., *J. Natl. Cancer Inst.* **49,** 493 (1972).

47. Baldwin, R. W., and Embleton, N. J., *Int. J. Cancer* **4,** 47 (1969).

48. Colnaghi, M. I., Menard, S., and Della Parta, G., *J. Natl. Cancer Inst.* **47,** 1325 (1971).

49. Burnet, F. M., in *Immune Surveillance* (R. T. Smith and M. Landy, eds.), Academic Press, New York, 1970, p. 512.

50. Mondal, S., Iype, P. T., Griesbach, L. M., and Heidelberger, C., *Cancer Res.* **30,** 1593 (1970).

51. Parmiani, G., Carbone, G., and Prehn, R. T., *J. Natl. Cancer Inst.* **46,** 261 (1971).

52. Parmiani, G., Carbone, G., and Lembo, R., *Cancer Res.* **33,** 750 (1973).

53. Basombrio, M. A., and Prehn, R. T., *Int. J. Cancer* **10,** 1 (1972).

54. Carbone, G., and Parmiani, G., *J. Natl. Cancer Inst.* **55,** 1195 (1975).

55. Warwick, G. P., *Fed. Proc.* **30,** 1760 (1971).

56. Bertram, J. S., and Heidelberger, C., *Cancer Res.* **34,** 526 (1974).

57. Marquardt, H., *Cancer Res.* **34,** 1612 (1974).

58. Prehn, R. T., *J. Natl. Cancer Inst.* **55,** 189 (1975).

59. Slemmer, G., *Natl. Cancer Inst. Monogr.* **35,** 57 (1972).

60. Lappe, M. A., *J. Reticuloendothel. Soc.* **10,** 120 (1971).

61. Lappe, M. A., *Natl. Cancer Inst. Monogr.* **35,** 49 (1972).

62. Andrews, E. J., *J. Natl. Cancer Inst.* **52,** 729 (1974).

63. Billingham, R. E., and Silvers, W. K., in *Ciba Found. Symp. Transplantation,* Little, Brown, Boston, 1962, p. 90.

64. Homburger, F., *Progr. Exp. Tumor Res.* **10,** 163 (1968).

65. Homburger, F., *Cancer* **23,** 313 (1969).

66. Homburger, F., *Progr. Exp. Tumor Res.* **16,** 152 (1972).

67. Friedell, G. H., Oatman, B. W., and Sherman, J. D., *Transpl. Bull.* **7,** 97 (1960).

68. Dunham, J. L., and Herrold, K. M., *J. Natl. Cancer Inst.* **29,** 1047 (1962).

69. Sabes, W. R., Chaudhry, A. P., and Gorlin, R. J., *J. Dent. Res.* **42,** 1118 (1963).

70. Shklar, G., *Cancer Res.* **26,** 2461 (1966).

71. Woods, D. A., *Nature* (London) **224,** 276 (1969).

72. Giunta, J. L., and Shklar, G., *Oral Surgery* **31,** 344 (1971).

73. Ghadially, F. N., and Illman, O., *J. Path. Bact.* **81,** 45 (1960).

74. Moore, C., and Christopherson, W. M., *Arch. Surg.* **84,** 425 (1962).

75. Hammer, J. E., III, *Oral Surgery* **22,** 114 (1966).

76. Ziegler, M. M., Lopez, V., and Barker, C. F., *J. Surg. Res.* **18,** 201 (1975).

77. Luginbuhl, H., Frankenhauser, R., and McGrath, J. T., *Progr. Neurol. Surgery* **2,** 85 (1968).

78. Wechsler, W., *Progr. Exp. Tumor Res.* **17,** 219 (1972).

79. Koestner, A., Swenberg, J. A., and Wechsler, W., *Progr. Exp. Tumor Res.* **17,** 9 (1972).

80. Druckery, H., Ivankovic, S., Preussman, S., Zulch, K. J., and Mendel, H. D., in *The Experimental Biology of Brain Tumors* (W. M. Kirsch, E. G. Paoletti, and P. Paoletti, eds.), Thomas, Springfield, 1972, p. 85.

81. Denlinger, R. H., Swenberg, J. A., Koestner, A., and Wechsler, W., *J. Natl. Cancer Inst.* **50,** 87 (1973).

82. Schmahl, D., Mundt, D., and Schmidt, K. G., *Z. Krebsforsch. Klin. Oncol.* (in press).

83. Prehn, R. T., and Lappe, M. A., *Transplant. Rev.* **7,** 26 (1971).

84. Prehn, R. T., *Science* **176,** 170 (1972).

85. Shearer, W. T., Philpott, G. W., and Parker, C. W., *Science* **182,** 1357 (1973).

86. Oettgen, H. F., in *Clinical Immunobiology,* Vol. 2. (F. H. Bach and R. A. Good, eds.), Academic Press, New York, 1974, p. 206.

87. Strickland, G. T., Ahmed, A., and Sell, K. W., *Clin. Exp. Immunol.* **22,** 167 (1975).

88. Hibbs, J. B., Jr., Lambert, L. H., and Remington, J. S., *Proc. Soc. Exp. biol. Med.* **139,** 1053 (1972).

89. Hersh, E. M., Whitecar, J. P.., Jr., McCredie, K. B., Bodey, G. P., Sr., and Freidreich, E. J. *N. Eng. J. Med.* **285,** 1211 (1971).

90. Malmgren, R. A., Bennison, B. E., and McKinley, T. W., *Proc. Soc. Exptl. Biol. Med.* **79,** 484 (1952).

91. Parfentjev, I. A., and Duran-Reynals, F., *Science* **113,** 690 (1951).

92. Dent, P. B., *Progr. Med. Virol.* **14,** 1 (1972).

93. Dent, P. B., in *The Immune System and Infectious Diseases,* Fourth Convoc. Immunol., Karger, Basel, 1975, p. 95.

94. Stutman, O., *Israel J. Med. Sci.* **9,** 217 (1973).

95. Defendi, V., and Roosa, R. A., in *The Thymus* (V. Defendi and D. Metcalf, eds.), Wistar Inst. Press., Philadelphia, 1964, p. 211.

96. Grant, G. A., and Miller, J. F. A. P., *Nature* (London) **205,** 1124 (1965).

97. Law, L. W., *Nature* (London) **205,** 672 (1965).

98. Law, L. W., *Cancer Res.* **26,** 1121 (1966).

99. Balner, H., and Dersjant, H., *J. Natl. Cancer Inst.* **36,** 513 (1966).

100. Johnson, S., *Brit. J. Cancer* **22,** 93 (1968).

101. Nomoto, K., and Takeya, K., *J. Natl. Cancer Inst.* **42,** 445 (1969).

102. Allison, A. C., and Taylor, R. B., *Cancer Res.* **27,** 703 (1967).

103. Trainin, N., Linker-Israeli, M., Small, M., and Boiato-Chen, L., *Intl. J. Cancer* **2,** 236 (1967).

104. Gillette, R. W., and Fox, A., *Cellular Immunol.* **19,** 328 (1975).

105. Cerilli, G. J., and Treat, R. C., *Transplantation* **8,** 774 (1969).

106. Rabbat, A. G.., and Jeejeebhoy, H. F.., *Transplantation* **9,** 164 (1970).

107. Balner, H., and Dersjant, H., *Nature* (London) **224,** 376 (1969).

108. Carbone, G., and Parmiani, G., *Tumori* **57,** 226 (1971).

109. Fisher, J. C., Davis, R. C., and Mannick, J. A., *Surgery* **68,** 150 (1970).

110. Fisher, B., Soliman, O., and Fisher, E. R., *Cancer Res.* **30,** 2035 (1970).

111. Wagner, J. L., and Haughton, G., *J. Natl. Cancer Inst.* **46,** 1 (1971).

112. Haran-Ghera, N., and Lurie, M., *J. Natl. Cancer Inst.* **46,** 103 (1971).

113. Rigdon, R. H., Neal, J., Anigstein, D., and Anigstein, L., *Cancer Res.* **27,** 2318 (1967).

114. Lappe, M., *Israel J. Med. Sci.* **7,** 52 (1971).

115. Baroni, C. D., Mingazzini, P., Pesando, P., Cavallera, A., Uccini, S., and Scelsi, R., *Tumori* **58,** 397 (1972).

116. Baroni, C. D., Scelsi, R., Peronace, M. L., and Uccini, S., *Brit. J. Cancer* **28,** 221 (1973).

117. Bolton, P. M., *Oncology* **27,** 520 (1973).

118. Mandel, M. A., and DeCosse, J. J., *J. Immunol.* **109,** 360 (1972).

119. Trainin, N., and Linker-Israeli, M., *J. Natl. Cancer Inst.* **44,** 893 (1970).

120. Rubin, B. A., *Progr. Exp. Tumor Res.* **14,** 138 (1971).

121a. Kroes, R., Berkvens, J. M., and Weisburger, J. H., *Cancer Res.* **35,** 2651 (1975).

121b. Weisburger, J. H., Madison, R. M., Ward, J. M., Viguera, C., and Weisburger, E. K., *J. Natl. Cancer Inst.* **154,** 1185 (1975).

122. Stutman, O., *Science* **183,** 534 (1974).

123. Stutman, O., in *Proceedings First International Workshop on Nude Mice* (J. Rygaard and C. O. Povlsen, eds.), Fischer Verlag, Stuttgart, 1974, p. 257.

124. Outzen, H. C., Custer, R. P., Eaton, G. J., and Prehn, R. T., *J. Reticuloendothel. Soc.* **17,** 1 (1975).

125. Frankel, H. H., Yamamoto, R. S., Weisburger, E. K., and Weisburger, J. H., *Toxicol. Appl. Pharmacol.* **17,** 462 (1970).

126. Barich, L. L., Schwarz, J., and Barich, D., *J. Invest. Dermatol.* **39,** 615 (1962).

127. Sheehan, R., and Shklar, G., *Cancer Res.* **32,** 420 (1972).

128. Dobson, R. L., *J. Invest. Dermatol.* **41,** 475 (1963).

129. Nemoto, N., Kato, N., Mizuno, D., and Takayama, S., *Gann* **62**, 293 (1971).

130. Arata, T., Tanaka, S., and Southam, C. M., *J. Natl. Cancer Inst.* **40**, 623 (1968).

131. Dargent, M., Bourgoin, J., Noel, P., and Weissbrod, R., *Eur. J. Cancer* **8**, 605 (1972).

132. Bolton, P. M., *Oncology* **27**, 525 (1973).

133. Trainin, N., *Cancer Res.* **23**, 415 (1963).

134. Gillman, T., Hathorn, M., and Penn, J., *Brit. J. Cancer* **10**, 394 (1956).

135. Schmahl, D., *Z. Krebsforsch. Klin. Oncol.* **8**, 211 (1974).

136. Anbari, N., Shklar, G., and Cataldo, E., *J. Dent. Res.* **44**, 1056 (1965).

137. Hoch-Ligetti, C., *J. Natl. Cancer Inst.* **15**, 1056 (1965).

138. Sulzberger, M. B., Herrmann, F., Piccagli, R., and Frank, L., *Proc. Soc. Exp. Biol. Med.* **83**, 673 (1953).

139. Spain, D. M., Molomut, N., and Novikoff, A. B., *Cancer Res.* **16**, 138 (1956).

140. Sherwin-Weidenriech, R., Herrman, R., and Rothstein, M. J., *Cancer Res.* **19**, 1150 (1959).

141. Qureshi, S. A., and Zaman, H., *Cancer Res.* **26**, 1516 (1966).

142. Nakai, T., *Cancer Res.* **21**, 221 (1961).

143. Baserga, R., and Shubik, P., *Cancer Res.* **14**, 12 (1954).

144. Engelbreth-Holm, J., and Asboe-Hansen, G., *Acta Pathol. Microbiol. Scand.*, **32**, 560 (1953).

145. Ghadially, F. N., and Green, H. N., *Brit. J. Cancer Res.* **8**, 291 (1954).

146. Lisco, H., Ducoff, H. S., and Baserga, R., *Bull. Johns Hopkins Hosp.* **103**, 101 (1958).

147. Foley, W. A., and Cole, J. J., *Cancer Res.* **23**, 1176 (1963).

148. Nowell, P. C., and Cole, L. J., *Radiation Res.* **11**, 545 (1959).

149. Duhig, J. T., *Arch. Path.* **79**, 177 (1965).

150. Heston, W. E., Lorenz, E., and Deringer, M. K., *J. Natl. Cancer Inst.* **13**, 573 (1953).

151. Vandeputte, M., *Ann. Inst. Pasteur* **122**, 677 (1972).

152. Grant, G. A., and Roe, F. J. C., *Nature* (London) **223**, 1060 (1969).

153. Weston, B. J., in *Contemporary Topics in Immunobiology,* Vol. 2 (A. J. S. Davies and R. L. Carter, eds.), Plenum Press, New York, 1973, p. 237.

154. Rabotti, G. F., in *Proceedings Third Quadr. Conf. on Cancer: Lung Tumors in Animals,* University of Perugia, Div. Cancer Res., Perugia, 1966, p. 239.

155. Burstein, N. A., and Law, L. W., *Nature* (London) **231**, 450 (1970).

156. Law, L. W., *Cancer Res.* **29**, 1 (1969).

157. Sanford, B. H., Kohn, H. I., Daly, J. J., and Soo, S. F., *J. Immunol.* **110**, 1437 (1973).

158. Cornelius, E. A., *Transplantation* **12**, 531 (1971).

159. Martinez, C., *Nature* (London) **203**, 1188 (1964).

160. Olivi, M., and Bolis, G. B., *Lav. Anat. Pat. Perugia* **27**, 77 (1967).

161. Sakakura, T., and Nishizuka, Y., *Gann* **58**, 441 (1967).

162. Heppner, G. H., Wood, P. C., and Weiss, D. W., *Israel J. Med. Sci.* **4**, 1204 (1968).

163. Yunis, E. J., Martinez, C., Smith, J., Stutman, O., and Good, R. A., *Cancer Res.* **29**, 174 (1969).

164. Squartini, F., Olivi, M., and Bolis, G. B., *Cancer Res.* **30**, 2069 (1970).

165. Papatestas, A. E., Osserman, K. E., and Kark, A. E., *Brit. J. Cancer* **25**, 635 (1971).

166. Vessey, M. P., and Doll, R., *Brit. J. Cancer* **26**, 53 (1972).

167. Simpson, E., and Nehlsen, S. L., *Clin. Exp. Immunol.* **9**, 79 (1971).

168. Rygaard, J., and Povlsen, C. O., *Transplantation* **17**, 135 (1974).

169. Heston, W. E., in *RNA Viruses and Host Genome in Oncogenesis* (P. Emmelot and P. Bentvelzen, eds.), North Holland, Amsterdam, 1972, p. 13.

170. Deringer, M. K., *J. Natl. Cancer Inst.* **35**, 1047 (1965).

171. Andervont, H. B., and Dunn, T. B., *J. Natl. Cancer Inst.* **8**, 235 (1948).

172. Madison, R. M., Rabstein, L. S., and Bryan, W. R., *J. Natl. Cancer Inst.* **40**, 683 (1968).

173. Ebbesen, P., *J. Natl. Cancer Inst.* **47**, 1241 (1971).

174. Smith, C. S., and Pilgrim, H. E., *Proc. Soc. Exp. Biol. Med.* **138,** 542 (1971).

175. Kiessling, R., Klein, E., and Wigzell, H., *Europ. J. Immunol.* **5,** 112 (1975).

176. Herberman, R., Nunn, M. E., and Lavrin, D. H., *Intl. J. Cancer* **16,** 216 (1975).

177. Stutman, O., *J. Immunol.* **114,** 1213 (1975).

178. Martin, W. J., and Martin, S. E., *Nature* (London) **249,** 564 (1974).

179. Haller, O., and Lindermann, J., *Nature* (London) **250,** 679 (1974).

180. Kirschstein, R. L., Rabson, A. S., and Peters, L. A., *Proc. Soc. Exp. Biol. Med.* **117,** 198 (1964).

181. Yohn, D. S., Funk, C. A., and Grace, J. T., *J. Immunol.* **100,** 771 (1968).

182. Vandeputte, M., Genys, P., Leyten, R., and DeSomer, P., *Life Sci.* **2,** 475 (1963).

183. Vandeputte, M., and DeSomer, P., *Nature* (London) **206,** 520 (1965).

184. Miller, J. F. A. P., Ting, R. C., and Law, L. W., *Proc. Soc. Exp. Biol. Med.* **116,** 323 (1964).

185. Malmgren, R. A., Rabson, A. S., and Carney, P. G., *J. Natl. Cancer Inst.* **33,** 101 (1964).

186. Law, L. W., and Ting, R. C., *Proc. Soc. Exp. Biol. Med.* **119,** 823 (1965).

187. Vandeputte, M., Eyssen, H., Sobis, H., and DeSomer, P., *Intl. J. Cancer* **14,** 445 (1974).

188. Allison, A. C., Monga, J. M., and Hammond, V., *Nature* (London) **252,** 746 (1974).

189. Allison, A. C., and Law, L. W., *Proc. Exp. Biol. Med.* **127,** 207 (1968).

190. Vandeputte, M., *Life Sci.* **7,** 855 (1968).

191. Ting, R. C., and Law, L. W., *Prog. Exptl. Tumor Res.* **9,** 165 (1967).

192. Allison, A. C., *Proc. Roy. Soc. Med.,* **63,** 1077 (1970).

193. Rowe, W. P., Huebner, R. J., and Hartley, J., *Perspect. Virol.* **2,** 177 (1961).

194. Huebner, R. J., *Ann. N.Y. Acad. Sci.* **108,** 1129 (1963).

195. Gaugas, J. M., Chesterman, F. C., Hirsch, M. S., Rees, R. J. W., Harvey, J. J., and Gilchrist, C., *Nature* (London) **221,** 1033 (1969).

196. Foster, A. G., and Moll, T., *Am. J. Vet. Res.* **29,** 1831 (1968).

197. Payne, L. N., in *Proc. Symp. Christ's College on Oncogenesis and Herpes Viruses* (P. M. Biggs, G. de The, and L. N. Payne, eds.), WHO, Geneva, 1972, p. 21.

198. Kenyon, A. J., Sevoian, M., and Horwitz, M., *Avian. Dis.* **13,** 585 (1969).

199. Payne, L. N., and Rennie, M., *J. Natl. Cancer Inst.* **45,** 387 (1970).

200. Sharma, J. N., *Nature* (London) **246,** 177 (1974).

201. Cotter, P. F., Jaworski, R. M., Fredrickson, T. N., Scierman, L. W., and McBride, R. A., *J. Natl. Cancer Inst.* **54,** 969 (1975).

202. Morris, J. R., Jerome, F. N., and Reinhart, B. S., *Poult. Sci.* **48,** 1513 (1969).

203. Smith, N. W., and Calnek, B. W., *J. Natl. Cancer Inst.* **52,** 1595 (1974).

204. Duquesnoy, R. J., in *Immunodeficiency in Man and Animals, Birth Defects Original Article Series,* The National Foundation, Vol. 9, No. 1 (1975), p. 536.

205. Hesten, W. E., and Valhakis, G., in *Carcinogenesis: A Broad Critique,* Williams & Wilkins, Baltimore, 1967, p. 347.

206. Toth, B., *Cancer Res.* **28,** 727 (1968).

207. Stutman, O., *Fed. Proc.* **33,** 2028 (1974).

208. Doll, R., and Kinlen, L., *brit. Med. J.* **4,** 420 (1970).

209. Metcalf, D., *Brit. J. Cancer* **15,** 769 (1961).

210. Krueger, G. R. F., Malmgren, R. A., and Beard, C. W., *Transplantation* **11,** 138 (1971).

211. Krueger, G. R. F., *Natl. Cancer Inst. Monogr.* **35,** 183 (1972).

212. Schwartz, R. S., *Lancet* **I,** 1266 (1972).

213. Gershwin, M. E., and Steinberg, A. D., *Lancet* **II,** 1174 (1973).

214. Matas, A. J., Simmons, R. L., and Najarian, J. S., *Lancet* **1,** 1277 (1975).

215. Hoover, R., and Fraumeni, J. F., *Lancet* **II,** 55 (1973).

216. Oleinick, A., *Blood* **29,** 144 (1967).

217. Oleinick, A., *J. Natl. Cancer Inst.* **43,** 775 (1969).

218. Fraumeni, J. F., *Natl. Cancer Inst. Monogr.* **32,** 221 (1969).

219. Gabrielsen, A. E., Cooper, M. D., Peterson, R. D. A., and Good, R. A., in *Textbook of Immunopathology* (P. Miescher and H. Muller-Eberhard, eds.), Grune & Stratton, New York, 1968, p. 385.

220. Douglas, S. D., Goldberg, L. S., and Fudenberg, H. H., *Am. J. Med.* **48,** 48 (1970).

221. Kersey, J. H., in *International Course on Transplantation, Lyon 1974* (J. L. Touraine, J. Traeger, and R. Triau, eds.), Simep Eds., Villeurbanne-France, 1975, p. 132.

222. Ten Bensel, R. W., Stadlam, E. M., and Krivit, W., *J. Pediat.* **68,** 769 (1966).

223. Epstein, W. L., Fudenberg, H. H., Reed, W. B., Boder, E., and Sedgwick, R. P., *Intl. Arch. Allergy* **30,** 15 (1966).

224. Reed, W. B., Epstein, W. L., Boder, E., and Sedgwick, R. P., *J. Am. Med. Assoc.* **195,** 746 (1966).

225. Knudson, A. G., *Adv. Cancer Res.* **17,** 317 (1973).

226. Miller, R. W., in *Transplacental Carcinogenesis* (L. Tomatis and U. Mohr., eds.), International Agency for Research on Cancer, Lyons, 1973, p. 175.

227. Turk, J. L., and Bryceson, D. M., *Adv. Immunol.* **13,** 209 (1971).

228. Purtillo, D. T., and Pangi, C., *Cancer* **35,** 1259 (1975).

229. Mitchell, D. N., Siltzbach, L. E., Sutherland, I., and Hart, P. D., in *Immunologic Deficiency Diseases in Man, Birth Defects Original Article Series,* Vol. 4, No. 1 (1968), p. 364.

230. Editorial, *Am. J. Med.* **57,** 847 (1974).

231. Brincker, H., and Wilbek, E., *Brit. J. Cancer* **29,** 247 (1974).

232. Canellos, G. P., DeVita, V. T., Arsenau, J. C., Whang-Peng, J., and Johnson, R. E. C., *Lancet* **I,** 947 (1975).

233. Starzl, T. E., Penn, I., Putnam, C. W., Growth, C. G., and Halgrimson, C. G., *Transplant. Rev.* **7,** 112 (1971).

234. Penn, I., in *International Course on Transplantation,* 1974 (J. L. Touraine, J. Traeger, and R. Triau, eds.), Simep Eds., Villeurbanne-France, 1975, p. 128.

235. Penn, I., *Transplant. Proc.* **7,** 553 (1975).

236. The Twelfth Report of the Human Renal Transplant Registry, *J. Amer. Med. Assoc.* **233,** 787 (1975).

237. The Eleventh Report of the Human Renal Transplant Registry, *J. Amer. Med. Assoc.* **226,** 1197 (1973).

238. Birkeland, S. A., Kemp, E., and Hauge, M., *Tissue Antig.* **6,** 28 (1975).

239. Simmons, R. L., Kjellstrand, C. M., Buselmeier, T. J., and Najarian, J. S., *Arch. Surg.* **103,** 290 (1971).

240. Woods, J. E., Anderson, C. F., Johnson, W. J., Donadio, J. V., Frohnert, P. P., Leary, F. J., DeWeerd, J. H., and Taswell, J. F., *Surg. Gynecol. Obst.* **137,** 393 (1973).

241. Delmonico, F. L., Cosimi, B., and Russell, P. S., *Arch. Surg.* **110,** 1107 (1975).

242. Damin, G. J., Couch, N. P., and Murray, J. E., *Ann. N.Y. Acad. Sci.* **64,** 967 (1957).

243. Wilson, W. E., Kirkpatrick, C., and Talmage, D. W., *Ann. Intern. Med.* **62,** 1)1965).

244. Matas, A. J., Simmons, R. L., Kjellstrand, C. M., Buselmeier, T. J., and Najarian, J. S., *Lancet* **I,** 883 (1975).

245. Lowrie, E. G., Lazarus, J. M., Mocelin, A. J., Bailey, G. L., Hampers, C. L., Wilson, R. E., and Merrill, J. P., *N. Eng. J. Med.* **288,** 863, 1973.

246. Tilney, N. L., Hager, E. B., Boyden, C. M., Sandberg, G. W., and Wilson, R. E., *Ann. Surg.* **182,** 108 (1975).

247. Burton, B. T., Kreuger, K. K., and Bryan, F. A., *J. Amer. Med. Assoc.* **218,** 718 (1971).

248. Scharer, K., Brunner, F. P., Dehn, H., Gurland, H. J., Harler, H., and Parsons, F. M., in *Dialysis, Transplantation, Nephrology* (J. F. Moorhead, ed.), Pitman Medical, London, 1973, p. 58.

249. Fiala, M., Payne, J. E., Berne, T. V., Moore, T. C., Henle, W., Mont-Gomerie, J. Z., Chatterjee, S. N., and Guze, L. B., *J. Infect. Dis.* **132,** 421 (1975).

250. Rapp F., *J. Natl. Cancer Inst.* **50,** 825 (1973).

251. Schnneck, S. A., and Penn, I., *Arch. Neurol.* **22,** 226 (1970).

252. Schnneck, S. A., and Penn, I., *Lancet* **I,** 983 (1971).

253. Littman, P., and Wang, C. C., *Cancer* **35,** 1412 (1975).

254. Pirofsky, B., Ramirez-Mateos, J. C., Bardana, E. J., and Reid, H., *Bhering Inst. Mitt.* **51,** 212 (1972).

255. Swanson, M., and Schwartz, R. A., *N. Eng. J. Med.* **277,** 163 (1967).

256. Lee, A. K. Y., Mackay, I. R., Rowley, M. J., and Yap, C. Y., *Clin. Exp. Immunol.* **9,** 507 (1971).

257. Harris, J., Jessop, J. D., and Chaput de Saintonge, D. M., *Brit. Med. J.* **4,** 463 (1971).

258. Skinner, M. D., and Schwartz, R. S., *N. Eng. J. Med.* **287,** 221 and 281 (two parts), 1972.

259. NIH Conference, Cytotoxic drugs in treatment of nonmalignant disease, *Ann. Intl. Med.* **76,** 619 (1972).

260. Wall, R. L., and Clausen, K. P., *N. Eng. J. Med.* **293,** 271 (1975).

Chapter Three

Mechanisms of Tumor Cell Destruction

CHRISTOPHER S. HENNEY

Department of Medicine, Johns Hopkins University School of Medicine and O'Neill Memorial Research Laboratories of Good Samaritan Hospital, Baltimore, Maryland

The possible involvement of the immune system in the destruction of tumor cells has been a matter of concern for several decades. Indeed, the subject was a recurring theme in the works of Ehrlich (1). Today, Ehrlich might be flattered to note that his ideas on the subject are still widely plagiarized, but he might express concern that the intervening time has yielded so little additional information. Certainly, the speculations of 70 years ago have been reinforced by convincing experimental evidence of the involvement of the immune system in the rejection of neoplastic tissue, but the manner of this participation remains in doubt.

In describing the infiltration of lymphoid cells that preceded the regression of a murine mammary carcinoma, Kidd and Toolan (1950) asked whether the lymphocytes could actually kill cancer cells (2). Some 10 years later an affirmative answer first came from Govaert's demonstration of the direct lytic activity of lymphoid cells in vitro (3). In the ensuing years a multiplicity of tumor-destructive pathways have been described in which cells of the immune system, or their products, play a salient role (4,5).

Our current knowledge of the tumor-destructive effects of the immune system has been derived almost exclusively from in vitro studies, and the material presented in this chapter represents a précis of some of this documentation. In many cases the studies reported deal with the destruction of nontumor cells, particularly

The author's original work reported here was supported by grant AI 10280 from the National Institute of Allergy and Infectious Disease, grant GB 36290 from the National Science Foundation, and by contract NO1-CB-43932 from the National Cancer Institute.

This is communication No. 203 from the O'Neill Memorial Research Laboratories of the Good Samaritan Hospital.

erythrocytes and lymphocytes. At this time it is difficult to know to what extent one can relate these studies to the mechanism of lysis of tumor cells.

In vitro observations have led to the delineation of at least four major pathways by which cells of the immune system contribute to tumor cell destruction:

1. Complement-mediated lysis in the presence of antitumor cell antibody.
2. Antibody-dependent, complement-independent, cell-mediated cytotoxicity.
3. The direct lytic action of "immune" thymus-derived (T) lymphocytes.
4. Macrophage-mediated cytotoxicity.

We shall discuss each of these pathways in turn, principally from a mechanistic standpoint, noting, where appropriate, experiments that have a bearing on the possible in vivo significance of each lytic pathway. We do not propose a discussion of other in vitro cytotoxic phenomena, such as lysis induced in the presence of plant mitogens, e.g., phytohemagglutinin (PHA) or concanavalin A (Con A), simply because these pathways appear patently artificial in terms of conceivable biological relevance.

An obvious shortcoming of in vitro approaches should be noted: these observations provide no information on the physiologic significance of the pathways under study. It does not follow that, because a tumor cell is destroyed under specified in vitro conditions, this is the manner in which the same tumor is killed in vivo. It may seem a rather pedantic argument to stress that an in vitro lytic pathway is no more than one of biologic feasibility, but this caveat is currently so often ignored in equating in vitro activities with in vivo significance that it seems necessary to reassert at the onset.

All of the pathways we will discuss result in the lysis of tumor target cells. Other in vitro effects of lymphocytes on tumor cells, such as those that result in cyto-stasis, or in tumor cell detachment from fixed surfaces, although they may well be relevant to tumor cell rejection in vivo, are less obviously related phenomena than is frank lysis and will not be discussed.

Some Initial Comments on Terminal Events in Cytolysis

From a historical perspective, the elucidation of multistaged biologic phenomena proceeds in a rather haphazard manner, some components inevitably being resolved before others. Such has certainly been the case with studies on the mechanism of tumor cell destruction by the immune system. The initial stages leading to lysis, e.g., the combination of effector cells with tumor cells, are still very poorly understood, but the terminal events have already been quite well characterized.

The rupture of the plasma membrane of tumor cells following interaction with the complement system, or with "immune" cells, occurs by colloid osmotic lysis (6,7). Immune interaction leads to the insertion of a lesion in the target cell membrane; water then enters the cell, which swells until the cell membrane is explosively ruptured. These observations have been shown to hold in such diverse systems as the complement-induced lysis of Ehrlich ascites tumor cells (6) and the T-cell-mediated lysis of mouse mastocytoma cells (7), leading to the assumption that the terminal stages in tumor cell destruction by the immune system are identical. A discussion of mechanisms of tumor cell destruction thus centers upon the manner in which a lytic lesion is initially inserted into the target cell. It is toward this end that the following descriptions of cytolytic pathways are directed.

COMPLEMENT-MEDIATED LYSIS IN THE PRESENCE OF ANTIBODY

The lysis of cells by antibody in the presence of complement is still the paradigm of cytodestruction by the immune system. Much of our knowledge of complement-induced lysis has been derived from studies on the destruction of erythrocytes, although there is evidence that the lysis of nucleated cells, including tumor cells, proceeds similarly (8).

It is not within the scope of this chapter to discuss the various components of the complement system in any detail, for this information has been succinctly presented elsewhere (9,10). It is appropriate, however, to consider several general features of lysis mediated by the complement system following its activation by antibody.

Characteristics of Cytolysis

Although Kalfayan and Kidd showed in 1953 that tumor cells swelled in the presence of antibody and complement (11), the first clear indications of events surrounding complement lysis came from a study of the release of various intrinsic labels from Krebs ascites cells by Green et al. in 1959 (6,12). These investigators found that in the presence of rabbit antibody and complement the ascites cells leaked ions, such as potassium, before they lost intracellular protein. In solutions of high osmolarity, cell membranes did not disrupt or leak protein. The authors concluded that complement induced "holes" of a discrete size in the cell membrane.

Following analysis of the kinetics of lysis of sheep erythrocytes, Mayer concluded that the production of a single irreparable lesion in the cell membrane was sufficient to cause lysis (13). His "one-hit" model of complement-induced lysis was an important conceptual advance. Since cell lysis occurred only at the late stage of the sequence of activation of successive complement components, the terminal lesion would presumably be that responsible for the loss of osmotic regulation by the cell membrane. It was immediately concluded by many that Green's functional "holes" corresponded to the lesions (or hits) predicted from Mayer's kinetic studies. Later, electron-microscopic studies produced direct experimental evidence that antibody and complement produced lesions, resembling "holes," in erythrocyte membranes (14). More recently, similar "holes" have been demonstrated in nucleated cells, including tumor cells (8,15).

Insertion of a Complement Lesion

Complement-induced membrane lesions are both uniform, as measured by electron microscopy, and stable, as assessed functionally by efflux measurements of

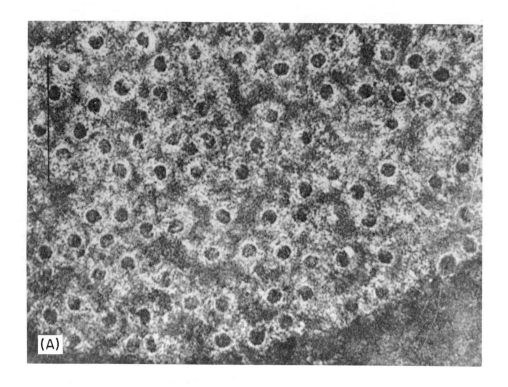

(A)

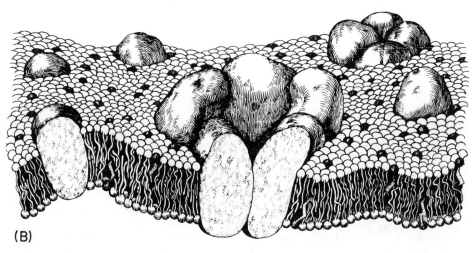

(B)

Figure 1. Electron micrograph of complement-induced "holes" in an erythrocyte membrane, and a diagrammatic representation of such lesions as suggested by Mayer (9). A: The photograph is of a human erythrocyte membrane treated with anti-I antibody and human complement, taken by Dr. R. R. Dourmashkin of the Clinical Research Centre, Harrow, England, and reproduced by kind permission of the author. The "holes" in the membrane approximate 100 Å in diameter. B: The diagram shows late-acting complement components assembled in the lipid bilayer of the plasma membrane into a "doughnut" shape. The hollow core that penetrates the bilayer is thought to form the lesion through which water flows into the cell until it bursts.

intracellular contents. The different size of the lesions reported in various cell types seems to reflect only the source of complement used (8). These findings have led to the hypothesis that complement-induced "holes" represent the insertion of terminal complement components (which are proteins) into the lipid matrix of the target cell membrane. This insertion, it is proposed, results in a rigid, hollow channel that connects the inside of the cell with the extracellular milieu (9). An electron micrograph of a complement-induced lesion is seen in Figure 1A. Mayer views the holes as "doughnuts," composed of several of the late-acting complement components arrayed in such a manner that the outside of the doughnut is composed of hydrophobic residues, the inner of polar, hydrophilic peptides. A diagrammatic representation of this view is shown in Figure 1B.

The "doughnut" model of complement lesions has received support from electron micrographs of freeze-fractured cells (16) and from chemical studies of erythrocyte membranes (17). Both of these approaches have demonstrated penetration of complement lesions into the lipid bilayer. The process by which soluble complement proteins become inserted into the lipid bilayer is yet to be determined.

Some Factors Affecting the Susceptibility of Tumor Cells to Complement-Induced Lysis

A major limitation in ascribing far-reaching in vivo significance to the complement-dependent lysis of tumor cells is that neoplastic cells differ markedly in their susceptibility to attack. For a considerable time it has been part of tumor immunology folklore that whereas leukemias are "sensitive" to cytotoxic antibody, sarcomas are "resistant." Such tales have led to the construction of a "hierarchy," in which neoplastic cells have been ranked in terms of their susceptibility to lytic attack.

Clearly there are many possible reasons why some cells would be more readily lysed than others: the density of distribution of antigenic determinants, a deficiency in complement binding sites, and differences in cell "repair" mechanisms are three that come readily to mind. In a recent series of studies (18,19,20) Borsos and his colleagues have begun, for the first time, a systematic analysis of factors affecting susceptibility to complement-induced lysis. Their studies have already yielded findings of considerable importance.

In one study employing two antigenically distinct hepatoma cells syngeneic to strain 2 guinea pigs, they found that in the presence of guinea pig complement and 19S rabbit anti-Forssman antibody, one hepatoma line was susceptible to attack, the other resistant (18). Variable susceptibility to antibody and complement could not be ascribed to antigen concentration, to antibody class, or to ability to "fix" complement components. In further studies these investigators found that susceptibility of both hepatoma cell lines to complement attack was enhanced following treatment with actinomycin D, with puromycin, and with a number of chemotherapeutic agents including methotrexate and cyclosphosphamide (19,20). While the drug effects were dose-related, two observations make it unlikely that enhancement was related to the well-known effects of these drugs on cell metabolism:

1.   The drug effects were always reversible; when the drugs were removed by washing, the cells displayed their original sensitivity to lytic attack. This was true even of drugs whose effects on cell metabolism are generally not reversible (e.g., the action of mitomycin C on DNA synthesis).

2.   The concentration of drugs required to enhance complement lysis was far greater than that needed to inhibit cell metabolism in any selective manner.

The way in which drugs affect the susceptibility of tumor cells to complement attack remains unknown. It may be that the drugs employed affected the synthesis of those portions of the cell membrane susceptible to the attack of terminal complement components, or that the drugs may have reduced the effectiveness of cell surface repair mechanisms. Alternatively, the drugs may have direct membrane effects that increase the incidence or rate of insertion of the complement components. Segerling et al. speculate (20) that the beneficial effect of various drugs in the treatment of cancer might be due, in part, to their ability to increase the susceptibility of tumor cells to killing by antibody and complement.

Some Considerations of the Biologic Significance of Complement-Mediated Cytolysis

Teleologically, it is difficult to suppose that the complex series of events that lead to complement-induced cytolysis would have evolved and survived in such a wide variety of vertebrate species if it did not have significant biologic value. This conclusion should, however, be tempered by several considerations: (1) the lytic action of complement is effective only when this system is activated at the surface of a susceptible cell; (2) all classes of antibody are not able to initiate the complement cascade, and those that are do so with differing degrees of efficiency (21,22). Thus, a single IgM antibody molecule is capable of "triggering" the complement system, while two or more antibody molecules of the IgG class are required, and even then they must be in close proximity to each other (21). As antigenic determinants on the cell surface are distributed in a relatively random fashion, the number of IgG molecules bound per cell must be much greater than twice the number of IgM molecules to achieve comparable lytic efficiency. Indeed, for the lysis of sheep erythrocytes by anti-Forssman antibody the relative effectiveness of IgM: IgG molecules has been calculated as 800:1. For practical purposes this would seem to limit the initiation of the complement sequence by IgG molecules to situations in which antigenic groups on the cell surface form a closely spaced, repeating pattern.

ANTIBODY-DEPENDENT CELL-MEDIATED CYTOTOXICITY

In addition to the direct cytotoxic activity of antibody in the presence of complement, antibody can also cooperate with a variety of normal cells to effect immunologically specific target cell destruction in vitro without the involvement of the complement system (4). This conclusion is difficult to assert unequivocally, because the cell populations employed may well synthesize and secrete complement components in vitro, but two sets of observations speak against complement involvement in cell-mediated cytotoxicity. The addition of a complement source neither initiates nor augments cytolysis (23), and the presence of antisera directed against complement components fails to affect the lytic reaction (24,25).

Antibody-dependent cell-mediated cytotoxicity was first described by Moller as a pathway by which murine methylcholanthrene-induced fibrosarcoma cells could be lysed in vitro (26). The mechanism of cytolysis by this pathway has been extensively studied by Perlmann and his collaborators using antibody-coated chicken erythrocytes as target cells (4,27). Such studies were undertaken on the premise that erythrocyte targets were comparable to tumor cells, but two recent observations question this assumption: Sanderson et al. have shown that the effector cells responsible for erythrocyte death may not be the same as those which lyse antibody-coated tumor cells (28). Golstein and Fewtrell suggest that the extracellular cation requirements for lysis may differ (29). Thus, the antibody-dependent lysis of erythrocytes may differ mechanistically from that of tumor cells. This consideration, as will become apparent, currently thwarts attempts at analyzing mechanisms of tumor cell destruction by this pathway, for Perlmann's elegant studies on erythrocyte destruction may simply not be germane. With this potentially important limitation in mind, we will consider several characteristics of antibody-dependent cell-mediated cytotoxicity.

Characterization of Components of the Reaction

Antibody.   The structural requirements on immunoglobulin molecules necessary for cell-mediated cytotoxicity are different from those needed for complement-dependent lysis. Several experimental observations warrant this conclusion:

1.   Antibody of the IgG class is the predominant, if not exclusive, immunoglobulin type which can serve in cell-mediated cytotoxicity. There is currently only one report that IgM antibody can support this mode of lysis (30). Further, the amounts of antibody required for cell-mediated lysis are far less than those required to demonstrate complement-dependent cytotoxicity (31). Indeed, in one study, a coating of as few as 100 IgG antibody molecules on the target cell served to render it susceptible to cell-mediated cytolytic attack (32).

2.   Inhibition studies using aggregated IgG myeloma proteins suggest that in man all IgG subclasses support cell-mediated cytotoxicity (32,33). In contrast, neither IgG_2 nor IgG_4 antibody molecules fix the first component of complement; thus they are ineffective in complement-mediated lysis, at least by the "classical" pathway.

3.   Cell-mediated cytotoxicity, like complement fixation, is dependent on the presence of an intact Fc portion of the IgG molecule. Within this domain, however, different sites appear to satisfy the two activities (33).

In summary, the antibody requirements for cooperation with effector cells in inducing tumor cell destruction are different from those required for complement fixation.

The Effector Cell.   Several distinct cell types can serve as effector cells in this lytic pathway; none of them need be derived from an immune animal. It is thus the antibody molecule which confers specificity to the cytodestructive process.

Several morphologically and developmentally distinctive cell types have been demonstrated to exert a cytotoxic capacity in vitro toward antibody-coated target cells (5,34). Among these are: polymorphonuclear leukocytes; macrophages; platelets; foetal liver cells; and a mononuclear cell of unknown lineage termed a K (for killer) cell. (Other investigators refer to the latter cell as a null cell because of its lack of those surface antigenic markers characteristic of B and T lymphocytes.) These heterogeneous effector cell populations share at least one common characteristic: a cell membrane with a capacity to bind the Fc fragment of IgG molecules (an Fc receptor) (34). The Fc receptor on the effector cell(s) appears to play a key role in cytolysis, for when effector and target cells are bridged together without accommodating this receptor (e.g., by the use of the plant lectin concanavalin A), then cell-cell interaction occurs, but it is not accompanied by lysis of the target cell (35). While Fc receptors are a common feature of effector cells, the receptor does not, of itself, endow cytotoxic potential. Many cells with functional Fc receptors are unable to lyse antibody-coated target cells. There appears, therefore, to be an additional cellular component, as yet undefined, which subclassifies Fc receptor-bearing cells into those with killer potential.

An earlier confusion regarding the nature of effector cells which can function in antibody-dependent cell-mediated cytotoxicity has been at least partially resolved. Holm suggests, in as yet unpublished work, that for a given target cell there is a predominant functional effector cell, even when several potential effector cells are present in the culture. Thus, when human peripheral leukocytes are used as effector cells against antibody-coated erythrocytes, the targets are killed predominantly by macrophages. When the same effector cell source is used to kill an antibody-coated human polyploid liver cell (Chang cell), nonphagocytic K cells effect lysis. Why for a given antibody-coated target cell there is a "preferred" effector cell is unknown. Perhaps it reflects an as yet undefined subspecificity of the Fc receptors. This would imply that a given set of target cell antigens preferentially stimulate antibody of a given IgG subclass (and thus of a restricted Fc type). These antibodies would then be preferentially served by a restricted range of Fc receptors, displayed only on a limited subpopulation of potential effector cells.

The Cytolytic Event

Cell-Cell Interaction.   Antibody-dependent cell-mediated cytotoxicity requires effector cell–target cell interaction (4). Target cells separated from effectors by a semipermeable membrane are not lysed. The key to cell bridging is the IgG molecule. Pepsin-digested antibody preparations readily coat target cells, but the cells are not lysed in the presence of effector cells. Similarly, when effector cells are mixed with antitarget cell antibody and then washed before target cell addition, lysis does not occur (27,31). These experiments argue forcibly that the cell-cell interaction required for lysis is bridged by IgG antibody molecules, with their Fab portions attached to the target cell and their Fc portions anchored by effector cell Fc receptors. This interaction is schematically represented in Figure 2.

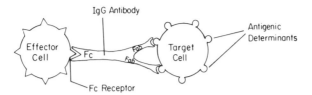

Figure 2. Schematic representation of cell-cell interaction leading to antibody-dependent cell-mediated cytotoxicity.

Kinetics.   The kinetics of lysis of antibody-coated target cells in vitro varies with the target cell. This variability is no doubt occasioned by a number of factors, including the inherent susceptibility of the target cell to lysis, the amount of antibody employed, and the incidence of effector cells present in the culture. A detailed comparison of the data reported from various laboratories using a variety of cell types is further complicated by the different methods used to assess cell death.*

In order to describe some principal features of antibody-dependent cell-mediated cytotoxicity in a meaningful way, therefore, we propose to confine our attention to lysis in one in vitro system: the destruction of Chang cells by lymphocytes from normal human peripheral blood in the presence of rabbit anti-Chang cell serum. The system is described diagrammatically in Figure 3. In this system the effector cell is a nonphagocytic, nonglass adherent cell sharing the morphologic characteristics of a small lymphocyte (36). This cell type, usually referred to as a K cell, will be referred to here as a lymphocyte, simply because the mononuclear cell fraction of peripheral blood leukocytes was used as the effector cell source. The observations to be discussed were made recently by Ziegler in this laboratory (37).

When varying numbers of lymphocytes were added to Chang cells internally labeled with sodium ^{51}chromate, the initial rate of cytolysis (^{51}Cr release) was directly related to the number of effector cells added (Figure 4A). Furthermore, the total number of target cells lysed during a 4-hour incubation was also directly proportional to lymphocyte number. When the percentage of target cells lysed was plotted as the ordinate against the number of lymphoid cells added, the curve obtained was entirely concave to the abcissa, suggesting that single events of collision lead to cytolysis (13,38). When the number of target cells specifically lysed was fitted to a Poisson probability distribution and plotted against the number of

---

*There are almost as many in vitro assay systems for cytotoxicity as there are investigative laboratories interested in the assessment. It is beyond the scope of this chapter to discuss these in detail. Most of the data reported in this chapter are derived from studies using the release of ^{51}chromium from target cells as the index of cell death. Conceptually, the technique is a simple one: cells are incubated in a solution of sodium ^{51}chromate in 0.15M NaCl; the ^{51}Cr becomes protein associated and leaks from the cell in a macromolecular form which is not reutilized. Significant leakage of radiolabel occurs concomitantly with plasma membrane destruction. In practice, some target cells leak ^{51}Cr in the absence of effector cells far more readily than do others. This places obvious limitations on the range of cells which can be used to study cell destruction by this technique.

[For a full discussion of assay systems and their limitations, the reader is referred to B. R. Bloom and P. R. Glade, eds., *In Vitro Methods in Cell-Mediated Immunity* (New York: Academic Press, Inc., 1971).]

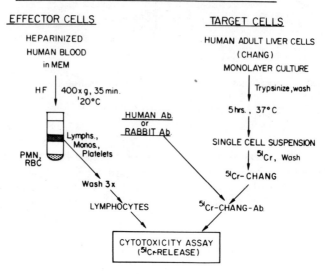

ASSAY OF HUMAN LYMPHOCYTE
MEDIATED ANTIBODY DEPENDENT CYTOTOXICITY

Figure 3.   Assay system used for detection of human lymphocyte-mediated destruction of antibody-coated Chang cells [after MacLennan et al. (36)].

effector cells added, the slope of a log/log plot approximated 1.0 (Fig. 4B). Thus, target cells were killed by a discrete process in which one "hit" with an effector cell was sufficient to induce lysis.

Although lysis of target cells proceeded linearly over short periods, during prolonged incubation ^{51}Cr release did not continue, and lysis evaluated after either 8 or 17 hours was no greater than that observed at 5 hours (Fig. 4C). It appeared likely that cessation of lysis resulted from effector cell inactivation. Support for this contention came from the experiment reported in Figure 5, in which effector cells were found to be almost completely inactivated following interaction with antibody-coated target cells but were unaffected by collision with uncoated target cells. The data presented in Figure 5 do not define how many target cells were destroyed by a single effector cell, but the simplest hypothesis would be that an effector cell killed only a single target prior to its inactivation. There is, however, as yet no definitive evidence that such is the case. As will be seen, the diminished activity of antibody-dependent effector cells following collision with their target cells contrasts markedly with that of effector T cells, whose lytic activity continues undiminished through many target cell interactions.

There are a number of possible reasons for the functional inactivation of effector cells following interaction with antibody-coated target cells. It is conceiv-

Figure 4.   The destruction of antibody-coated Chang cells by human peripheral lymphocyte populations. A and C: Lymphocytes (10^4 to 6×10^5) were added to 10^4 ^{51}Cr target cells to give the indicated lymphocyte-target cell ratios. Percent specific cytolysis was calculated by subtracting ^{51}Cr released from target cells treated with preimmune serum at each lymphocyte concentration. B: Lymphocytes were added to 10^4 ^{51}Cr target cells and lysis evaluated 2 hours (■) and 4 hours (●) later. The number of target cells specifically lysed was fitted to a Poisson probability distribution. The slopes in each case are 1.0. [Data from Ziegler and Henney (37).]

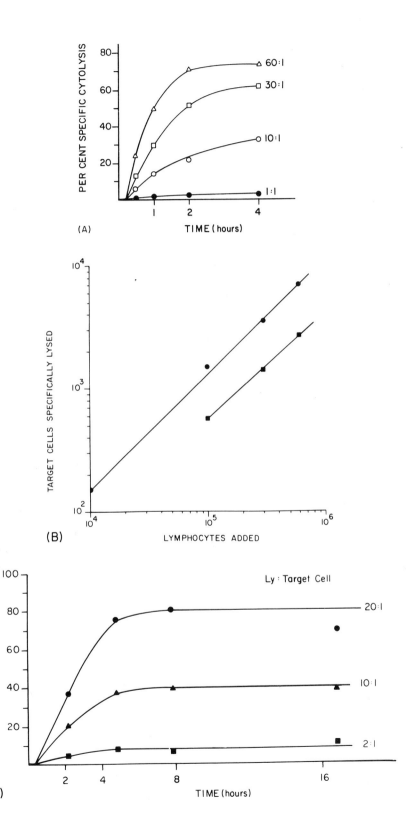

(A)

(B)

(C)

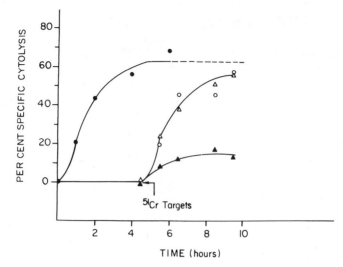

Figure 5.   Functional inactivation of effector cells following interaction with antibody-coated target cells. Lymphocytes (10^5) were added to 10^4 antibody-coated ^{51}Cr Chang cells at time zero (●). Parallel cultures contained 10^5 lymphocytes alone (○); 10^5 lymphocytes and 10^4 unlabeled Chang cells treated either with preimmune serum (△) or with antibody (▲). To each of these cultures (○, △, and ▲) 10^4 antibody-coated ^{51}Cr-labeled Chang cells were added at time 4½ hours. As can be seen, lymphocytes incubated with antibody-coated target cells (▲) become inactivated. [Data from Ziegler and Henney (37).]

able that the effector cells are themselves destroyed concomitantly with target cells. Vital dye exclusion data (37) have to date found no support for this, but such procedures may be too insensitive to detect the death of a small percentage of the lymphocyte population. If the effector cells do not die after target cell interaction, they are certainly inactivated for very prolonged periods, for Ziegler and Henney did not observe restoration of lytic activity even after culturing the cells for an additional 24 hours (37).

Functional inactivation of the effector cell could occur by "blocking" of its Fc receptor sites. If, following target cell destruction, the Fc receptors of the effector cell remained unoccupied, this would incapacitate the cell's ability to initiate new lytic cycles. This argument would seem to be predicated on the assumption that all of the Fc receptor sites on an effector cell become occupied following interaction with an antibody-coated target cell. While there is no direct evidence that this occurs, observations that cytotoxicity is inhibited by aggregated IgG (32,33) and by immune complexes (39) suggest that blocking of Fc receptor sites does inhibit cytolytic expression.

Thus, the principal features of cytolysis via this pathway are: (1) lysis occurs following single events of collision between an antibody-coated target cell and an effector cell; (2) such interaction eventually leads to the functional inactivation of the killer cell. It is not known to what extent the kinetics of destruction of Chang cells by human peripheral lymphocytes reflects other antibody-dependent cytotoxic phenomena. There is already some preliminary evidence that the killing of antibody-coated EL4 lymphoma cells by polymorphonuclear leukocytes may differ in the extent to which inactivation of effector cells occurs (40).

Metabolic Requirements for Lysis

All available evidence suggests that the effector cell must be alive in order to be cytotoxic. Thus, X-irradiation, the presence of sodium azide, or treatment of effector populations with antimycin A (a potent inhibitor of electron transport processes) all result in inhibition of lysis (4). It is unlikely that either protein synthesis or DNA synthesis is required for cytotoxicity, as puromycin, cyclohex-imide, and mitomycin all fail to affect lysis (41,42). Pactamycin, an irreversible inhibitor of protein synthesis, is similarly ineffective. Cytochalasin B, a fungal metabolite with a wide variety of biologic activities, including that of microfilament disruption, inhibits cytolysis of several target cells (32) but perhaps not all (43). Agents which augment cAMP levels in a variety of cells have also been reported to inhibit lysis (44).

It is difficult to interpret these metabolic inhibition studies incisively, particu-larly as they largely preceded our current knowledge of the heterogeneity of effector cells which can function in antibody-dependent cell-mediated cytotoxi-city. Thus, many of the studies were made in in vitro systems in which several different lytic pathways might have been concomitantly expressed. Further, it is often impossible to decide whether the drugs inhibited lysis by suppressing effector cell function or by "protecting" target cells from lysis. These problems will be addressed further when we consider how similar approaches have been used to study the mechanism of T-cell-mediated lysis.

Biologic Significance of Antibody-Dependent Cell-Mediated Cytotoxicity

Most attempts to define a possible biologic significance for antibody-dependent cell-mediated cytotoxicity have used modifications of a local adoptive transfer method originally described by Winn (45). Tumors are grown subcutaneously in sublethally irradiated animals and the effect on growth rate of antibody and/or various cell types mixed with the tumor prior to inoculation is assessed.

A number of studies of this type, notably those of Shin et al. (46,47,48) using a murine lymphoma, have shown that the growth of tumor in irradiated mice is unaffected by the presence of alloantibody. In contrast, when the tumor cells, treated with alloantibody, were mixed with peritoneal exudate macrophages and subsequently transferred to an X-irradiated host, lymphoma cell growth was markedly retarded (46). Less pronounced suppression of tumor cell growth was seen when non-θ-bearing lymphocytes or platelet populations were substituted for macrophages (47). Neither T lymphocytes nor polymorphonuclear leukocytes were found to be growth-inhibitory in this system (47,48). Most surprisingly, both freeze-thawed and heat-killed macrophages retained their inhibitory activity, although lymphocytes and platelets treated in this manner did not (47,48).

A number of problems are associated with an evaluation of these in vivo data. The problems principally revolve around the assay system used. When exogen-ous cells restore the suppressive capacity of an irradiated host, the effect may be due to the direct suppressive action of the transferred cells upon the target cell (the viewpoint usually taken), but it may also reflect, at least in part, a "helper" function of these cells which enables radioresistant host elements to suppress tumor growth. With these caveats in mind, it can still be stated that there is a broad concordance between in vivo and in vitro studies in this area. Both the antibody-dependent suppression of tumor cell growth in vivo and cytolysis in vitro are mediated by a variety of cell types, of which the principal elements appear to be macrophages, nonlymphoid cells, polymorphonuclear leukocytes, and, perhaps, platelets.

It is obviously premature to pass judgment on the in vivo significance of this lytic pathway, but observations that killing is a very rapid process, that very small amounts of antibody support cytolysis, and that several cell types have the capacity to serve as effector cells, would all argue that antibody-dependent cell-mediated cytotoxicity represents a potentially significant arm of immune defenses.

CYTOLYSIS BY THYMUS-DERIVED LYMPHOCYTES

So far in this chapter we have dealt exclusively with antibody-dependent pathways of tumor cell destruction. It is apparent, however, that some lymphoid cells can express a direct lytic action without the involvement of either antibody or the complement system. Lymphocytes with this capacity belong to a group of cells which have a characteristic mode of differentiation, involving passage through the thymus. The resulting cells are consequently termed thymus-derived lymphocytes or, more simply, T cells.

The lytic activity of lymphocytes was first shown by Govaerts, when he observed that thoracic duct cells from dogs which had rejected kidney allografts killed donor kidney cells in vitro (3). Cerottini et al. (49) subsequently showed that thymus-derived lymphocytes were responsible for cytotoxicity, when they selectively removed T cells from alloimmunized mouse spleen cell populations and abrogated cytolytic activity. It is currently recognized that cytotoxic T cells are produced as a normal component of a host's immune response to cell-associated antigens. As discussed in Chapter 2, Thomas, Burnett, and others have suggested that this lytic activity has a general biologic role—that of "immune surveillance" (50,51). In this hypothesis, killer T cells "guard" against neoplastic growth by lysing cells which exhibit "nonself" antigens. In this light lytically active T cells have been championed as a major factor in the destruction of tumor cells in vivo. Most of the current information on how killer T cells function has been derived, however, not in the context of tumor cell destruction, but from studies of in vitro correlates of allograft rejection.

From a mechanistic standpoint probably more is known about the mode of action of effector T cells than of any other cell-mediated cytotoxic process. This is due to a powerful analytic tool: an in vitro model which measures the cytolytic activity of T cells exclusively. This system, first described by K. T. Brunner and his colleagues in 1968 (52), and depicted diagrammatically in Figure 6, was developed to study the lysis of a murine mastocytoma (P815 of the DBA/2 strain) by spleen cells from alloimmunized C57BL/6 mice. While the antigens that elicit killer T cell production in this model are therefore allogeneic to the host, there is reason to believe that, from a mechanistic standpoint, tumor cell destruction by syngeneic killer T cells is identical. Many of the generalizations that follow are predicated on this assumption.

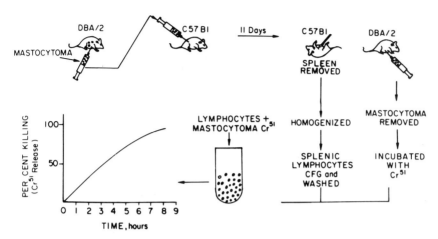

Figure 6. Diagrammatic representation of model system used to measure the T-cell-mediated lysis of a mouse mastocytoma target cell. [After Brunner et al. (52).]

Some General Characteristics of Cytolysis

T-cell-mediated cytolysis is an exquisitely specific phenomenon. In circumstances where a variety of antigenically distinctive target cell types are concurrently employed, only those cells bearing antigens against which the host is immune are lysed (5). Lysis is independent of the complement system (23,24).

Kinetics. T-cell-mediated cytolysis occurs as a linear function of time, and the number of target cells destroyed is directly proportional to the number of effector lymphocytes (38,53) and is related to the number of target cells present in the assay system (38,54). Kinetic analyses of target cell destruction have shown that cytolysis results from events of collision between a single lymphocyte and a single target cell (38,53). Thus, the "one-hit" model applies to T-cell-mediated lysis as it does to antibody-dependent cell-mediated cytotoxicity and to the insertion of complement lesions. Unlike those antibody-dependent events, however, several observations suggest that the T-cell-mediated destruction of target cells is a cyclic phenomenon: the T lymphocyte has the capacity to kill more than one target cell (5,54). Thus, circumstances have been described in which more target cells were killed than there were lymphocytes in the culture (5,54). In this respect the mode of action of killer T cells differs from that of the K cells which mediate the lysis of antibody-coated Chang cells (37).

Metabolic Requirements for Cytolysis. Using a time-honored approach of biochemists and pharmacologists, the molecular basis of the T cell's cytotoxic activity has been pursued by the employment of selective metabolic inhibitors.

Cytolysis requires a viable effector cell (52,55). Cytochalasins A and B are potent inhibitors of cytolysis (56,57), leading to suggestions that microfilamentous structures may be involved in the lytic event. Colchicine, vinblastine, and vincristine also inhibit lysis (56,58). The well-known antimitotic action of these vinca alkaloids is not the basis of their ability to inhibit cytolysis, for DNA synthesis is not required during the lytic event (52). It is possible that the ability of colchicine to inhibit T-cell-mediated lysis is related to the drug's affinity for microtubule subunits, with a subsequent disruption of the T cell's microtubular network (56). Drugs which modulate lymphocyte cyclic adenosine $3'5'$-monophosphate (cAMP) levels also inhibit cytolysis (59,60), a phenomenon which we will discuss in detail later.

Although inhibitors of protein synthesis have repeatedly been shown to suppress T-cell-mediated lysis (52,61), in a recent study using emetine and pactamycin we observed no effect on lysis at drug concentrations which totally abrogated amino acid incorporation (62). We also observed that effector cells prevented from protein synthesis continued to kill target cells over a 24-hour period with an efficiency comparable to that of protein synthesizing controls (62). There is thus firm evidence that the earlier findings were based on drug effects unrelated to protein synthesis and that, consequently, *de novo* protein synthesis is not required for T-cell-mediated lysis.

While a viable effector cell is necessary, there is no evidence that the target cell needs to be metabolically active in order to be subjected to lytic attack. Indeed, recent observations of Bubbers and Henney using glutaraldehyde-fixed target cells, suggest that the target cell is a passive partner in cytolysis, serving merely to display antigen (63).

It is currently difficult to interpret data on the suppression of cytolysis by metabolic inhibitors. In part this is due to two general shortcomings of such studies: (1) the metabolic inhibitors are not usually as selective as one would wish, and (2) the fact that a viable cell is necessary for cytolysis ensures, almost by definition, that metabolic inhibitors will compromise lytic function. The problem is thus one of distinguishing the diminished function of a "sick" cell from the inhibition of a process essential for the expression of lytic activity. An excellent example of the pitfalls of this approach has already been alluded to in the case of inhibitors of protein synthesis (62). Despite these caveats, there are a number of reproducible observations with inhibitors whose effects are entirely reversible and which any hypothesis on the mechanism of T-cell-mediated cytolysis must satisfactorily take into account. In order to place these inhibitor studies into a mechanistic framework, it is perhaps useful to consider the T-cell-mediated lytic cycle in three somewhat arbitrary phases: cell-cell interaction, the insertion of a lesion in the target cell membrane, and lysis of the target cell.

The Lytic Cycle

Cell-Cell Interaction.   The initiation of lysis by effector T cells is conceptually a simple one: the interaction of a killer lymphocyte with an antigen-bearing target cell. This process remains, however, largely uncharacterized, for neither the antigenic determinants, nor their homologous lymphocyte receptor sites, have been defined in molecular terms. The nature of the antigen receptor site on the T cell has proved a particularly fascinating problem for cellular immunologists. While it can be argued on teleologic grounds that this should be an immunoglobulin molecule—for T cell receptors appear to exhibit the same range of antigenic specificity as do antibody molecules, and it would be "wasteful" of Nature to devise two independent systems of comparable scope—there is no firm evidence that such is the case. The best evidence to date is the demonstration of Binz and Wigzell that T and B cell receptors directed against alloantigens share a common idiotypic specificity (64). In contrast, there stands a body of evidence which is difficult to accommodate into an immunoglobulin receptor hypothesis [see, e.g., the review of Crone et al. (65)]. It is not within the scope of this chapter to discuss this issue further, except from one standpoint: experiments in which killer T cells were shown to have antigen receptors considerably influenced our understanding of effector-target cell interactions.

Effector T cells bind avidly, and specifically, to cell monolayers bearing antigenic determinants against which the T cell donor is immune (66,67). This binding is usually studied in an allogeneic setting, using primary embryonic fibroblasts as the monolayer. It is widely regarded that such adsorption is analogous to the first stage in T-cell-mediated lysis, for it has frequently been shown that cytolysis requires intimate cell-cell interaction (53,68). In this regard, both the insertion of a semipermeable membrane between effector and target cell or the suspension of the interacting cells in a viscous medium, e.g., dextran or agarose, result in the complete inhibition of cytolysis.

The binding of cytolytically active T cells onto allogeneic monolayers has been shown to be inhibited by low temperatures, by azide, and by dinitrophenol, implying that the cell-cell interaction is an energy-requiring process (66). In recent studies from this laboratory, the adhesion of effector cells to their targets has also been shown to be inhibited by cytochalasin B, implying, perhaps, that accommodation of antigen into its T cell receptor site is accompanied by membrane modulatory movement (67). T cell-target cell interaction has also been shown, by several investigators, to require the presence of Mg^{++} (69,70,71).

Berke and Fishelson have suggested that the binding of a killer cell to its homologous target is accompanied by a polar localization of target cell surface components to the site of binding (72). Whether this phenomenon is germane to the subsequent insertion of a lytic lesion is unknown but seems unlikely, as glutaraldehyde-fixed target cells, which presumably could not manifest "capping" of surface antigens, can be lysed by effector T cells (63).

Lesion Insertion.   In contrast to the energy requirements of effector cell-target cell conjugation, the subsequent lytic phase of cytolysis is apparently energy independent (73,74).

Membrane permeability changes in the target cell occur within minutes of effector cell addition (75,76); thus, in ^{51}Cr release assays most of the time is consumed by extrusion of macromolecular ^{51}Cr from the target cells rather than in the establishment of a lytic lesion. It is not known how long the lymphocyte "sits" on the target cell before moving on to effect more damage, but those events following lesion insertion, and which occur prior to membrane disruption, can proceed without the lymphocyte. Thus, Martz and Benacerraf have shown that shortly after cell mixing, the lysis of lymphocytes, or the separation of effector cells from target cells by a mixture of dextran-EDTA, is still followed by target cell destruction (73,77).

A number of inhibitors of cytolysis do not interfere with effector cell adherence to target cell monolayers (67). Such inhibitors thus apparently prevent lysis at a stage following cell-cell interaction, and it is convenient to suppose that they affect lesion insertion. Principal among these agents are those drugs which augment cAMP levels (59,67).

An inverse relationship between lymphocyte cAMP levels and cytolytic activity was first observed during studies with a stimulator of adenylate cyclase, isoproterenol, and a phosphodiesterase inhibitor, theophylline (78). The relationship was strengthened considerably by studies involving a number of prostaglandin congeners (79). These drugs, which exhibited a wide range of adenylate cyclase stimulatory activities (Fig. 7A), also showed a great variability in their inhibitory activity in lytic assays (Fig. 7B). There was a close correlation between the increased cAMP levels seen in the presence of the prostaglandins and the inhibition of cytolysis observed. Thus, prostaglandins E₁ and E₂ were found to be potent adenylate cyclase stimulating agents and important inhibitors of cytolysis. Prostaglandins F₁α and F₂α, on the other hand, caused little or no rise in the cAMP

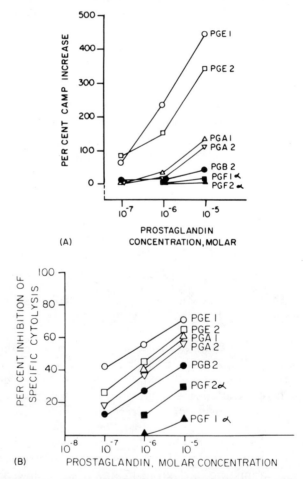

Figure 7. A: The effect of prostaglandins on the intracellular cAMP level of mouse C57BL/6 spleen cells. The control level of cAMP was 4.3 pm/10⁷ cells. B: Prostaglandin inhibition of the specific cytolysis of mouse DBA/2 mastocytoma cells by immune C57BL/6 spleen cells. [Both A and B reproduced from *Prostaglandins* **2**, 519 (1972), by the kind permission of Geron-X, Los Altos, Calif.]

content of spleen cell suspensions and interfered only very poorly with cytolysis (72).

It appears that increased cAMP levels in lymphocyte populations, resulting from adenylate cyclase stimulation, is mediated via specific membrane-associated hormone receptors closely linked to the enzyme. This inference is drawn from the exquisite specificity shown by hormone antagonists. Thus, propranolol, a beta-adrenergic antagonist, specifically reversed the augmentation of cAMP and the inhibition of cytolysis caused by isoproterenol, but had no effect on activities mediated by prostaglandin E_1 (PGE$_1$) (59). Similarly, we have shown that the ability of histamine to increase cAMP levels, and to inhibit the cytolytic activity of spleen cells, was reversed by the antihistamine burimamide (but not, interestingly enough, by other antihistamines, e.g., diphenhydramine or pyrilamine, which antagonize different histamine receptor site specificities) (80). Burimamide had no effect on the augmentation of lymphocyte cAMP levels or on the inhibition of cytolysis caused by PGE$_1$ (80).

These earlier studies were all made with drugs which inhibited cytolysis, and increased cAMP levels, in a reversible manner. It was thus difficult to decide whether the inhibition of cytolysis was mediated via the effector or target cell. In investigations employing cholera enterotoxin, which stimulates adenylate cyclase in a very protracted manner, we were able to show that augmented cAMP levels in the effector cell population were associated with a depressed cytolytic activity (81). On the other hand, cholera toxin treatment of target cells had no effect on their susceptibility to lymphocyte-induced lysis (81). These findings clearly strengthen the evidence relating lymphocyte cAMP levels to the expression of cytolytic activity. Perhaps the only weak link in this chain of association lies in the cell populations employed for cAMP assays. The cells used for such measurements have invariably been extremely heterogenous, including only a small proportion of effector T cells. To equate increased cAMP levels in this population with changes in the biological activity of a small fraction of the cells is thus clearly a questionable practice. The isolation of purified effector cell populations would obviously be useful in resolving the validity of these suppositions.

Recently Goldberg and his colleagues (82,83) have demonstrated that events mediated by augmented cAMP levels are often antagonized by agents which augment intracellular guanosine cyclic 3'5'-monophosphate (cGMP). Thus, while elevation of cAMP levels had an antimitotic role in various cell types, a rise in cGMP was reported to have a proliferative effect (83). In an apparent confirmation of this phenomenon in cytolytically active rat lymphocyte populations, Strom et al. (44) showed that while β-adrenergic agents suppressed cytolysis (presumably by augmenting cAMP levels), cholinergic agents (which augment cGMP in some tissues) increased the cytolytic activity of lymphocyte populations. This finding was not reproduced in two other laboratories (5,84); indeed, there is currently much difficulty in demonstrating the presence of cholinergic receptors on T lymphocytes (85). Despite our own current inability to implicate cGMP in the cytolytic process, interrelationships between this cyclic nucleotide and cAMP seem worthy of further study.

The stage in the cytolytic pathway inhibited by increased cAMP levels awaits definition. We have previously argued that the inhibitory effects of the cAMP-active drugs, cytochalasin B and colchicine, collectively suggest that the T cell must be able to secrete in order to kill (61). The evidence for this assertion is, of course, circumstantial, but is based on the antisecretory effects of these drugs in a wide variety of cell types. We will consider later the implications of T cell "secretion" during the lytic event.

Destruction of the Target Cell Membrane.   The terminal stages of the lytic cycle are perhaps the best understood. As a result of the collision with an effector T lymphocyte, the target cell undergoes a progressive series of membrane permeability changes, ending in rupture of the cell membrane (75). The progressive changes in the target cell membrane which herald lysis of the cell have perhaps been most clearly demonstrated using markers of varying molecular size as indicators of target cell destruction (75). Typical results are shown in Figure 8.

Using the P815 mastocytoma as target cell, and effector lymphocytes from alloimmunized C57BL/6 mice, changes in the permeability of the target cell membrane (as measured by ATP and ^{86}Rb efflux) were specifically induced within 10 minutes of lymphocyte addition. Protein-bound ^{51}C- or ^{3}H- thymidine DNA effluxed from target cells only later, after lag periods which were related to the effective molecular size of the indicator (Fig. 8). These findings suggest that the initial lesion allows rapid exchange of inorganic ions and small molecules, but not of macromolecules (75). It seems likely that the latter become able to pass the cell membrane only after secondary effects on the cell, resulting from disordered osmotic regulation. The eventual demise of the target cell appears to be caused by colloid osmotic forces resulting from water influx. This conclusion is based on observations that both macromolecular efflux from the damaged target cell and plasma membrane destruction can be prevented by the addition of exogenous

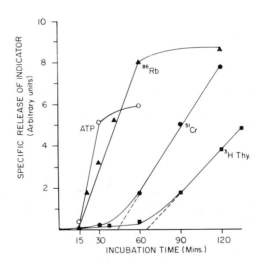

Figure 8.   T-lymphocyte-mediated release of various indicators from mastocytoma target cells. 10^{5} DBA/2 mastocytoma (P815) cells internally labeled with ^{86}Rb, ^{51}Cr, or ^{3}H thymidine were incubated with 10^{7} splenic lymphocytes derived from C57BL/6 mice which had been immunized 10 days earlier with 10^{7} mastocytoma cells intraperitoneally. The specific release of each indicator was calculated by subtraction of the amount of indicator released in the presence of 10^{7} normal C57BL/6 splenic lymphocytes. [Reproduced from the *Journal of Immunology* **110**, 73 (1973), by the kind permission of the Williams and Wilkins Company, Baltimore, Md.]

high-molecular weight dextrans (7). The minimal size of dextran molecules which we found to afford such protection was approximately 40,000 mol. wt., leading to a suggestion that the initial T-cell-induced lesion was approximately 90 A° in diameter (7).

The progressive nature of the lytic lesion induced by T cells, the suppression of its development by solutions of high osmotic pressure, and the apparent initial size of the lesion, all parallel remarkably the nature of the complement-induced membrane permeability changes in tumor cells (6,12). As stated earlier, however, it seems very unlikely that T-cell-induced lesions can be attributed to complement components.

In sum, we have a fairly good overall appreciation of the events involved in T-cell-mediated lysis (these are summarized in Fig. 9), but we have so far not considered the issue of overriding importance: how is the lesion inserted in the target cell membrane?

Role of Soluble Mediators in T-Cell-Mediated Lysis.   Of the suggestions offered to account for lesion insertion, most attention has been paid to the proposition that target cell destruction is caused by a soluble mediator released from the lymphocyte in response to an antigen "trigger." This hypothesis, which is discussed also in Chapter 4, was initially proposed by Granger and his collaborators (86). It has received support principally for two reasons: (1) it is conceptually attractive, making T-cell-mediated cytolysis dependent upon the product of an "activated" lymphoid cell in the same manner as are so many other cellular immune phenomena, and (2) there is a body of supportive experimental evidence, most notably the observation that stimulated lymphoid cell cultures produce a cytotoxic factor, "lymphotoxin" (86). Although there is much to commend the

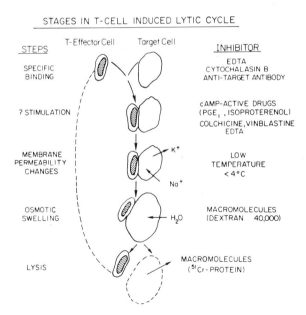

Figure 9.   Stages in the T-cell-mediated lytic cycle. [After Henney, C. S., *J. Reticuloendothelial Society* **17**, 4 (1975). Reproduced by the kind permission of Edwards and Broughton Company, Raleigh, N. C.]

candidature of lymphotoxin as the mediator of T-cell-induced cytolysis, its acceptance has not been universal, for there remain a number of experimental observations that are difficult to explain.

First, kinetic evidence shows that target cell destruction results from single collisions with an effector lymphocyte (38,53,54). If a soluble mediator were being secreted into the milieu, lysis would eventually be independent of such collision. It is not, even after extensive incubation periods.

Second, when cultures containing mixed target cell populations are employed, effector cells kill only those cells bearing homologous antigen; there is no lysis of "innocent bystander" cells (5). Lymphotoxin, on the other hand, is nonspecific in its action.* Furthermore, medium obtained from cultures in which large numbers of target cells have been destroyed is not lytic toward other targets cells, nor does it enhance the activity of effector T cell populations (87).

A series of recent observations on the relationship between mediator production and the cytolytic potential of lymphocytes casts further doubts on the role of lymphotoxin in T-cell-mediated lysis. It was found that the cytolytic activity of a lymphoid cell population could readily be dissociated experimentally from its ability to produce soluble mediators (88). Thus, treatment of lymphocytes with a number of drugs (e.g., cholera enterotoxin, colchicine, and vinblastine) ablated the direct lytic activity of these populations but left unaffected their ability to produce soluble mediators (including lymphotoxin) in the presence of antigen or mitogen (88).

Although not speaking against the role of soluble mediators per se, a recent observation of Gately et al. makes it unlikely that lymphotoxin itself plays an important role in T-cell-mediated lysis (89). These investigators, using a potent rabbit antilymphotoxin antiserum [which effectively neutralized both antigen- and mitogen-induced guinea pig lymphotoxin (90)] failed to affect cytolysis in vitro in systems employing guinea pig effector cells generated by mixed lymphocyte culture.

Another question continues to bother advocates of lymphotoxin's central role: why don't killer cells get destroyed during the lytic process? Unless there are cytoplasmic connections between the interacting cells—an unlikely proposition —the effector cell membrane should be as equally exposed to mediator action as is the target cell membrane. The activity of effector cells persists, however, through many lytic cycles (5), and their membranes are not inherently resistant to lymphocyte attack. Killer cells of one specificity can serve as target cells for other effector lymphocytes (91,92).

The latter observation poses an intriguing question: what role does the T cell's antigen receptor play in cytolysis? On the evidence currently available one can view a cytolytically active T cell in one of two distinctive ways: it may be either an intrinsically lytic cell or one which expresses its lytic activity only after "triggering" by antigen. A cell which has gained an inherent lytic activity during differentiation would be expected to kill other cells indiscriminately and to be limited in expressing this function only by factors governing proximity to other cells. In this case

---

*Lymphotoxin does appear to exert some selectivity in the spectrum of cells which it kills. L cell monolayers are by far the most susceptible cells to attack. This factor in itself has led some to query a broad biologic significance for lymphotoxin.

Table 1   Lysis of One Set of Killer T Cells by Another: A Search for Reciprocal Cell Death

Effector Cell Population	Percent Target Cell Death	
	b cells	*d* cells
a anti-*d*	4	27
d anti-*b*	53	0
Mixture of *a* anti-*d* and *d* anti-*b* incubated together for 4 hr before assessing effector function	5	31

The *a* anti-*d* effector cells were mixed at a ratio of 4:1 with *d* anti-*b* cells. After 4 hours at 37°C the lytic activity of this cell mixture was assessed by using ^{51}Cr-labeled *b*- and *d*-type target cells. As can be seen, following incubation, all *d* cells (and the resulting anti-*b* activity) were destroyed, but the effector activity of the anti-*d* effector cells was fully maintained. See ref 92 for further details.

the antigen-receptor site would serve only to bring the target cell into close enough approximation with the killer cell. Alternatively, if the effector T cell were only potentially a lytically active cell and acquired the activity only after antigen "triggering," the antigen receptor would clearly play a more crucial role in lytic expression. We have recently begun experiments to distinguish between these possibilities. The results obtained by R. Kuppers and reported in Table 1 suggest that killer cells become lytically active only after accommodation of their antigen receptor sites (92). Two sets of killer cells were raised by mixed lymphocyte culture: one of H-2a cells with anti-H-2d specificity, the other of H-2d cells with anti-H-2b specificity. When these two killer populations were mixed, the anti-H-2b activity was ablated while the anti-H-2d activity remained intact. These data suggest that during killer-killer cell interaction there is not reciprocal killing, but the effector cell whose antigen receptor is engaged becomes the killer, the partner cell the target.

While all of these observations seem to speak against the involvement of a freely permeating soluble mediator in the T-cell-mediated lytic process, it is premature to discount such a possibility. It is conceivable that a mediator is involved, but that it is delivered, and is effective, only over very short distances. With this in mind two mechanisms are currently receiving considerable attention. One of these proposes that the event is a totally membrane phenomenon; a recent observation that isolated lymphoid cell membranes can exhibit lytic activity (93) is certainly consistent with this but is difficult to associate with the data presented in Table 1. Another hypothesis suggests that tight junctions occur between effector and target cell (94), allowing the transfer of mediator from lymphocyte to target without contamination of the *milieu exterieur*. While the latter model would account for the specificity of T-cell-mediated lysis, it is an extremely demanding hypothesis, for it requires junctions between heterologous cell types over very short periods. These liaisons, if they occur, would create major precedents in cell biology.

Biologic Significance of Killer T Cells

Initial evidence that thymus-derived lymphocytes play a role in rejection of neoplasms came from findings that neonatally thymectomized animals develop more primary tumors after infection with oncogenic viruses than do control animals (95). Thymectomized mice were also found to be more susceptible to some forms of chemical carcinogenesis (96). In light of our current knowledge of the "helper" role of T cells in antibody formation, however, neither of these observations can be said to argue very forcibly that the absence of killer T cells is responsible for increased neoplasia.

Perhaps the best evidence that lytically active T cells are of in vivo significance comes from studies of cells sensitized to the major transplantation antigens. For example, neonatally thymectomized mice demonstrate accelerated skin graft rejection following injection of a purified population of T cells from syngeneic mice immunized against the graft alloantigens (97). Similar T cell pools, but not B cell or macrophage populations, prevent allogeneic tumor growth in X-irradiated syngeneic recipients (98).

There have been few in vivo studies involving tumor cells in a syngeneic environment in which the effector cells have been well characterized. In his study of the development of tumors in adult-thymectomized, antilymphocyte serum-treated mice infected with polyoma virus, Allison (99) found that tumor formation could be prevented by transfer of syngeneic lymphoid cells from specifically immunized donors. Pretreatment of the lymphoid cells with anti-θ serum and complement abolished their ability to prevent tumor development. Rouse et al. (100) found that spleen cells from mice immunized against a syngeneic plasma cell tumor were no longer able to inhibit tumor growth in sublethally irradiated mice following treatment with anti-θ serum and complement. In contrast, treatment of the same spleen cells with a rabbit antiserum against mouse immunoglobulin light chains in the presence of complement, which specifically killed B cells, had no effect. Similar results have been found with lymphoid cells from mice immunized with syngeneic cells transformed by the papovavirus SV 40 (101).

While the number and extent of these studies remain small, when collectively considered they make a forceful argument that killer T cells can play an important role in in vivo tumor destruction.

MACROPHAGE-MEDIATED CYTOTOXICITY

There has been much recent interest in the role of the macrophage as an effector cell in immune processes, particularly in defense against microbial infection. This interest has stemmed principally from the elegant studies of Mackaness, who has shown that macrophages become "activated" on exposure to soluble factors derived from immune T cells (102,103,104). The "activated" macrophage expresses at least two activities that the normal cell does not: (1) it is able to destroy intracellular facultative parasites (e.g., Listeria monocytogenes), and (2) it is cytotoxic toward a variety of cell types. The latter activity is thought by some to be of importance in allograft rejection (105), and it may also be significant in tumor cell rejection in vivo.

Although the well-documented phagocytic activity of macrophages is undoubtedly one means of effecting cytotoxicity, recent evidence suggests that there are at least two additional pathways by which macrophages can be induced to effect cell destruction. One of these is analogous to the pathway which gives the cell its antibacterial effects. In this, a normal macrophage is "activated" to a cytolytically active cell by a number of agents, including soluble product(s) synthesized following antigen "triggering" of an immune T lymphocyte (106). The other route to effector macrophage production, termed an "arming" process, requires direct contact between immune lymphoid cells and macrophages (107). The nature of the "arming" process is still undefined, but neither supernatants from cultures of immune cells nor immune T cells separated from macrophages by a Millipore membrane are able to produce this effect (108). These demonstrations would speak against cytophilic antibody being the key to arming, although this viewpoint still has some proponents.

The specificity of action of macrophages in effecting cell destruction reflects the two routes of "sensitization" ("activation" or "arming"); we will discuss each of these processes separately.

The Cytotoxicity of "Activated" Macrophages

The Mechanism of "Activation." The stimuli inducing macrophage "activation" still await characterization, as do the biochemical changes induced by the activation process. Consequently, one can currently define activation only in functional terms: it is a process by which a number of agents convert normal macrophages into cells which exhibit cytotoxicity in vitro.

Functional activation can be induced in vitro either directly, by agents such as polyinosinic-polycytidylic acid and endotoxin (109), or indirectly by exposure to soluble nonimmunoglobulin factor(s) elaborated by immune T cells on exposure to homologous antigen (110,111). Activation can also be readily induced in vivo, e.g., following immunization with BCG (106). In this case functional activation appears to require an immune response and does not occur simply as a *sequela* of inflammation, because macrophages harvested from the mouse peritoneal cavity following administration of thioglycollate, proteose peptone, and mineral oil are not cytotoxic (112).

Specificity of the Cytotoxic Action of "Activated" Macrophages. Hibbs et al. have demonstrated that mice chronically infected with intracellular protozoa or immunized with complete Freund's adjuvant showed increased resistance to a range of autochthonous and allogeneic tumors (113,114). Peritoneal macrophages from the infected mice were cytotoxic in vitro to a similar spectrum of tumor cells (113,114). The cytotoxic process was thus an entirely nonspecific one in an immunological sense—although, interestingly, there was selectivity: only cells with abnormal growth characteristics (e.g., tumorigenic cells) were killed (115). Activated macrophages did not destroy allogeneic fibroblasts but were markedly cytotoxic to both syngeneic and allogeneic tumor cell lines (115). Similarly, other studies have shown that activated macrophages were cytotoxic to EMT-6 mouse mammary adenocarcinoma cells but did not affect the growth of secondary cultures of mouse kidney cells (116). The activated macrophage has also been shown to kill neoplastic cells across species barriers: murine macrophages derived from animals chronically infected with BCG destroyed human HeLa and VA-13 cells but not normal foreskin fibroblasts (106).

These experiments suggest that cells with abnormal growth characteristics (including tumor cells) show an increased susceptibility to destruction by the activated macrophage. The basis for this increased susceptibility appears to be an undefined cell membrane change in the tumor cell. It is possible that such changes are a feature of in vitro culture, but one might speculate that they may be related to neoplastic transformation.

Mechanism of Cytotoxicity by "Activated" Macrophages.   "Activated" macrophages do not kill tumor cells by phagocytosis, for cytochalasin B, a potent inhibitor of phagocytosis, has no effect on cytotoxicity (117). Inhibitors of nucleic acid synthesis (mitomycin C, actinomycin D) and protein synthesis (puromycin, cyclohex-imide) have also been reported to be incapable of suppressing macrophage-mediated cytolysis (118).

Hibbs has recently presented a hypothesis for the mechanism of cytolysis by macrophages which is compatible with these observations (119). He suggests that the cytotoxicity is caused by lysosomal enzymes secreted directly from the acti-vated macrophage into the cytoplasm of the target cell. There is experimental evidence for this assertion of both a biochemical and morphologic nature: (1) hydrocortisone, an inhibitor of lysosomal exocytosis, inhibits lysis, as does trypan blue, an inhibitor of lysosomal enzyme action. (2) Phase contrast microscopy has demonstrated the transfer of a lysosomal marker (dextran sulfate stained with toluidine blue) into target cells. In this study there was a positive correlation between transfer of marker to a target cell and its subsequent lysis (119). Direct transfer of lysosomal products into the target cell was inferred by the total absence of cytotoxic factor(s) in the milieu of the cultured cells. Hibbs favors the possibility that lysis occurs because of direct membrane fusion between the attacking mac-rophages and the target cell, but the experimental evidence for this proposition is so far lacking.

Cytolysis by the "Armed" Macrophage

Far less is known about the "armed" macrophage and its mode of action. It is clear, however, that its cytotoxic potential differs from that of the "activated" mac-rophage, for, most strikingly, "armed" macrophages kill in an immunologically specific manner (107,108,109). Thus, Evans and Alexander have shown that peritoneal cells from mice hyperimmunized with an X-irradiated syngeneic lym-phoma were able to inhibit the growth of the same tumor cells in vitro but had no effect on allogeneic lymphomas (108).

The specificity of tumor cell destruction by "armed" macrophages suggests that they bear specific recognition structures. The most likely candidates for such receptors appear to be either cytophilic antibody or immune complexes. As detailed in an earlier section of this chapter, macrophages bear surface receptors for the Fc portion of immunoglobulin molecules, thus providing a possible anchor for the attachment of cytophilic antibody to the macrophage surface. Experimental evidence in keeping with the supposition that cytophilic antibody is the key to the cytotoxic activity of "armed" macrophages has been put forward by Granger and Weiser (120). These investigators showed that antibody could be eluted from the surface of "armed" cells either by heating at 56°C for 30 minutes or by treatment with trypsin. Such treatment was associated with abrogation of cytotoxic potential. Cytolytic activity was restored by incubation of the denuded cells in immune serum. It should be pointed out that Evans and Alexander failed to reproduce these findings and have offered an alternative explanation of the "arming" process (121). They suggest that "arming" is mechanistically similar to one of the routes leading to macrophage "activation" and is caused by a soluble factor derived from T cells. However, unlike those soluble T-cell-derived factors which prime the macrophage to exert nonspecific cytotoxicity, this factor endows specificity and has been termed "specific macrophage-arming factor" (SMAF) (122). Recent experimental evidence from Alexander's laboratory suggests that the specific arming factor is composed of two components: one cytophilic for the macrophage membrane, the other possessing a specific recognition site (122). Presumably both sites are on the same molecule. In view of its specificity for antigen, it has been suggested that SMAF may contain specific T cell receptors. There is some precedent for this: Feldmann has reported that T cell receptors are shed during in vitro incubation with homologous antigen (123).

The mechanisms by which "armed" cells exhibit cytotoxicity has so far not been studied, and the question of the biologic significance of macrophage "arming" is an open one. Particularly intriguing is the relationship between "armed" and "activated" macrophages: do they coexist in vivo? Do they cooperate synergistically? What is the relationship between "armed" macrophages and those Fc-receptor bearing monocytes which function as effector cells in antibody-dependent cell-mediated cytotoxicity? Answers to these questions should aid considerably in evaluating the biologic significance of cytotoxic macrophages.

SUMMARY

We have detailed a number of pathways by which the immune system and its products can lead to tumor cell destruction in vitro. In all cases, except those in which the "activated" macrophage serves as the effector cell, cell death is an immunologically specific event. It is clear that no cytotoxic pathway has yet been defined in molecular terms, but a number of requirements for cytolysis have been delineated. These can be summarized briefly as follows:

1. Complement-mediated lysis following antibody activation is primarily of significance when IgM antibody is involved. The lytic lesion appears to be formed by an insertion of several of the terminal complement components (or their partial degradation products) into the lipid bilayer of the plasma membrane, forming a structure conveniently regarded as a "doughnut"—a rigid cylinder connecting the cytoplasm with the *milieu exterieur*.

2.   Antibody-dependent cell-mediated cytotoxicity: This is due to effector cells bearing receptors for the Fc portion of IgG molecules, which interact with IgG antibody bound to the target cell surface. Effector cells are a heterogeneous group, but for a given target cell type one effector cell type appears to predominate. The effector cells are present in normal (unimmunized) individuals.

Operationally this lytic process is inhibited by aggregated IgG and by soluble antigen-antibody complexes. Lysis is an energy-requiring process, dependent on a viable effector cell but independent of protein synthesis.

3.   T-cell-mediated lysis is effected by cells with a membrane-associated antigen receptor. Under optimal conditions these cells effect lysis rapidly in vitro (less than 1 hour), and each effector cell can kill more than one target. The overall reaction is energy dependent, most of this requirement apparently being involved in effector cell-target cell conjugation. Cytolysis is inhibited by EDTA, by the cytochalasins A and B, and by drugs which augment lymphocyte cAMP levels. *De novo* protein synthesis is unnecessary for lytic expression, as is DNA synthesis. Lysis is dependent on intimate association between effector and target cell rather than on the secretion of soluble lytic mediators.

4.   Macrophages can also effect tumor cell destruction. In addition to phagocytosis, there are two pathways by which macrophages can be primed to become cytolytically active. One of these, referred to as an "arming" process, may be due to the adsorption of cytophilic antibody onto the macrophage surface or to an acquisition of T cell receptors. Although the mechanism by which these cells effect destruction is unknown in detail, "armed" macrophages kill in an immunologically specific manner which depends upon intimate contact between macrophage and target cell.

The other pathway by which macrophages acquire cytotoxic potential has been termed "activation." A number of agents (e.g., endotoxin, polyinosinic-polycytidilic acid) can "activate" macrophages directly in vitro, while activation can also occur in vivo following immunization with some microbial products, e.g., BCG. The "activated" macrophage kills target cells with no immunologic specificity, though, interestingly, it shows selectivity, preferentially killing cells with abnormal growth characteristics (e.g., tumor cells). There is evidence that the "activated" macrophages effect cell destruction by direct secretion of lysosomal enzymes into the cytoplasm of the target cell.

Despite the many pathways leading to the insertion of lesions in a target cell's membrane, the terminal events in cell destruction seem to be very similar. In all cases, water influx through the membrane lesion leads to disordered osmotic regulation, and the resulting colloid osmotic forces cause disruption of the plasma membrane.

Another feature of lytic attack by the immune system appears to be common to several pathways: the offense is directed against the lipid moiety of the plasma membrane. The case for this assertion cannot be made with total assurance at this time, but the circumstantial evidence is good. Antibody in the presence of complement can cause the lysis of synthetic membranes called liposomes, which contain no protein. Furthermore, the lesions inserted in the liposome membrane appear, from electron micrographs, to be identical to those in erythrocytes. In a recent study Henkart has observed changes in electrical conductance across synthetic lipid bilayers following the addition of a lymphocyte source and antibody directed against a component of the membrane (124). Neither lymphocytes nor antibody caused such changes when used alone. It is tempting to view Henkart's model as an analogue of antibody-dependent cell-mediated cytotoxicity and to conclude that lysis of plasma membranes by this pathway is effected via its lipid component.

In this chapter we have tried to bring together a large body of data obtained from studies in many in vitro systems. The aim was to establish some general guidelines for viewing cytotoxic pathways mediated by the immune system. In the interests of simplicity there have been several deliberate overextrapolations of published data. No defense is offered for this practice, and only time will tell whether it was justified.

The last year has seen the demonstration of yet another cell-mediated cytotoxic pathway (125,126,127,128). The effector cell is present in neonatal lymphoid tissues in a vareity of mouse strains (125,126), and because it can kill a wide variety of cell types it has been termed a "natural killer" or NK cell (127). NK cells lack both surface immunoglobulin and Thy 1.2 antigens, although they are purportedly of lymphoid cell origin. Little is yet known about the mechanism of action or of the significance of NK cells, nor indeed what stimulus initiates their development. They seem to be characterized, however, by a marked lability (125,128) and a susceptibility to proteolytic enzymes (127,128). NK-mediated cytotoxicity is unaffected by the presence of immune complexes and is independent of the presence of antitarget cell antibody.

Interestingly, Wolfe et al. have been able to induce NK cells in the mouse peritoneal cavity by administration of viable BCG organisms, but not by other irritants (128). These investigators have suggested that NK cells might be responsible for the tumor regression frequently reported following the local administration of BCG. There is currently much speculation that NK cells may be involved in immune surveillance.

ACKNOWLEDGMENTS

The author wishes to thank Dr. Richard Thorn for much of the literature search that led to the section on complement-mediated lysis. He also wishes to thank Drs. Marshall Plaut and Daniel Tracey for critical readings of the manuscript. Drs. Manfred Mayer and Robert Dourmashkin kindly allowed reproduction of figures from their published work.

REFERENCES

1. *The Collected Papers of Paul Ehrlich* (B. Himmelweit, ed.), Pergamon Press, New York, 1957.
2. Kidd, J. G., and Toolan, H. W., *Am. J. Pathol.* **26,** 672 (1950).
3. Govaerts, A., *J. Immunol.* **85,** 516 (1960).
4. Perlmann, P., and Holm, G., *Adv. Immunol.* **11,** 117 (1969).
5. Cerottini, J.-C. and Brunner, K. T., *Adv. Immunol.* **18,** 67 (1974).
6. Green, H., Barrow, P., and Goldberg, B., *J. Exp. Med.* **110,** 669 (1959).
7. Henney, C. S., *Nature* **249,** 456 (1974).
8. Humphrey, J. H., and Dourmashkin, R. R., *Adv. Immunol.* **11,** 75 (1969).

9. Mayer, M. M., *Proc. Nat. Acad. Sci. USA* **69**, 2954 (1972).

10. Muller-Eberhard, H., *Adv. Immunol.* **8**, 1 (1968).

11. Kalfayan, B., and Kidd, J. G., *J. Exp. Med.* **97**, 145 (1953).

12. Green, H., Fleischer, R. A., Barrow, P., and Goldberg, B., *J. Exp. Med.* **109**, 511 (1959).

13. Mayer, M. M., in *Immunochemical Approaches to Problems in Microbiology* (M. Heideiberger and O. Plescia, eds.), Rutgers University Press, New Brunswick, N.J., 1961, p. 268.

14. Humphrey, J., *Third International Symposium of Immunopathology*, Schwabe, Basel, 1963, pp. 369.

15. Humphrey, J. H., and Dourmashkin, R. R., *Ciba Foundation Symposium on Complement*, Churchill, London, 1965, p. 175.

16. Iles, G. H., Seeman, P., Naylor, D., and Cinader, B., *J. Cell Biol.* **56**, 528 (1973).

17. Bhakdi, S., Knuferman, H., Schmidt-Ullrich, R., and Fischer, H., *Protides of the Biological Fluids* (H. Peeters, ed.), Permagon Press, Oxford, 1974, Vol. 21, p. 331.

18. Ohanian, S. H., Borsos, T., and Rapp, H. J., *J. Nat. Cancer Inst.* **50**, 1313 (1973).

19. Segerling, M., Ohanian, S. H., and Borsos, T., *J. Nat. Cancer Inst.* **53**, 1411 (1974).

20. Segerling, M., Ohanian, S. H., and Borsos, T., *Science* **188**, 55 (1975).

21. Borsos, T., and Rapp, H. J., *Science* **150**, 505 (1965).

22. Ishizaka, T., Ishizaka, K., Borsos, T., and Rapp, H. J., *J. Immunol.* **97**, 716 (1966).

23. Canty, T. G., and Wunderlich, J. R., *J. Nat. Cancer Inst.* **45**, 761 (1970).

24. Henney, C. S., and Mayer, M. M., *Cell. Immunol.* **2**, 702 (1971).

25. Henney, C. S., Clayburgh, J., Cole, G. A., and Prendergast, R. A., *Immunol. Comm.* **1**, 93 (1972).

26. Moller, E., *Science* **147**, 873 (1965).

27. Perlmann, P., and Perlmann, H., *Cell. Immunol.* **1**, 300 (1970).

28. Sanderson, C. J., Clark, I. A., and Taylor, G. A., *Nature* (London), **253**, 377 (1975).

29. Golstein, P., and Fewtrell, C., *Nature* **255**, 491 (1975).

30. Lamon, E. W., Whitten, H. D., Lidin, B., and Fudenberg, H. H., *J. Exp. Med.* **142**, 542 (1975).

31. MacLennan, I. C. M., Loewi, G., and Howard, A., *Immunol.* **17**, 887 (1969).

32. Perlmann, P., Perlmann, H., and Wigzell, H., *Transpl. Rev.* **13**, 91 (1972).

33. MacLennan, I. C. M., *Transpl. Rev.* **13**, 67 (1972).

34. MacLennan, I. C. M., and Harding, B., *Progress in Immunol.*, II (L. Brent and J. Holborrow, eds.), North Holland American Elsevier, New York, 1974, Vol. 3, p. 347.

35. Forman, J., and Moller, G., *Transpl. Rev.* **17**, 108 (1973).

36. MacLennan, I. C. M., Loewi, G., and Howard, A., *J. Immunol.* **17**, 897 (1969).

37. Ziegler, H. K., and Henney, C. S., *J. Immunol.* **115**, 1500 (1975).

38. Henney, C. S., *J. Immunol.* **107**, 1558 (1971).

39. MacLennan, I. C. M., *Clin. Exp. Immunol.* **10**, 275 (1972).

40. Granger, R. P., and Ziegelboim, J., *J. Immunol.* **114**, 1047 (1975).

41. MacLennan, I. C. M., and Harding, B., *Immunol.* **18**, 405 (1970).

42. Wunderlich, J. R., Rosenberg, E. B., and Connolly, J. M., in *Progress in Immunology* (B. Amos, ed.), Academic Press, New York, 1971, p. 473.

43. Henney, C. S., *Fed. Proc.* **32**, 997 (abst.), 1973.

44. Strom, T. B., Carpenter, C. B., Garovoy, M. R., Austen, D. F., Merrill, J. P., and Kaliner, M., *J. Exp. Med.* **138**, 381 (1973).

45. Winn, H. J., *J. Immunol.* **84**, 530 (1960).

46. Shin, H. S., Kaliss, N., Borenstein, D., and Gately, M. K., *J. Exp. Med.* **136**, 375 (1972).

47. Shin, H. S., Hayden, M. L., and Gately, C. L., *Proc. Nat. Acad. Sci.* **71**, 163 (1974).

48. Shin, H. S., Hayden, M. L., Langley, S., Kaliss, N., and Smith, M. R., *J. Immunol.* **114**, 1255 (1975).

49. Cerottini, J.-C., Nordin, A. A., and Brunner, K. T., *Nature* (London) **228**, 1308 (1970).

50. Thomas, L., in *Cellular and Humoral Aspects of the Hypersensitive State* (H. S. Lawrence, ed.), Harper (Hoeber), New York, 1959, pp. 529.

51. Burnet, F. M., *Brit. Med. J.* **1,** 779 (1957).
52. Brunner, K. T., Mauel, J., Cerottini, J.-C., and Chapuis, B., *Immunol.* **14,** 181 (1968).
53. Wilson, D. B., *J. Exp. Med.* **122,** 143 (1965).
54. Berke, G., Ax, W., Ginsburg, H., and Feldman, M., *Immunol.* **16,** 643 (1969).
55. Rosenau, W., and Moon, H. D., *J. Immunol.* **96,** 80 (1966).
56. Plaut, M., Lichtenstein, L. M., and Henney, C. S., *J. Immunol.* **110,** 771 (1973).
57. Bubbers, J. E., and Henney, C. S., *J. Immunol.* **115,** 145 (1975).
58. Strom, T. B., Garovoy, M. R., Carpenter, C. B., and Merrill, J. P., *Science* **181,** 171 (1973).
59. Henney, C. S., Bourne, H. R., and Lichtenstein, L. M., *J. Immunol.* **108,** 1526 (1972).
60. Strom, T. B., Deisseroth, A., Morganroth, J., Carpenter, C. S., and Merrill, J. P., *Proc. Nat. Acad. Sci. USA* **69,** 2995 (1972).
61. Henney, C. S., *Transpl. Rev.* **17,** 37 (1973).
62. Thorn, R., and Henney, C. S., *J. Immunol.* **116,** 146 1976.
63. Bubbers, J. E., and Henney, C. S., *J. Immunol.* **114,** 1126 (1975).
64. Binz, H., and Wigzell, H., *J. Exp. Med.* **142,** 197 (1975).
65. Crone, M., Koch, C., and Simonsen, M., *Transpl. Rev.* **10,** 36 (1972).
66. Werkele, H., Lonai, P., and Feldman, M., *Proc. Nat. Acad. Sci. USA* **69,** 1620 (1972).
67. Henney, C. S., and Bubbers, J. E., *J. Immunol.* **111,** 85 (1973).
68. Rosenau, W., *Fed. Proc.* **27,** 34 (1968).
69. Mauel, J., Rudolf, H., Chapuis, B., and Brunner, K. T., *Immunol.* **18,** 517 (1970).
70. Stulting, R. D., and Berke, G., *J. Exp. Med.* **137,** 932 (1973).
71. Plaut, M., Bubbers, J. E., and Henney, C. S., *J. Immunol.* **116,** 150 (1976).
72. Berke, G., and Fishelson, Z., *J. Exp. Med.* **142,** 1011 (1975).
73. Martz, E., *J. Immunol.* **115,** 261 (1975).
74. Berke, G., and Gabison, D., *Eur. J. Immunol.* **5,** 671 (1975).
75. Henney, C. S., *J. Immunol.* **110,** 73 (1973).
76. MacDonald, H. R., *Eur. J. Immunol.* **5,** 521 (1975).
77. Martz, E., and Benacerraf, B., *J. Immunol.* **111,** 1538 (1973).
78. Henney, C. S., and Lichtenstein, L. M., *J. Immunol.* **107,** 610 (1971).
79. Lichtenstein, L. M., Gillespie, E., Bourne, H. R., and Henney, C. S., *Prostaglandins* **2,** 519 (1972).
80. Plaut, M., Lichtenstein, L. M., Gillespie, E., and Henney, C. S., *J. Immunol.* **111,** 398 (1973).
81. Lichtenstein, L. M., Henney, C. S., Bourne, H. R., and Greenough, W. B., *J. Clin. Invest.* **52,** 691 (1973).
82. George, W. J., Polson, J. B., O'Toole, A. G., and Goldberg, N. D., *Proc. Nat. Acad. Sci. USA* **66,** 398 (1970).
83. Hadden, J. W., Hadden, E. M., Haddox, M. K., and Goldberg, N. D., *Proc. Nat. Acad. Sci. USA* **69,** 3024 (1972).
84. Henney, C. S., in *Cyclic AMP, Cell Growth and the Immune Response* (W. Braun, C. W. Parker, and L. M. Lichtenstein, eds.), Springer-Verlag, New York, 1974, p. 195.
85. Wedner, H. J. Dankner, R., and Parker, C. W., *J. Immunol.* **115,** 1682 (1975).
86. Granger, G. A., and Kolb, W. P., *J. Immunol.* **101,** 111 (1968).
87. Henney, C. S., unpublished observations, 1973.
88. Henney, C. S., Gaffney, J., and Bloom, B. R., *J. Exp. Med.* **140,** 837 (1974).
89. Gately, M. K., Mayer, M. M., and Henney, C. S., *Cell. Immunol.*, in press 1976.
90. Gately, M. K., Gately, C., Henney, C. S., and Mayer, M. M., *J. Immunol.* **115,** 817 (1975).
91. Golstein, P., *Nature* **252,** 81 (1974).
92. Kuppers, R. K., and Henney, C. S., *J. Exp. Med.* **143,** 684 (1976).
93. Ferluga, J., and Allison, A. C., *Nature* **255,** 708 (1975).
94. Ferluga, J., and Allison, A. C., *Nature* **250,** 673 (1974).
95. Wagner, J. L., and Haughton, G., *J. Nat. Cancer Inst.* **46,** 1 (1971).

96. Ting, R. C., and Law, L. B., *Progr. Exp. Tumor Res.* **9,** 165 (1967).

97. Sprent, J., and Miller, J. F. A. P., *Nat. New Biol.* **234,** 195 (1971).

98. Freedman, L. R., Cerottini, J.-C., and Brunner, K. T., *J. Immunol.* **109,** 1371 (1972).

99. Allison, A. C., *Ann. Inst. Pasteur, Paris* **122,** 619 (1972).

100. Rouse, B. T., Rollinghoff, M., and Warner, N. L., *Nat. New Biol.* **238,** 116 (1972).

101. Zarling, J. M., and Tevethia, S. S., *J. Nat. Cancer Inst.* **50,** 137 (1973).

102. Mackaness, G. B., *J. Exp. Med.* **116,** 105 (1964).

103. Mackaness, G. B., *J. Exp. Med.* **129,** 973 (1969).

104. Mackaness, G. B., *J. Exp. Med.* **120,** 105 (1964).

105. Gorer, P. A., *Adv. Cancer Res.* **4,** 149 (1956).

106. Hibbs, G. J., *J. Nat. Cancer Inst.* **53,** 1487 (1974).

107. Evans, R., and Alexander, P., *Nature (London)* **236,** 168 (1972).

108. Evans, R., and Alexander, P., *Nature (London)* **228,** 620 (1970).

109. Evans, R., and Alexander, P., *Nature (London)* **232,** 75 (1971).

110. Nathan, C. F., Karnovsky, M. L., and David, J. R., *J. Exp. Med.* **133,** 1356 (1971).

111. Krahenbuhl, J. L., Rosenberg, J. T., and Remington, J. S., *J. Immunol.* **111,** 992 (1973).

112. Hibbs, J. B., Lambert, L. H., and Remington, J. S., *Nature* **235,** 48 (1972).

113. Hibbs, J. B., Lambert, L. H., and Remington, J. S., *J. Infect. Dis.* **124,** 587 (1971).

114. Hibbs, J. B., Lambert, L. H., and Remington, J. S., *Proc. Soc. Exp. Biol. Med.* **139,** 1053 (1972).

115. Hibbs, J. B., *Proc. Soc. Exp. Biol. Med.* **139,** 1049 (1972).

116. Hibbs, J. B., *Science* **180,** 868 (1973).

117. Temple, A., Loewi, G., Davies, P., and Howard, A., *Immunol.* **24,** 655 (1973).

118. Keller, R., *Immunol.* **27,** 285 (1974).

119. Hibbs, J. B., *Science* **184,** 468 (1974).

120. Granger, G. A., and Weiser, R. S., *Science* **151,** 97 (1966).

121. Evans, R., and Alexander, P., *Immunol.* **23,** 627 (1972).

122. Evans, R., Grant, C. K., Cox, H., Steele, K. and Alexander, P., *J. Exp. Med.* **136,** 1318 (1972).

123. Feldmann, M., *J. Exp. Med.* **136,** 737 (1972).

124. Henkart, P., and Blumenthal, R., *Proc. Nat. Acad. Sci. (USA),* **72,** 2789 (1975).

125. Herberman, R., Nunn, M. and Lavrin, D., *Int. J. Cancer* **16,** 216, (1975).

126. Herberman, R., Nunn, M., Holden, H. and Lavrin, P., *Int. J. Cancer* **16,** 230 (1975).

127. Kiessling, R., Klein, E. Pross, H. and Wigzell, H., *Eur. J. Immunol.* **5,** 117 (1975).

128. Wolfe, S. A., Tracey, D. E. and Henney, C. S., *Nature* **262,** 586 (1976).

Chapter Four

Lymphokines in Tumor Immunity

TAKESHI YOSHIDA* AND STANLEY COHEN

Department of Pathology, University of Connecticut Health Center, Farmington, Connecticut

The role of cell-mediated immunity in mechanisms of host defense against tumors is described throughout this volume and in many other recent reviews (1–6) and needs no further justification here. Rather, we will discuss some ways in which this role may manifest itself. As introduction, it should be pointed out that the term cell-mediated immunity is now generally recognized to be something of a misnomer. Many of the manifestations of this form of immunologic reactivity do not involve direct cell-cell interactions but rather are due to the actions of soluble effector (mediator) substances called lymphokines. This understanding is based firmly upon a large variety of in vitro studies (7,8). In addition, a number of recent in vivo observations have confirmed the importance of lymphokines in cell-mediated immunity (9,10) and have also led to the suggestion that they represent one aspect of a general biologic process which is not confined to immunologic events (11). In spite of this mass of data, and the association of cell-mediated tumor immunity, there is as yet no convincing direct evidence for the role of lymphokines in defense against tumors. Only a limited literature on this subject is available, and most of it deals with lymphokines as tools for assay, insofar as they represent detectable parameters of the immune response that appear during the evolution of neoplastic disease either in experimental animals or in clinical states.

In the present review we will not attempt a complete survey of the literature but rather will try to bring together some of the available experimental data which suggest a potentially important role for lymphokines in defense against tumor growth. In so doing, we will inevitably touch on some topics described elsewhere in this book. Such repetition is unavoidable and, indeed, may be beneficial.

Some of the work reported here was supported by N.I.H. Grant No. AI-12225.

*Recipient of Public Health Service Career Development Award, AI-00082.

BACKGROUND

As discussed in Chapter 1, two more or less concurrent lines of investigation set the stage for the discovery of the lymphokines. It was shown in a number of laboratories (reviewed in 12) that the cellular infiltrate at sites of delayed hypersensitivity reactions consists predominantly of nonsensitized cells. Only small numbers of specifically sensitized lymphocytes, which do not appear to accumulate preferentially, are sufficient to initiate a series of events which then lead to a slowly evolving, nonspecific inflammatory response. The second set of experiments demonstrated that the migration of mononuclear cells in vitro could be inhibited by the interaction of sensitized lymphocytes and antigen (13–15), provided that the cells were obtained from animals with delayed hypersensitivity. It was soon discovered that only a small number of specifically sensitized cells are sufficient to initiate this reaction, in analogy with the situation in vivo (14,15).

These two lines of investigation showed clearly that the delayed hypersensitivity reaction, and by extension cell-mediated immunity in general, is a cascade phenomenon with at least two stages. Activation of a small number of sensitized cells by antigen (first stage) somehow results in the accumulation of large numbers of inflammatory cells (second stage). A clue to the coupling of these two stages came from an elegant series of experiments, performed independently and simultaneously by Bloom (15) and David (16) as described in Chapter 1. These investigators showed that the migration inhibition reaction was mediated by a soluble factor (MIF) elaborated by the antigen-triggered lymphocytes. Subsequently, a large number of lymphokine activities were described by many workers in many laboratories (reviewed in 7 and 8). These, in general, fall into three main categories: lymphokines that exert toxic effects on target cells, lymphokines that exert proliferative effects on target cells, and lymphokines that modulate the inflammatory response. This latter category includes substances that affect migration properties of inflammatory cells, modify surface properties of such cells, influence biochemical activity, and activate various cells for phagocytosis and killing functions.

It was soon postulated that the lymphokines, though defined in terms of in vitro activity, were the responsible factors for many of the in vivo manifestations of cell-mediated immunity. In recent years much evidence has accumulated in support of this contention (reviewed in 9 and 10). This includes the detection of various lymphokines at sites of in vivo reactions of cell-mediated immunity (17,19), the induction of biologically significant in vivo reactions by administration of exogenous lymphokines (18,20–22), and the recent demonstration that antibody prepared against lymphokines has suppressive effects on cell-mediated immunity in vivo (23,24).

Thus, the available evidence strongly suggests important biological roles for the lymphokines, although specific details regarding these roles are not yet fully available. It should be noted that this evidence was obtained in the face of a very difficult technical limitation: none of the lymphokines has been completely characterized in physicochemical terms, and none has been completely isolated or purified. This has hampered studies aimed at clarifying their mechanism of action and protective function, not only in tumor immunity but in all forms of immune response.

LYMPHOKINES PRODUCED BY "TUMOR-IMMUNE" LYMPHOCYTES

As indicated in the previous section, a large body of literature has accumulated on the production of lymphokines in a variety of experimental settings involving many different kinds of antigenic and nonantigenic challenge. It is therefore surprising that only a small number of studies are available dealing with the production of lymphokines by lymphocytes stimulated with tumor antigens.

Macrophage Migration Inhibition Factor (MIF)

The first description of the macrophage migration inhibition phenomenon in a system involving tumor antigen was given by Kronman et al. (25) and also by Bloom and Bennett (26). Kronman et al. have demonstrated that the in vitro migration of peritoneal exudate cells from strain 2 guinea pigs immunized by injections of diethylnitrosamine-induced hepatoma lines could be inhibited by the presence of specific live tumor cells. These were introduced into the test capillary tubes in numbers equal to those of the indicator cells (macrophages). This inhibition was tumor specific; thus, line 1 tumor cells could inhibit the migration of peritoneal exudate cells from guinea pigs immunized with transplanted line 1 tumor but could not inhibit the migration of cells from animals immunized with line 7, and vice versa. These investigations involved the direct migration inhibition reaction; the investigators did not study production of MIF by lymphocytes in this system.

Bloom et al. (26) have published independently a similar set of observations. They have shown that peritoneal exudate cells from guinea pigs immunized with soluble antigens from methylcholanthrene- or dimethylbenzanthracene-induced sarcoma could be inhibited in in vitro migration by specific antigen. There was no cross-reactivity among the three different tumor lines studied. In addition, these workers showed that it was possible to produce MIF-containing supernatants when they incubated lymph node cells from the immune guinea pigs with specific soluble tumor antigen. Subsequent studies (27) showed that the migration inhibition test was useful in distinguishing various tumor-specific surface antigens from different tumor lines obtained from chemically induced sarcomas in inbred guinea pigs. It was claimed in these reports that the migration inhibition assay is more sensitive than skin testing in terms of the amount of antigen required to give a positive reaction. Thus, it was suggested that this direct assay system may be useful in monitoring the fractionation of soluble antigens from various tumor tissues.

Churchill et al. (28), using diethylnitrosamine-induced hepatoma in strain 2 guinea pigs, have shown that peritoneal exudate lymphocytes from tumor-bearing guinea pigs could produce MIF when stimulated by tumor cells. Instead of soluble antigens, they employed either live or irradiated hepatoma cells to stimulate lymphocytes for MIF production. Another difference between their experimental design and that of Bloom et al. (26,27) was that they immunized guinea pigs by repeated inoculations of tumor cells without using adjuvant. These differences are significant, since in the natural state all the antigens possessed by tumor cells may not be exposed or immunogenic, and thus the protocol of

Churchill et al. (28) is a more accurate reflection of what might occur in vivo in an animal or man bearing a tumor. It is entirely possible that experimental results obtained with cell extracts, used as immunizing agents or test substances, may not entirely parallel results when whole cells are used. The point here is that in any experiments involving immunization it is important to distinguish between immunogenic potency, relative ability of test materials to elicit a response in a test assay, and relative protective effect. There is no a priori reason to suppose absolute correlation among these three parameters. Although a comparative study to clarify this point should be feasible, no systemic investigation along these lines has been reported.

In another species, Halliday and Webb (29) have reported that the migration of peritoneal cells of CBA mice bearing methylcholanthrene-induced tumors could be inhibited by the presence of tumor cells with the peritoneal cells in capillary tubes. Confirming the results by others, it was shown that such inhibition was tumor antigen specific. Further studies by Halliday (30,31) have shown that tumor-specific soluble antigen, as well as whole tumor cells, were effective in inhibiting the migration of peritoneal cells. A most interesting observation in this system relates to the ability to correlate migration inhibition with the "clinical" status of the experimental animals. For these experiments Halliday used either Moloney sarcoma virus-induced or methylcholanthrene-induced tumors. He found that peritoneal exudate cells from mice with growing tumors could not be migration inhibited by tumor-specific antigens. In contrast, cells from "regressor" mice, with spontaneously regressed tumor, or from mice in which the tumor was surgically removed could readily be inhibited by the antigen.

In analogy to the blocking factor in serum from tumor-bearing mice which blocks the oncocidal capacity of immune lymphocytes (reviewed in 3), Halliday was able to show that the serum from such mice growing tumors ("progressor" mice) can reverse the inhibition of macrophage migration by specific tumor antigen in "regressor" mice. The similarity of such "blocking factors" in both migration inhibition and lymphocyte cytotoxicity assays does not necessarily prove their identity. More definite studies have to be done to clarify this point as well as to explore the existence of the blocking factor in other experimental models, since many studies on migration inhibition assays in tumor-immune systems by others (25,28,32–34) have indicated that peritoneal exudate cells from tumor-bearing or tumor-immunized (therefore, so-called "progressor") animals could be inhibited by antigen, as mentioned above.

These conflicting results could have several explanations. First, cell-mediated immune reactions to tumors may be different from species to species. Even in mice, however, Blasecki and Tevethia (34) have reported that macrophage migration of mice bearing SV 40 virus-induced tumors was inhibited by tumor-specific soluble antigen from SV 40 transformed cells. In this case, species differences can not account for the discordant results. In hamsters (34) the peritoneal exudate cells from animals which were inoculated neonatally with SV 40 virus and did not develop tumors were inhibited in migration by soluble antigen extracted from SV 40-induced tumor cells. Conversely, there was a failure of the soluble tumor-specific antigen to inhibit the migration of peritoneal cells from hamsters themselves bearing primary SV 40 virus-induced tumors. Thus the migration inhibition of peritoneal cells from tumor-bearing animals is most likely affected by different tumor systems (origins, antigenicity, etc.) rather than by species. Which specific factors are involved remains an open issue. It is clearly of the utmost importance to determine the conditions under which macrophage migration is inhibited in any given species of animals with regressing tumors and the conditions under which migration cannot be inhibited in animals with growing tumors. If the pattern of events described by Halliday (30,31) proves to have general applicability, the migration inhibition assay may prove to have important prognostic value.

In these studies, some technical problems must be solved before reports from various laboratories can be fully evaluated in relation to each other. One of the problems most frequently encountered in macrophage migration inhibition assay studies, even in commonly used nontumor antigen systems, has been the inconsistency of peritoneal exudate cell populations, especially in terms of macrophage content in some species of animals. Mice, for example, are known to be poor producers of macrophage-rich peritoneal exudates, and rats are little better. In addition to their lower content of macrophages, the number of cells obtainable from a single animal is low, thus making it an absolute requisite to combine peritoneal cells from many animals (sometimes more than 10) in order to perform well-controlled migration inhibition assays. It is entirely possible that various peritoneal cell populations from different individual animals (even in inbred animals) may interreact with each other, resulting in a not readily controllable variation in experimental conditions.

One of the early studies on migration inhibition in a tumor-antigen system may be instructive in this regard. Thus, Steiner and Watne (35) have obtained peritoneal exudate cells in Wistar rats bearing Walker 256 tumor and DBA/1J mice bearing sarcomas, 24 hours after the intravenous injection of gelatin. In vitro migration of these peritoneal cells was inhibited in a quite inconsistent manner and was sometimes enhanced instead by the presence of tumor-specific soluble antigen. This may be attributed equally as well to the various technical problems discussed above as to the fluctuating and spontaneous appearance of putative "blocking factors" for MIF or of specific enhancing substances.

In addition to these studies in experimental animals, a few reports (36,37) have shown the feasibility of macrophage migration inhibition assay studies in human tumor immunity. In one such study Hillberg et al. (36) have demonstrated that MIF could be produced by peripheral blood lymphocytes from cancer patients when stimulated with tumor extract. The assay system was a modification of the procedure employed in detecting delayed hypersensitivity to soluble antigens such as purified protein derivative (PPD), streptokinase-streptodornase (SKSD), or *Candida albicans* antigen, utilizing guinea pig peritoneal macrophages as indicator cells (38–40).

In the years following the above-mentioned study only a few papers describing the use of the MIF assay for detection of cell-mediated immunity to tumor-associated antigens were published (41–46). Unfortunately, most of these studies did no more than demonstrate the usefulness of the assay for detection of immunity, in confirmation of previous reports; they failed to show any real advantage or value of the MIF assay over other in vitro assays for evaluating tumor immunity. Thus, a number of important questions remain to be answered in this area. First, as already indicated, the migration inhibition assay was shown to be very useful and sensitive in detecting specific tumor antigens when various antigenic fractions were tested using cells from guinea pigs immunized with such soluble antigens in complete Freund's adjuvant (26,27). While this gives us a strong tool to fractionate or purify the antigenic substances in this system, it is not yet clear whether sensitivity to such various antigens detectable by the MIF assay correlates in any clinically or pathogenically meaningful way with tumor growth in the animals. As a related question, does the assay have any diagnostic or prognostic value in tumor growth or rejection? Although some studies on "blocking factors" have indicated the prognostic value of the assay at least in some experimental tumors (30,31), more systematic studies have to be done in human disease as well as animal models. Most of the assays reported in the early literature were "direct" migration inhibition tests without examining for production and release of MIF. It should be noted that direct assay may be misleading or technically difficult, since the antigens one deals with are often cells themselves or crude, relatively insoluble fractions and since the mobility of macrophages is easily affected nonspecifically by such particulate matter. Finally, there seems to be no valid reason for limiting attention to MIF, whose preeminence among the lymphokines is mainly based on historical grounds, and for which there is no evidence for special biologic importance in these various models of tumor immunity.

Leukocyte Migration Inhibition Factor (LIF)

The most convenient source of indicator cells in man for lymphokine assays is peripheral blood leukocytes. These are rich in neutrophils rather than macrophages. Bendixen and Soborg (46) first described a migration inhibition assay which involved packing of capillary tubes with peripheral blood leukocytes rather than peritoneal exudate cells. Soborg (47,48), and Bendixen and Soborg (46) demonstrated that Brucella antigen could inhibit the migration of leukocytes obtained from patients with delayed skin reactivity to this antigen. Initially, this phenomenon was difficult to interpret in terms of its correlation with delayed hypersensitivity because most investigators encountered difficulty in obtaining reproducible results with PPD. Furthermore, in patients with immediate-type hypersensitivity, such as hay fever, one could also obtain inhibition of leukocyte migration (49). Recently, however, Rocklin et al. (50) have reported comparative studies of leukocyte migration inhibition which provide convincing evidence for lymphokine participation. These authors could show that supernatants obtained from human lymphocyte cultures stimulated by PPD contained mediators which inhibited neutrophils as well as macrophages. More importantly, they could find the substances responsible to be physicochemically distinguishable. The factor responsible for the inhibition of leukocyte migration was defined as a new "lymphokine," leukocyte inhibition factor (LIF).

In any event, even prior to the definition of this lymphokine, many studies on clinical applications of the assay have been reported by Soborg and Bendixen co-workers (53–60) and by other groups of investigators (49,61–64). A number of reports deal with applications to cancer patients (65–78). The number of papers in this field is increasing exponentially.

Andersen et al. (66) have reported that extracts of mammary tumor tissue (100

μg/ml) inhibited autologous leukocyte migration in vitro in 8 out of 22 patients with mammary carcinoma studies. The autologous or heterologous extracts did not inhibit leukocytes from control patients. Wolberg (76) has reported that, in 19 of 21 patients with various tumors, extracts of those tumors induced inhibition of leukocyte migration. Interestingly, he could also observe the migration inhibition of lymphocytes utilizing lymphocyte-rich cell suspensions separated from whole leukocytes to the same extent as total leukocyte migration inhibition. Cochran et al. (77) have studied this assay in patients with cystic melanoma. In 11 out of 22 patients the migration of leukocytes was inhibited by cystic fluid obtained from the lesion. However, inhibition was also observed in 2 of 16 normal subjects or patients with nonmalignant diseases. Furthermore, they found a higher incidence of positive findings (10/16) in patients with no recurrence; in patients with metastatic tumor, only 1 out of 6 showed the inhibition. Specificity with respect to tumor antigen was observed in many similar studies. In one such study Segall et al. (70) have reported that in 58% of 57 patients examined the migration of leukocytes was inhibited by autologous extracts. In most of these patients, extracts from different types of tumors or tumors of the same type obtained from different individuals could not inhibit leukocyte migration, showing very low cross-reactivity among individual tumors. However, high cross-reactivity of antigenicity was found in patients with melanoma.

Instead of using the capillary tube migration system, Claussen (79) has described a technique involving leukocyte migration in agarose. This assay also has been shown to correlate well with delayed cutaneous hypersensitivity to a variety of skin test antigens (80). The usefulness of the assay in the investigation of human tumor antigens has been demonstrated in studies involving melanoma and lung cancer patients (81,82). In one of these studies Boddie et al. (81) have shown that KCl extracts of allogeneic lung cancer could inhibit leukocyte migration in 17 out of 22 lung cancer patients (77%), suggesting that common lung cancer antigens do exist. They have negated the possibility that they were merely detecting HLA antigens in this system, since the migration was inhibited by extracts of allogeneic lung tumors but not by that of allogeneic normal lung tissue.

The evaluation of the leukocyte migration inhibition assay in studies on tumor immunity depends upon answers to a number of questions. It seems to be of the utmost importance to develop a system for detecting LIF in supernatants from peripheral lymphocytes cultured with extracts of tumors, rather than relying on direct inhibition of migration of neutrophil-rich suspensions cultured with those preparations. No matter what currently available procedures are used for antigen solubilization or isolation, the extracts are relatively crude antigen preparations which may contain HLA antigen as well as tumor antigens, and they may be potentially contaminated with toxic products of cell lysis, bacterial antigens, organ-specific antigens, and so forth. For instance, Wolberg (83) suggested that nonspecific toxicity to tumor extracts might play a role in inhibition of leukocyte migration, even though most of the previous studies had included a control culture in which the extracts failed to inhibit various control leukocytes, including normal subjects and patients with nonmalignant diseases. If one uses the supernatants from lymphocyte cultures activated by tumor extracts for LIF assay, such problems will be reduced considerably if not completely. One may argue against this proposal simply because such an indirect assay system is more complicated and laborious. Such experimentation is essential, however, in order to establish that this assay is truly reflecting a cell-mediated hypersensitivity reaction to tumor antigens. In this context, comparative studies on MIF and LIF in the same patients with cancer may well be meaningful, since at the present time the MIF assay is better established as a correlate of delayed hypersensitivity. One of the few studies on this point was recently reported by Jones and Turnbull (46). They have shown that both macrophage migration and (peripheral blood) leukocyte migration in mammary carcinoma patients were inhibited by tumor antigens. Although the leukocyte migration test appeared to be more sensitive and simpler than the macrophage migration test in their study, they have suggested that further studies of this kind in different tumor systems would provide us with clinically important information.

On the basis of presently available data it is still difficult to judge the clinical value of the LIF assay in cancer patients, because only very limited numbers of patients have been serially examined by this assay. Some of those studies (66,77,81) appeared to indicate that the result of the LIF assay would have prognostic value, since a shift from inhibition to noninhibition or rather enhancement was noted with progressive or recurrent disease. These results, however, are far from conclusive. Leukocyte inhibition assay has been almost exclusively studied in human subjects. Strict evaluation of the assay would seem to require animal experimentation using the peripheral leukocyte migration phenomenon in experimental animals with various tumors.

Miscellaneous Lymphokine Assays in Cancer

As has been discussed, direct or indirect assays for MIF and LIF represent the bulk of the work involving assessment of lymphokine activity in experiment and clinical neoplastic disease. There have been no comparable studies involving detection of cytotoxic mediators, chemotactic factors, mitogenic factors, or lymphokine inhibitors of DNA or protein synthesis. This is unfortunate, reflecting not only major lack of knowledge about the potential role of such factors but also a failure to clinically exploit a number of well worked-out and reproducible assays.

Two in vitro assay systems which may involve new lymphokines similar to MIF have been recently introduced. Although their biological significance has yet to be determined, we will briefly discuss them here. One is leukocyte adherence inhibition, described by Halliday et al. (84–87). The test is based on the observation that when blood leukocytes from tumor-bearing mice or patients with cancer are mixed with the corresponding specific tumor antigen, the tendency of the leukocytes to adhere to glass is inhibited. Serum from such patients or animals interferes with or "blocks" this inhibition. Patients with malignant melanoma and primary hepatoma have shown leukocyte adherence inhibition with tumors of the same histologic type. No normal tissues have given positive reactivity. The presence of blocking serum factor was correlated well with the presence of tumor, as was also shown in experimental macrophage migration inhibition tests to tumor-associated antigens. In one of these studies (84) a positive result in this assay preceded the clinical appearance of tumor by up to three years in two patients, suggesting the assay's diagnostic value.

Halliday et al. (86) have suggested that the leukocyte adherence inhibition may be due to a lymphokine produced by immune lymphocytes reacting with tumor-associated antigens. Although total leukocyte populations were utilized in the assay system, it was also suggested that the majority of indicator cells which adhere to the glass were macrophages. More recently Malnish and Halliday (88) have described the production of a lymphokine by peripheral blood leukocytes stimulated with tumor antigen in mice which had the required properties. This lymphokine could inhibit leukocyte adherence and had properties similar to those of MIF. However, the production of maximal titers within 60 minutes is not consistent with the known kinetics of MIF production, which continues to be released into the culture medium for several days. The leukocyte adherence inhibitory factor is thus suggested to be a preformed, stored factor, liberated shortly after antigenic stimulation and not renewed for at least several hours. Holan et al. (89), on the other hand, could not produce any soluble factor or mediator with leukocyte adherence inhibitory activity by incubating sensitized cells with antigen. Thus, these studies remain inconclusive. Furthermore, the effect of humoral antibody or antigen-antibody complexes must be examined to confirm that this assay is actually measuring cell-mediated immunity to tumor antigens.

Another technique recently reported is an application of the method originally described by Turk and Diengdoh (90) as an in vitro model of delayed hypersensitivity. This method was developed on the basis that the interaction of immune lymphocytes with specific antigen might result in the release of a substance which would change the surface charge of macrophages. Turk and Diengdoh found the slowing of macrophage electrophoretic mobility when normal indicator macrophages and immune lymphocytes were placed into electrophoretic apparatus together with specific antigen. The phenomenon was confirmed by Caspary (91) in studies involving delayed hypersensitivity to tuberculin antigen. Since then, Caspary and Field have applied this technique to various clinical studies, especially for various neurological diseases including multiple sclerosis, using myelin basic protein [of encephalitogenic factor (EF)] as an antigen (92). Field et al. (93) also demonstrated that in patients with Graves' disease, macrophage electrophoretic mobility was slowed by the presence of the patient's lymphocytes and either thyroglobulin or long-acting thyroid stimulator antigen. In applying this technique to tumor immunity in man, these authors have obtained results (94) that seem quite different from those observed with the MIF or LIF assays described previously.

Thus, most patients with various neoplasms have reacted to an antigen, myelin basic protein (or EF), which is not only found in normal nervous tissues but common in a wide variety of tumors. More specifically, the electrophoretic mobility of guinea pig macrophages is diminished when EF is added to a mixture of normal guinea pig peritoneal exudate cells and peripheral lymphocytes of cancer patients. According to Caspary (95), this phenomenon could be observed when cell-free supernatants from lymphocytes cultured with EF were added to the macrophage electrophoresis system. A responsible soluble factor was named macrophage slowing factor (MSF). MSF was suggested to be the same factor as MIF, but no direct evidence has yet been reported.

Some comparisons are available, since cell-mediated immunity to myelin basic protein has been studied by macrophage migration inhibition test in man and in animal model systems (96). Sensitization to EF was demonstrated in 71% of patients with various forms of neoplastic disease. More importantly, 31% of patients with nonneoplastic diseases such as warts, chronic bronchitis, and hernia had shown a positive reaction to EF. Other studies with macrophage electrophoretic mobility testing have shown sensitization to EF in patients with multiple sclerosis, Crohn's disease, ulcerative colitis, asthma, and sarcoidosis (97). It is, therefore, clear that sensitization to EF is not confined to patients with neoplastic diseases but is part of a more general immune reaction. This is not surprising, since, as stated previously, this test antigen is present in nonneoplastic tissue. If, as claimed by Shelton et al. (96), the macrophage electrophoretic mobility test gives inconsistent findings and is complex and difficult to standardize, this assay does not seem to have any advantage over the traditional MIF assay. Nevertheless, further studies with a variety of animal models would seem justified. As before, careful comparative evaluation with respect to known mediator activity, such as MIF activity, would seem essential.

Other lymphokine assays involving cell surface alterations such as changes in glucosamine content (98) or changes in surface tension (99) have not yet been exploited in studies of tumor immunity.

RECOVERY OF LYMPHOKINES FROM TUMOR-BEARING HOSTS

If cell-mediated immune reactions against tumor-associated antigens occur in tumor-bearing animals (or man), lymphokines should be released in vivo. It should therefore be possible to recover such factors from appropriate tissues or tissue fluids. This has proven possible in a variety of experimental and clinical situations not involving tumor immunity. In particular, MIF or substances with MIF-like activity have been found in joint fluid of patients with rheumatoid arthritis (100), peritoneal exudates of immunized guinea pigs (19), draining lymph of immunized sheep (101), and sera of immunized and challenged mice (102) and guinea pigs (18,103). Furthermore, chemotactic factors for macrophages and skin reactive factor were found in peritoneal exudate fluid (19) and in delayed skin reaction sites of immunized guinea pigs (17).

Similar detection of lymphokines or lymphokine-like substances in tumor-bearing animals or man, however, has been a subject of very few papers. In one of these studies Cohen et al. (104) have reported that macrophage migration inhibitory activity can be detected in the sera of the majority of patients with lymphoproliferative diseases but in less than 3% of controls. This activity was found in 14 of 16 patients with non-Hodgkin's lymphoma, 10 of 13 with Hodgkin's disease, and four of five with chronic lymphocytic leukemia. The preliminary physicochemical characterization of this material shows properties similar to those of conventional MIF obtained from antigen-stimulated lymphocyte cultures. The presence of such substances in the sera of these patients did not seem to be related to any of the clinical or laboratory data, with the possible exception of duration of disease. The authors pointed out that in addition to immunologic activation, possible stimuli for the production of migration inhibition factors in these patients may include (a) virus infection, (b) the presence of nonspecific mitogenic factors, and (c) the proliferative response of the neoplastic cells itself. The first possibility is conceivable, because MIF has been shown to be produced by viral infection of various cells in vitro (105–107). Although these human lymphoproliferative diseases have never directly been attributed to viral infection, some types of animal leukemias have been so implicated. The second possibility is suggested by the many studies reporting that nonspecific mitogenic stimulation of lymphocytes leads to the production of MIF, though, again, such mitogenic activity has never been reported in these diseases. The last possibility may hold true, since human lymphoid cell lines have been shown to be a good producer of MIF or MIF-like substances in vitro, without the requirement for further in vitro stimulation (108–110). The observations by Yoshida et al. (111) on patients with Sezary syndrome are consistent with this possibility. They not only showed MIF activity in sera of most patients with Sezary syndrome but also found that peripheral lymphocytes obtained from these patients could spontaneously generate and release MIF-like substances into the culture medium when incubated for more than 24 hours in vitro without any stimulating agents. In this study the investigators also found skin reactive factor in the supernatants, thereby demonstrating yet another lymphokine activity.

At the time of this writing no other report has appeared concerning the detection of any of the known lymphokine activities in serum or tissues of humans or animals with spontaneous or experimental neoplasms. To further our understanding of tumor immunity, it would appear important to do a systematic survey of lymphokines in tumor-bearing hosts. In this context one must bear in mind the possibility that the concomitant presence of regulating factors could make analysis difficult. One example of such a regulator is a chemotactic factor inhibitor (CFI) described by Ward et al. (112–114), which can be extracted from tumor tissues, and which is also present in various normal tissues as well as serum. This substance can inhibit not only chemotactic activity but also MIF (115). It may represent a "protective" mechanism for the tumor cells themselves and serve to counter the attack by host defense mechanisms, which require the local accumulation and retention of inflammatory cells. The substance itself appears to be an enzyme and is not related to any of the known lymphokines. Such abnormal substances, or normal substances in excess quantity generated by tumor cells, may intervene in immunologic reactions and modify both the accumulation of inflammatory cells and the effect of various mediators. In another set of studies Sylven (116) could find large amounts of a cathepsin B-like substance in interstitial fluid of various solid tumors. Such proteolytic enzymes and inhibitory factors would be expected to have definite effects not only on various in vivo cell-mediated reactions in situ, but also on nonimmunologic inflammatory reactions.

Some recent observations point to an in vivo role for CFI. Thus, following intraperitoneal administration, the P815 mastocytoma can grow in ascitic form in DBA/2 mice and kill the host within 1 to 2 weeks. In other strains, such as C57BL/6, the tumor is rejected and the animal survives. The intraperitoneal inflammatory infiltrate associated with this process consists mainly of neutrophils. In the DBA/2 mouse, which cannot reject the tumor, there is only a transient neutrophil response, which rapidly disappears. Cohen et al. (117) have shown that this disappearance correlates precisely with the appearance of detectable CFI in the peritoneal fluid. It is not yet known whether the mechanism for neutrophil accumulation in this model involves a lymphokine. However, the histocompatibility requirements between tumor and host which determine survival or death strongly suggest that the mechanisms involved are immunologic in nature. In any case, these considerations indicate the importance of further research concerning both lymphokine activity and the regulation of lymphokine activity in vivo.

IN VITRO EFFECTS OF LYMPHOKINES ON TUMOR CELLS

Direct Effects of Lymphokines

In addition to the several in vitro assays mentioned in previous sections, assays of cytotoxicity of growth inhibition have been the most extensively used methods for st'idy of cell-mediated immunity to tumors. Different from other assays, these cytotoxicity assays measure directly the effects of interactions between immune lymphocytes and tumor antigens on the target tumor cells. A large number of experimental studies have proved these assays useful for the detection of cell-mediated immunity in a wide variety of animal and human tumor systems, and these have been the subject of many previous reviews (1–6), including various chapters in this book. The specific question to be discussed here is whether or not any lymphokines, especially cytotoxic lymphokines, play a role in the so-called lymphocyte-mediated cytotoxicity (or tumor cell killing).

Evidence to support a role of lymphotoxins in lymphocyte-mediated cell killing in tumor immunity has been provided by Granger and associates (118–121), and this topic has been critically reviewed in the previous chapter. It has been shown that lymphotoxins produced by lymphocytes stimulated with specific antigen or with nonspecific mitogens could kill or at least damage various cell lines in culture. Like other lymphokines, lymphotoxins, though induced by specific immunologic or mitogenic stimuli, are themselves capable of acting in a nonspecific manner. Although lymphotoxins are thus usually cytotoxic to a variety of both normal and malignant cultured cells, a few reports show that tumor cells are more susceptible to lymphotoxins than normal cells. Thus, Meltzer and Bartlett (122) have shown that supernatants obtained from PPD-stimulated spleen cells of BCG-immunized mice could destroy tumor cell monolayers but not normal cell monolayers. Weedon et al. (123) have shown that lymphotoxins obtained by PHA stimulation of human lymphocytes could be cytotoxic to various tumor cells as well as their normal counterpart, although, for example, glioma was more susceptible than normal nervous tissue. Although studies by other investigators (124–126) in addition to those mentioned above confirm the nonspecific tumor cell destruction by lymphotoxins which are produced by reacting lymphocytes with a variety of antigens (or mitogens), there are almost no data available on the production of lymphotoxins by immune lymphocytes stimulated with tumor-associated antigen.

Most studies on lymphocyte-mediated cytotoxicity for tumor cells seem to have excluded the possibility of involving any nonspecific factors (such as lymphotoxins) in the mechanism of cytotoxicity. Thus, the majority of results suggest that cytotoxic effects of lymphocytes are highly specific, and adjacent nonspecific target cells remain intact (4,5,127,128). Furthermore, close contact or even fusion between attacking and target cells is necessary for the effect. However, some studies did demonstrate that innocent bystander cells were also affected by a specific interaction between immune lymphocytes and target cells (129,130). On the basis of these observations Holm et al. (131) have suggested the following interpretation: specialized membrane contacts between activated lymphocytes and target cells are either necessary for target cell lysis or needed to facilitate lysis. In the contact area nonspecific toxic products may accumulate and induce cell damage.

In any event, it has been almost impossible to recover cell-free lymphotoxins after the specific reactions between immune lymphocytes and target cells. Therefore, one has to assume that lymphotoxins, if generated by such interactions, must be in smaller quantity than that usually generated by antigen- or mitogen-stimulated lymphocytes, or that the production and consumption of lymphotoxin must occur at the limited area adjacent to the area of contact. Recent experiments have demonstrated that target cell cytolysis by immune lymphocytes requires continued protein synthesis and an active secretory system (132,133). Furthermore, Walker and Lucas (134) have recently demonstrated that rabbit antiserum prepared against human lymphotoxin inhibits target cell destruction by PHA-activated nonimmune and PPD-activated immune lymphocytes and by lymphocytes sensitized in vivo to renal transplants and tumor tissue. These indirect data seem to indicate the role of soluble toxic materials in the so-called direct cell-mediated cytotoxicity. However, in view of the data presented here and in the previous chapter, it remains for future experimentation to determine directly and unequivocally whether lymphocyte-mediated tumor cell killing does or does not involve a nonspecific cytotoxic substance (e.g., lymphotoxin).

As another possible direct effect of lymphokines in addition to cytotoxic killing of tumor cells, one can consider the effects of lymphokines on the mobility of tumor cells. It has been thought for many years that the mobility of individual tumor cells may be important in local tumor spread and in the establishment of metastasis (135–138). More recently, a relationship between the loss of contact inhibition, as a specific characteristic of malignant cells, and the motility of in vitro tumor cells has been suggested (138,139). It has, however, proved difficult to examine the mobility of tumor cells in in vitro systems. Recently, murine lymphoma cells, mastocytoma cells, and various human tumor cells have been shown capable of migration from a capillary tube (140–142). This is a simple system which allows a quantitative approach to the examination of the motility of tumor cells en masse. The technique is similar to that used in studies on macrophage migration in vitro as a model for in vivo delayed hypersensitivity.

Most murine and human tumor cells obtained from in vivo tumors or from tissue culture cells so far studied have been shown to migrate well in this system, although some of the cells from solid and ascitic tumors have been reported not to be motile (140). The migration of these tumor cells out of capillary tubes is known to be inhibited by various biological and chemical substances, such as concanavalin A or sera from tumor-bearing mice or man (143–145). In addition to these agents, we have recently shown that lymphokines can be inhibitory to the migration of tumor cells. Thus, Cohen et al. have demonstrated that the migration of P815 mastocytoma cells out of capillary tubes was inhibited by the MIF-rich supernatants of antigen-stimulated human lymphocytes and of SV 40-infected monkey kidney cells (142). Antigen-stimulated guinea pig lymphocyte supernatant was not effective. This fact may suggest limited species specificity of the responsible factor, as in the case of the MIF effect on macrophages. Recent studies in our laboratory have revealed that supernatants from human lymphoid cell lines could also inhibit the migration of mastocytoma cells. Another important finding in this initial study was that the inhibition of tumor cell migration was not associated with cytotoxicity, suggesting that this migration system is not measuring simple killing of the cells.

These studies are still preliminary, and many additional experiments are suggested by the data already obtained: (1) Can immune lymphocytes from tumor-bearing animals produce such tumor migration inhibitory factors? (2) What is the range of tumor cell types sensitive to its effect? (3) Is this factor different from MIF? (4) Can this material in any way effect contact inhibition or its loss? (5) Can one recover this factor from tumor-bearing animals in any stage? (6) Does this factor change the metastatic capacity of tumors when administered exogeneously?

In this context, recent studies on tumor cell chemotaxis could also be of potential importance. These studies are reviewed in Chapter 12. In brief, a component derived from complement has been found to be chemotactic for various tumor cells. It would be of great interest if lymphokines from antigen-stimulated lymphocyte could produce such effects as well.

Indirect Effects of Lymphokines

There is much evidence that animals injected with microorganisms show an increased nonspecific resistance to certain other microorganisms or tumors and that this effect is mediated by "activated" macrophages (146–155). These macrophages have been reported to kill cells with malignant growth potential. For instance, it was shown that fibroblasts were killed by activated macrophages only after their spontaneous or induced transformation in vitro (156,157). At present it is clear that there are at least two mechanisms by which normal macrophages can be rendered cytotoxic for tumor cells: "arming" and "activation." These have been defined in Chapter 3.

Cytotoxicity by macrophages armed with a product of activated lymphocytes called "specific macrophage arming factor (SMAF)" was described by Evans and Alexander (158). SMAF is a product of thymus-dependent lymphocytes stimulated by antigen (159,160). The SMAF produced by stimulating specifically immune lymphocytes with one tumor specifically arms macrophages to kill that tumor but not others. The arming factor is cytophilic and can be absorbed by the macrophages. It can also be absorbed by the specific tumor used to produce it. It may be a cytotoxic receptor shed into the culture medium by activated lymphocytes (160) or a cytophilic antibody (161). Although there is no direct evidence, it is very tempting to consider that SMAF is another version of the antigen-specific MIF reported by Amos et al. (162). In any event, SMAF is yet another lymphokine.

Churchill et al. have shown that supernatants from cultures of lymphocytes stimulated by an antigen (ortho-chlorobenzoyl-bovine gamma globulin, OCB-BGG) activate normal macrophages, either as monolayers (163) or in suspension culture (164). The responsible lymphokine was called macrophage activating factor (MAF). These "activated" macrophages exhibit enhanced cytotoxic capacity against syngeneic strain 2 hepatoma and MCA-25 sarcoma cells. As compared to SMAF, MAF may thus be induced by unrelated antigens, and it enhances the cytotoxicity of macrophages in the absence of the specific eliciting antigen. The enhancing factor which was generated by the antigen (OCB-BGG) was removed from the lymphocyte supernatants by Churchill using gel filtration on Sephadex G100 columns. This procedure did not cause loss of activity. The factor is not cytophilic and, further, activated macrophages can be trypsinized without losing cytotoxic capacity.

Little is known of the mechanism underlying the interaction of the lymphocyte mediator with the surface of the macrophage which results in enhanced cytotoxicity by the activated cells. However, a number of morphologic, biochemical, and functional alterations have been described when macrophages are activated by MAF. These include (1) increased adherence to glass and plastic (165,166), (2) increased ruffled membrane movement (165), (3) increased phagocytotic activity (165), (4) increased glucose oxidation (165), (5) decrease in lysosomal enzyme, acid phosphatase, cathepsin D, and B-glucuronidase (167), (6) increase in membrane enzyme adenylate cyclase (168), (7) increase in incorporation of glucosamine (98), (8) enhanced bacteriostasis to Listeria (169,170). It is interesting that present physicochemical characterization studies cannot distinguish MAF from MIF, although there still remains the possibility that several different factors affecting macrophages exist. As stated above, MAF described by Churchill et al. was produced by an antigen unrelated to tumor antigens. It may be interesting to see if one could produce MAF by tumor-antigen-stimulated lymphocytes.

In summary, it has been shown that a lymphokine, MAF, generated by antigen-stimulated lymphocytes can activate macrophages for nonspecific cytotoxicity against tumor cells, while SMAF, another lymphokine, can arm macrophages to be specifically cytotoxic to tumor cells. In other words, both factors require for their generation interaction of specifically sensitized lymphocytes with antigen. However, once formed, MAF can exert nonspecific effects, whereas SMAF is effective only against a target cell containing the antigen used to induce it.

LYMPHOKINES AS THERAPEUTIC AGENTS

As discussed above, lymphokines may have direct cytotoxic or migration inhibitory effects on tumor cells and may have an indirect effect via the inflammatory cells. The cell type which has received the most attention to date in this regard is the macrophage. Immunotherapeutic approaches which involve local contact sensitization or local injection of BCG at a cutaneous tumor site may well involve one or more of these lymphokine-dependent mechanisms. If so, one could in theory use lymphokine preparations as therapeutic agents. A number of recent studies suggest that this may be possible. Thus, Bernstein et al. have demonstrated that the growth of tumor was suppressed when MIF-containing lymphocyte supernatants were injected at the site of syngeneic tumor grafts (171). In their experiments, MIF was produced by the incubation of Mycobacterium tuberculosis-immunized guinea pig (strain L) lymph node cells with PPD. Such culture supernatants were partially purified by Sephadex G75 gel filtration, followed by polyacrylamide gel electrophoresis. The purified MIF fraction was dissolved in a volume of medium equal to the original supernatant fluid. This material was mixed with diethylnitrosamine-induced hepatoma cells to the concentration of 10^7 cells/ml. One-tenth milliliter of the mixture was injected intradermally. Control mixtures were made similarly from lymphocyte cultures without antigen or with unrelated (coccidioidin) antigen. It was observed that tumor growth was inhibited in the injection sites of the mixture of MIF fraction and tumor cells, but not at the sites injected with control fraction and tumor cells. The effect was limited to the actual intradermal injection sites; a tumor adjacent to a rejected tumor remained unaffected. In further studies (171) tumor cells were inoculated into skin sites where MIF or control supernatants had been injected 24 hours earlier. Tumor cell growth was inhibited at sites where an inflammatory reaction induced by MIF-containing supernatants was present. This observation favors the view that tumor rejection was due to host cells, rather than to a direct cytotoxic effect by MIF.

Mann et al. (172) have reported that an MIF-containing fraction derived from the sensitized lymphocytes of guinea pigs can delay the appearance of palpable subcutaneous tumors when injected at the time of implantation of L1210 tumor subcutaneously in BDF1 mice. In addition, a prolonged mean survival time from 9.42 days in control animals to 13.19 days in the MIF-treated group was found.

Recently, Salvin et al. (173) have reported that the injection of lymphokine-containing fluids into mice resulted in suppression of tumor growth. These fluids were obtained from serum rather than lymphocyte culture supernatants. Salvin et al. (102) had previously shown that lymphokines such as migration inhibitory factor and type-II interferon were released into the circulation of tuberculin-sensitive mice after intravenous injection of old tuberculin. Daily administration of such sera into the tumor sites of mice given implants of sarcoma MC-36 was effective in suppressing tumor growth. It was suggested that the activity was due to a lymphokine. However, these investigators used unfractionated whole serum for the treatments, and it is difficult to conclude which of the many substances contained in such serum had antitumor effects. Gresser et al. (174) reported that 1–2 months repeated injections of mouse brain interferon increased the survival times of several strains of mice after intraperitoneal challenge with Ehrlich ascites tumor. A further possibility is the presence of nonspecific toxic factors, which are known to occur in mouse serum. It is possible that the process of immunization or some other effect resulting from the presence of bacterial products in the experimental animals could have augmented the appearance of such toxic factors. Further studies characterizing this phenomenon in relation to the results using culture supernatants reported by others (171,172), and in relation to the various in vitro effects of lymphokines on tumor cells described above, should provide information as to whether the effect observed by Salvin et al. is due to a lymphokine.

Data for a therapeutic role of lymphokines in man are even less clear. In human subjects, Papermaster et al. (175) have utilized supernatants from human lymphoid cell lines which are known to contain various lymphokine activities. They have injected such supernatants into sites of mammary carcinoma, reticulum cell sarcoma, multiple squamous cell carcinomas (175). Clinical regressions were induced in 16 out of a total of 18 lesions injected with supernatants ultrafiltered and concentrated by lyophilization. Of 12 lesions treated with the lower molecular weight fractions, which do not contain lymphokine activities (used in those experiments as controls), none showed regression clinically or microscopically. Results by other investigators have shown regression of cutaneous neoplasms or mammary tumors when injected by lymphokine-containing materials induced by Con A or PPD stimulated lymphocytes (176,177). These human experiments are still very preliminary and must be cautiously interpreted, since, owing to ethical considerations, appropriately controlled double-blind studies with strict attention to all variables are difficult to perform. For example, the effects of associated or adjunctive treatment such as chemotherapy cannot be dissected out in these studies. Nevertheless, the results obtained thus far suggest that lymphokines may exert significant in vivo effects on tumors in man. A great deal of work with fractionated and purified lymphokine preparations in animal models is clearly necessary before widespread applicability to man can be considered.

For completeness, the role of transfer factor should be mentioned. Transfer factor may be considered to be an agent capable of conferring immunocompetence upon recipients with respect to those antigens to which the donor had been sensitized. This competence seems to be confined to an initiation and/or augmentation of cell-mediated immunity. Transfer factor thus seems to play a role in the affector loop of the immune response; it is not itself an effector molecule in the same sense that the lymphokines are. Other details relating to the generation and release of transfer factor, its biochemistry, and biologic behavior, all of which are beyond the scope of this book, serve to exclude transfer factor from the set of mediators collectively defined as lymphokines. This is important to an understanding of the possible therapeutic effects of transfer factor therapy. The mechanism of such effect, if any, relates to an induction of the capacity for an immune response or an augmented immune response in the tumor-bearing host. Presumably, once that initial event occurs, tumor destruction is via the usual effector immunologic mechanisms available to the organism, including those described in this chapter. Specific approaches to immunotherapy and an analysis of results to date may be found in Chapter 9.

SUMMARY

Many of the manifestations of cell-mediated immunity appear to depend on the activity of soluble lymphocyte-derived mediators called lymphokines. The ability of lymphocytes from experimental animals, either bearing tumors or immunized with tumor antigens, to produce certain lymphokines, most notably MIF and LIF, has been repeatedly confirmed. Similar data are available in human disease. These findings have provided suggestive evidence for a role of lymphokines in tumor immunity and also provided the rationale for clinical tests of competence for cell-mediated immunity in neoplastic disease. These findings are complemented by studies demonstrating the presence of lymphokines in vivo, an example of which is the detection of MIF in the serum of patients with various lymphoproliferative disorders.

The specific mechanisms whereby lymphokines might exert protective effects are still unclear. However, at least two kinds of direct effects of lymphokines on tumor cells are known. Certain lymphokines (lymphotoxins) can directly kill tumor cells. Related lymphokine activities involving the inhibition of growth or proliferation of target cells may be due to similar factors and, indeed, may represent the effects of limiting dilutions of lymphotoxin itself. Also, it has recently been shown that a lymphokine (possibly related to MIF) can inhibit the migration of at least one kind of tumor cell (P815 mastocytoma) without killing it. In addition to these direct effects, lymphokines can destroy tumors by initiating, focusing, and amplifying inflammatory responses. The most direct evidence here comes from studies on the activation and arming of macrophages by soluble lymphocyte products. The results of a number of in vivo experiments can be best explained in terms of these lymphokine activities, as has been discussed.

These considerations suggest the possibility that lymphokines might find a role as therapeutic agents. Several animal experiments are available to support this contention, and a small number of clinical trials have already begun. Efforts in this direction, however, are hampered by a lack of information as to the relative importance of any of the known lymphokines on protection against tumors and by a lack of appropriately isolated, characterized, and purified preparations for study. Thus, further definition of the role of lymphokines in tumor immunity, and their therapeutic manipulation, await further advances in the "state of the art" of lymphokine biology and biochemistry.

REFERENCES

1. Herberman, R. B., *Int. J. Med.* **9**, 300 (1973).
2. Herberman, R. B., in *Pathobiology Annual* (H. L. Ioachim, ed.), Vol. 3, Appleton, New York, 1973, p. 291.
3. Hellstrom, K. E., and Hellstrom, I., *Adv. Immunol.* **18**, 209 (1974).
4. Cerottini, J. C., and Brunner, K. T., *Adv. Immunol.* **18**, 67 (1974).
5. Green, I., and Shevach, E. M., in *Mechanisms of Cell-mediated Immunity (R. T. McCluskey and S. Cohen, eds.) John Wiley & Sons, New York, 1974, p. 221.*
6. Herberman, R. B., *Adv. Cancer Res.* **19**, 207 (1974).
7. Bloom, B. R., *Adv. Immunol.* **13**, 102 (1971).
8. David, J. R., and David, R. A., *Progr. Allergy* **16**, 300 (1972).
9. Yoshida, T., and Cohen, S., in *Mechanisms of Cell-Mediated Immunity* (R. T. McCluskey and S. Cohen, eds.), John Wiley & Sons, New York, 1974, p. 43.
10. Yoshida, T., and Cohen, S., in *The Immune System and Infectious Diseases,* Fourth International Convoc. Immunology (E. Neter and F. Milgrom, eds.), S. Karger, Basel, 1975, p. 512.
11. Cohen, S., Ward, P. A., and Bigazzi, P. E., in *Mechanisms of Cell-Mediated Immunity* (R. T. McCluskey and S. Cohen, eds.), John Wiley & Sons, New York, 1974, p. 331.
12. McCluskey, R. T., and Leber, P. D., in *Mechanisms of Cellular Immunity* (R. T. McCluskey and S. Cohen, eds.), John Wiley & Sons, New York, 1974, p. 1.
13. David, J. R., Al-Askari, S., Lawrence, H. S., and Thomas, L. *J. Immunol.* **93**, 264 (1964).
14. David, J. R., Lawrence, H. S., and Thomas, L. *J. Immunol.* **93**, 274 (1964).
15. Bloom, B. R., and Bennett, B. *Science* **153**, 80 (1966).
16. David, J. R., *Proc. Natl. Acad. Sci. U.S.A.* **56**, 72 (1966).
17. Cohen, S., Ward, P. A., Yoshida, T., and Burek, C. L., *Cell. Immunol.* **9**, 363 (1973).

18. Yoshida, T., and Cohen, S. *J. Immunol.* **112,** 1540 (1974).

19. Sonozaki, H., Papermaster, V., Yoshida, T., and Cohen, S. *J. Immunol.* **115,** 1657 (1975).

20. Bennett, B., and Bloom, B. R., *Proc. Natl. Acad. Sci. U.S.A.* **59,** 756 (1968).

21. Pick, E., Krejci, J., Cech, K., and Turk, J. L., *Immunol.* **17,** 741 (1969).

22. Yoshida, T., Nagai, R., and Hashimoto, T. *Lab. Invest.* **29,** 329 (1973).

23. Yoshida, T., Bigazzi, P. E., and Cohen, S. *J. Immunol.* **114,** 688 (1975).

24. Geczy, C. L., Friedrich, W., and de Weck, A. L., *Cell. Immunol.* **19,** 65 (1975).

25. Kronman, B. S., Wepsic, H. T., Churchill, W. H., Jr., Zbar, B., Borsoo, T., and Rapp, H. J., *Science,* **165,** 296 (1969).

26 Bloom, B. R., Bennett, B., Oettgen, H. F., McLean, E. P., and Old, L. J., *Proc. Natl. Acad. Sci. U.S.A.* **64,** 1176 (1969).

27. Suter, L., Bloom, B. R., Wadsworth, E. M., and Oettgen, H. F. *J. Immunol.* **109,** 766 (1972).

28. Churchill, W. H., Zbar, B., Belli, J. A., and David, J. R., *J. Natl. Cancer Inst.* **48,** 541 (1972).

29. Halliday, W. J., and Webb, M., *J. Natl. Cancer Inst.* **43,** 141 (1969).

30. Halliday, W. J., *J. Immunol.* **106,** 855 (1971).

31. Halliday, W. J., *Cell. Immunol.* **3,** 113 (1972).

32. Malmgren, R. A., Holmes, E. C., Morton, D. L., Yee, C. L., Marrone, J., and Myers, M. W., *Transpl.* **8,** 485 (1969).

33. Pekarek, J., Svejcar, J., Vonka, V., and Zavadova, H., *Z Immunforsch. Allergie Klin. Immun.* **134,** 449 (1968).

34. Blasecki, J. W., and Tevethia, S. S., *J. Immunol.* **110,** 590 (1973).

35. Steiner, T., and Watne, A. L. *Cancer Res.* **30,** 2265 (1970).

36. Hilberg, R. T., Balcerzak, S. P., and LoBuglio, A. F., *Cell. Immunol.* **7,** 152 (1973).

37. Churchill, W. H., Jr., and Rocklin, R. E., *Natl. Cancer Inst. Monogr.* **37,** 135 (1973).

38. Thor, D. E., *Science,* **157,** 1567 (1967).

39. Thor, D. E., Jureziz, R. E., Veach, S. R., Miller, E., and Dray, S. *Nature* (London) **219,** 755 (1968).

40. Rocklin, R. E., Myers, O. L., and David, J. R., *J. Immunol.* **104,** 95 (1970).

41. Medzihradsky, J., and Kalafut, F., *Neoplasma,* **19,** 147 (1972).

42. Kenjo, T. *Keio J. Med.* **23,** 1 (1974).

43. Vaage, J., Jones, R. D., and Brown, B. W., *Cancer Res.* **32,** 680 (1972).

44. Rees, R. C., and Potter, C. W., *Eur. J. Cancer* **9,** 497 (1973).

45. Harrington, J. T., *Cell Immunol.* **12,** 476 (1974).

46. Jones, B. M., and Turnbull, A. R., *Br. J. Cancer* **32,** 339 (1975).

47. Bendixen, G., and Soborg, M., *Acta Med. Scand.* **181,** 247 (1967).

48. Soborg, M., *Acta. Med. Scand.* **182,** 167 (1967).

49. Soborg, M., *Acta Med. Scand.* **184,** 135 (1968).

50. Brostoff, J., and Roitt, I. M., *Lancet* **ii,** 1269 (1969).

51. Rocklin, R. E., *J. Immunol.* **112,** 1461 (1974).

52. Chess, L., Rocklin, R. E., MacDermott, R. P., David, J. R., and Schlossman, S. F., *J. Immunol.* **115,** 315 (1975).

53. Bendixen, G., *Scand. J. Gastroent.* **2,** 214 (1967).

54. Bendixen, G., *Acta Med. Scand.* **184,** 99 (1968).

55. Bendixen, G. *Gut.* **10,** 631 (1969).

56. Soborg, M. and Bertram, V., *Acta Med. Scand.* **184,** 319 (1968).

57. Soborg, M. and Halberg, P. *Acta. Med. Scand.* **183,** 101 (1968).

58. Nerup, J., Andersen, V., and Bendixen, G., *Clin. Exp. Immunol.* **4,** 355 (1969).

59. Nerup, J., Andersen, V., and Bendixen, G., *Clin. Exp. Immunol.* **6,** 733 (1970).

60. Hardt, F., Nerup, J., and Bendixen, G., *Lancet* **i,** 730 (1969).

61. Aalund, O., Hoerlein, A. B., and Adler, H. C., *Acta Vet. Scand.* **11,** 331 (1970).

62. Brostoff, J., *Proc. Roy. Soc. Med.* **63,** 905 (1970).

63. Brostoff, J., Roitt, I. M., and Doniach, D., *Lancet* **i,** 1212 (1969).

64. Eddleston, A. L. W. F., Williams, R., and Calne, R. Y., *Nature* (London) **222,** 674 (1969).

65. Andersen, V., Bendixen, G., and Schiodt, T., *Act. Med. Scand.* **186,** 101 (1969).

66. Andersen, V., Bjerrum, O., Bendixen, G., Schiodt, T. and Dissing, I., *Int. J. Cancer* **5,** 357 (1970).

67. Wolberg, W. H., and Goelzer, M. L., *Nature* **229,** 632 (1971).

68. Braun, M., Sen, L., Bachmann, A. E. and Pavlovsky, A. *Blood* **39,** 368 (1972).

69. Cochran, A. J., Spilg, W. G. S., Mackie, R. M., and Thomas, C. E., *Brit. Med. J.* **4,** 67 (1972).

70. Segall, A., Weiler, O., Genin, J., Lacour, J., and Lacour, F. *Int. J. Cancer* **9,** 417 (1972).

71. Bull, D. M., Leibach, J. R., Williams, M. A., and Helms, R. A., *Science* **181,** 957 (1973).

72. McCoy, J. L., Jerome, L. F., Dean, J. H., Cannon, G. B., Alford, T. C., Doering, T., and Herberman, R. B., *J. Natl. Cancer Inst.* **53,** 11 (1974).

73. Cochran, A. J., Grant, R. M., Spilg, W. G., Mackie, R. M., Ross, C. E., Hoyle, D. E., and Russell, J. M., *Int. J. Cancer,* **14,** 19 (1974).

74. Black, M. M., Leis, H. P., Jr., Shore, B., and Zachran, R. E., *Cancer* **33,** 952 (1974).

75. Kjaer, M., *Eur. J. Cancer* **10,** 523 (1974).

76. Wolberg, W. H., *Cancer Res.* **31,** 798 (1971).

77. Cochran, A. J., Jehn, U. W., and Grohoskar, B. P., *Lancet* **i,** 1340 (1972).

78. Char, D. H., Jerome, L., McCoy, J. L., and Herberman, R. B., *Amer. J. Ophthol.* **79,** 812 (1975).

79. Claussen, J. E., *Acta. Allerg.* **26,** 56 (1971).

80. Astor, S. H., Spitler, L. E., Frick, O. L., and Fudenberg, H. H., *J. Immunol.* **110,** 1174 (1973).

81. Boddie, A. W., Jr., Holmes, E. C., Roth, J. A., and Morton, D. L., *Int. J. Cancer* **15,** 823 (1975).

82. Spitler, L. E., *Clin. Res.* **21,** 654 (1974).

83. Wolberg, W. H., *Arch. Surg.* **109,** 211 (1974).

84. Halliday, W. J., Halliday, J. W., Campbell, C. B., Malnish, A. E., and Powell, L. W., *Brit. Med. J.* **2,** 349 (1974).

85. Malnish, A., and Halliday, W. J., *J. Natl. Cancer Inst.* **52,** 1415 (1974).

86. Halliday, W. J., Malnish, A. E., and Isbister, W. H., *Br. J. Cancer* **29,** 31 (1974).

87. Halliday, W. J., Malnish, A. E., Little, J. H., Davis, N. C. *Int. J. Cancer* **16,** 645 (1975).

88. Malnish, A. E., and Halliday, W. J., *Cell. Immunol.* **17,** 131 (1975).

89. Holan, V., Hasek, M., Bubenik, J., and Chutna, J., *Cell. Immunol.* **13,** 107 (1974).

90. Turk, J. L., and Diengdoh, J. V., *Int. Arch. Allergy* **34,** 297 (1968).

91. Caspary, E. A., *Nat. New Biol.* **231,** 24 (1971).

92. Caspary, E. A., and Field, E. J., *Europ. Neurol.* **4,** 257 (1971).

93. Field, E. J., Caspary, E. A., Hall, R., and Clark, F., *Lancet* **i,** 1144 (1970).

94. Field, E. J., and Caspary, E. A., *Lancet* **ii,** 1337 (1970).

95. Caspary, E. A., *Clin. Exp. Immunol.* **11,** 305 (1972).

96. Shelton, J. B., Potter, C. W., and Carr, I., *Br. J. Cancer* **31,** 528 (1975).

97. Field, E. J., Caspary, E. A., and Smith, K. S., *Br. J. Cancer,* **28,** Suppl. I, 208 (1973).

98. Hammond, M. E., and Dvorak, H. F., *J. Exp. Med.* **136,** 1518 (1972).

99. Thrasher, S. G., Yoshida, T., van Oss, C. J., Cohen, S., and Rose, N. R., *J. Immunol.* **110,** 321 (1973).

100. Stastny, P., and Ziff, M., in *Immunopathology of Inflammation,* Excerpta Medica, Amsterdam, 1971, p. 66.

101. Hay, J. B., Lachmann, P. J., and Trnka, Z., *Proc. Seventh Leucocyte Culture Conference,* Academic Press, New York, 1973, p. 341.

102. Salvin, S. B., Youngner, J. S., and Lederer, W. H., *Infect. Immunity* **7,** 68 (1973).

103. Yamamoto, K., and Takaheshi, Y., *Nat. New Biol.* **233,** 261 (1971).

104. Cohen, S., Fisher, B., Yoshida, T., and Bettigole, R. E., *N. Engl. J. Med.* **290,** 882 (1974).

105. Flanagan, T. D., Yoshida, T., and Cohen, S., *Infect. Immunity* **8,** 145 (1973).

106. Hammond, M. E., Roblin, R. O., Dvorak, A. M., Selvaggio, S. S., Black, P. H., and Dvorak, H. F., *Science,* **185,** 955 (1974).

107. Bigazzi, P. E., Yoshida, T., Ward, P. A., and Cohen, S., *Am. J. Pathol.* **80,** 69 (1975).

108. Papageorgious, P. S., Henley, W. L., and Glade, P. R., *J. Immunol.* **108,** 494 (1972).

109. Tubergen, D. G., Feldman, J. D., Pollock, E. M., and Lerner, R. A., *J. Exp. Med.* **135,** 255 (1972).

110. Yoshida, T., Kuratsuji, T., Takada, A., Takada, Y., Minowada, J., and Cohen, S. Submitted for publication.

111. Yoshida, T., Edelson, R., Cohen, S., and Green, I. *J. Immunol.* **114,** 915 (1975).

112. Ward, P. A., and Talamo, R. C., *J. Clin. Invest.* **52,** 516 (1973).

113. Berenberg, J. L., and Ward, P. A., *J. Clin. Invest.* **52,** 1200 (1973).

114. Ward, P. A., and Berenberg, J. L., *N. Engl. J. Med.* **290,** 76 (1974).

115. Ward, P. A., and Rocklin, R. E., *J. Immunol.* **115,** 309 (1975).

116. Sylven, B., *Schweiz Med. Wochenschr.* **104,** 258 (1974).

117. Cohen, M. C., Brozna, J., Ward, P. A., and Cohen, S., *Fed. Proc.* **35,** 388 (1976).

118. Williams, T. W., and Granger, G. A., *Nature* (London) **219,** 1076 (1968).

119. Williams, T. W., and Granger, G. A., *J. Immunol.* **102,** 911 (1969).

120. Granger, G. A., and Williams, T. W., *Progr. Immunol.* **1,** 438 (1971).

121. Kramer, S. L., and Granger, G. A., *Cell. Immunol.* **15,** 57 (1975).

122. Meltzer, M. S., and Bartlett, G. L., *J. Natl. Cancer Inst.* **49,** 1439 (1972).

123. Weedon, D. D., Meester, L. J., Elveback, L. R., and Shorter, R. G., *Mayo Clin. Proc.* **48,** 556 (1973).

124. Ruddle, N. H., and Waksman, B. H., *J. Exp. Med.* **128,** 1237 (1968).

125. Heise, E., and Weiser, R., *J. Immunol.* **103,** 570 (1969).

126. Walker, S. M. and Lucas, Z. J., *J. Immunol.* **109,** 1233 (1972).

127. Perlmann, P., and Holm, G., *Adv. Immunol.* **11,** 117 (1969).

128. Brunner, K. T., and Cerottini, J. C., *Prog. Immunol.* **1,** 385 (1971).

129. Cohen, I. R., and Feldman, M., *Cell. Immunol.* **1,** 521 (1971).

130. Blomgren, H., and Svedmyer, E., *Cell. Immunol.* **2,** 285 (1971).

131. Holm, G., Stejskal, V., and Perlmann, P., *Clin. Exp. Immunol.* **14,** 169 (1973).

132. Plant, M., Lichtenstein, L. M., and Henney, C. S., *J. Immunol.* **110,** 771 (1973).

133. Henney, C. S., *Transpl. Rev.* **17,** 37 (1973).

134. Walker, S. M., and Lucas, Z. J., *Transpl. Proc.* **5,** 137 (1973).

135. Lambert, R. A., *J. Cancer Res.* **1,** 169 (1916).

136. Coman, D. R., *Cancer Res.* **4,** 625 (1944).

137. Rosenaw, W., *Oncology* **24,** 21 (1969).

138. Burk, R. R., *Proc. Nat. Acad. Sci. U.S.A.* **70,** 369 (1973).

139. Abercrombie, M., *Eur. J. Cancer,* **67** (1970).

140. Cochran, A. J., *Eur. J. Clin. Biol. Res.* **16,** 44 (1971).

141. Cochran, A. J., Kiessling, R., Klein, E., Gunven, P., and Foulis, A. K., *J. Nat. Cancer Inst.* **51,** 1109 (1973).

142. Cohen, M., Zeschke, R., Bigazzi, P. E., Yoshida, T., and Cohen, S., *J. Immunol.* **114,** 1641 (1975).

143. Friberg, S., Golub, S. H., and Lilliehook, B., *Exp. Cell. Res.* **73,** 101 (1972).

144. Currie, G. A., *Nat. New Biol.* **241,** 284 (1973).

145. Cochran, A. J., *J. Nat. Cancer Inst.* **51,** 1431 (1973).

146. Old, L. J., Clarke, D. A., and Benacerraf, B. *Nature* (London) **184,** 291 (1959).

147. Mathe, G., Pouillant, P., and Lapeyraque, F., *Brit. J. Cancer* **23,** 814 (1969).

148. Scott, M. T., *J. Natl. Cancer Inst.* **53,** 855 (1974).

149. Zbar, B., Berstein, I. D., and Rapp, H. J., *J. Natl. Cancer Inst.* **46,** 831 (1971).

150. Hibbs, J. B., Jr., Lambert, L. H., Jr., and Remington, J. S., *J. Infect. Dis.* **124,** 587 (1971).

151. Keller, R., *J. Exp. Med.* **138,** 625 (1973).

152. Mackaness, G. B., *J. Exp. Med.* **116,** 381 (1962).

153. Mackaness, G. B., *J. Exp. Med.* **129,** 973 (1969).

154. Remington, J. S., and Merigan, T. C., *Proc. Soc. Exp. Biol. Med.* **131,** 1184 (1969).

155. Hibbs, J. B., Jr., Lambert, L. H., Jr., and Remington, J. S., *Proc. Soc. Exp. Biol. Med.* **139,** 1053 (1972).

156. Hibbs, J. B., Jr., Lambert, L. H., Jr., and Remington, J. S. *Science* **177,** 998 (1972).

157. Hibbs, J. B., Jr., *Science* **180,** 868 (1972).

158. Evans, R., and Alexander, P., *Nature* (London) **228,** 620 (1970).

159. Evans, R., Grant, C. K., Cox, H., Steele, K., and Alexander, P. *J. Exp. Med.* **136,** 1318 (1972).

160. Lohmann-Matthes, M. L., Ziegler, F. G., and Fischer, H., *Eur. J. Immunol.* **3,** 56 (1973).

161. Pels, E., and Den-Otter, W., *Cancer Res.* **34,** 3089 (1974).

162. Amos, H. E., and Lachmann, P. J., *Immunol.* **18,** 269 (1970).

163. Piessens, W. F., Churchill, W. H., Jr., and David, J. R., *J. Immunol.* **114,** 293 (1975).

164. Churchill, W. H., Jr., Piessens, W. F., Sulis, C. A., and David, J. R., *J. Immunol.* **115,** 781 (1975).

165. Nathan, C. F., Karnovsky, M. L., and David, J. R., *J. Exp. Med.* **133,** 1356 (1971).

166. Mooney, J. J., and Waksman, B. H., *J. Immunol.* **105,** 1138 (1970).

167. Remold, H. G., and Mednis, A., *Fed. Proc.* **31,** 753 (abs.), (1972).

168. Remold-O'Donnell, E., and Remold, H. G., *J. Biol. Chem.* **249,** 3622 (1974).

169. Leibowitch, J. L., and David, J. R., *Ann. d'Immunol.* (Paris) **124c,** 441 (1973).

170. Fowles, R. E., Fajardo, I. M., Leibowitch, J. L., and David, J. R., *J. Exp. Med.* **138,** 952 (1973).

171. Bernstein, I. D., Thor, D. E., Zbar, B., and Rapp, H. J., *Science,* **172,** 729 (1971).

172. Mann, J., Leichner, J. P., and Affronti, L. F., *Fed. Proc.* **33,** 782 (abs.), (1974).

173. Salvin, S. B., Youngner, J. S., Nishio, J., and Neta, R., *J. Natl. Cancer Inst.* **55,** 1233 (1975).

174. Gresser, I., and Bourali, C., *J. Natl. Cancer Inst.* **45,** 365 (1970).

175. Papermaster, B. W., Holtermann, O. A., Rosner, D., Klein, E., Dao, T., and Djerassi, I., *Res. Communic. Cham. Path. Pharmacol.* **8,** 413 (1974).

176. Djerassi, I., and Kim, quoted in ref. 175 (unpublished).

177. Holtermann, O. H., Papermaster, B. W., Rosner, D., Milgrom, H., and Klein, E., *J. Med. Expt. Clin.* (in press).

Chapter Five

Tumor-Associated Antigens

SANDRA RISTOW AND CHARLES F. McKHANN

Departments of Biochemistry, Surgery, and Microbiology, University of Minnesota, Minneapolis, Minnesota

The first positive identification of an immune response specific for a tumor set in motion a sequence of studies that will continue for several years to come. These studies will continue to depend heavily on developments in two other areas: our general understanding of the immune response, and techniques of biochemistry. Isolation and biochemical and biological characterization of tumor antigens are early in development and must borrow from both of these disciplines. The methods of isolation and purification of potentially antigenic materials are entirely those of the biochemist and only subsequently to be applied to tumor systems. Toward this goal major steps have already been accomplished in the purification of normal transplantation antigens, using techniques that appear to be largely applicable to tumor antigens. Similarly, any hope for manipulating the immune interaction between host and tumor will depend on continuing progress in our understanding of the entire field of immunology.

The rewards for isolation and purification of tumor antigens may be considerable. They include a better understanding of the relationship of the tumor antigen to the cell surface membranes and other cellular components, the relationship of the tumor antigens to normal transplantation antigens, the mechanism by which immunization takes place (or does not take place) in vivo, the significance of free antigen or antigen-antibody complex in the circulation, the use of purified antigen for development of sensitive assays to diagnose and monitor the growth of tumors, and, ultimately, the potential use of specific antigen for immunotherapy.

The following review is in no way comprehensive; rather, it attempts to provide a background for understanding the current approaches to purification and immunologic identification of tumor-associated antigens and to indicate the role that these antigens may play in the tumor-host interaction.

ISOLATION OF TUMOR ANTIGENS

Extraction and characterization of tumor-associated antigens have borrowed heavily from the methods developed in the past for preparation of normal transplantation antigens involved in the rejection of tissue allografts, the H-2 antigens of mice and the HLA antigens of humans. Several reviews cover the immunogenetics and the immunochemistry of these complex glycoproteins (1–5). The methods used for isolation of both murine and human histocompatibility antigens include ultrasound, nitrogen cavitation, detergent extraction, proteolytic digestion, and hypertonic salt extraction.

H-2 antigens recovered by *papain digestion* were from 30,000 to 55,000 in molecular weight, with carbohydrate contents of approximately 10% (6). Since proteolytic digestion fragmented the antigenic molecules, other means were sought to remove antigens from the plasma membranes of cells. One such method is *detergent extraction*. Nathenson extracted H-2 antigens from tumor cells with Non-Idet P40, obtaining 80–100% yields (7). Further purification was accomplished by direct immunoprecipitation. Polyacrylamide gel electrophoresis subsequently revealed that there was a 6,000 molecular weight difference between one of the NP40-solubilized specificities and its papain-cleaved counterpart, indicating that proteolytic digestion did remove portions of the antigenic molecules (8). In the case of H-2 antigens solubilized by papain, several different specificities were shown to reside on the same molecule (9). NP40 extraction has recently revealed a new set of membrane molecules on normal lymphoid cells, the Ia antigens, which are clearly distinct from the H-2D and H-2K antigens (10).

Hypertonic salt extraction is another favored method for extraction of histocompatibility antigens from lymphoid cells, since it is more efficient than high-frequency sonication for removing antigens from the plasma membrane. It is believed that hypertonic salt causes a change in the structure of the membrane and of the antigen, thus releasing the antigen from its lipid milieu. It has been established that most inorganic salts may be arranged in an order referred to as the Hoffmeister, or lyotropic series, according to their ability to stabilize or destabilize protein conformation. These electrolytes vary in their ability to alter electrostatic interactions in macromolecules, react with dipolar groups, and affect hydrophobic areas of protein. Potassium chloride lies approximately in the middle of this series, possessing equal power to form helical structures or to denature a protein. This phenomenon has been reviewed (11). Some investigators believe that it is not perturbation of protein structure by KC1 which solubilizes antigens, but rather that proteolytic enzymes may be active in the hypertonic salt solutions, releasing the antigens by an autolytic action (12).

Human HLA antigens are obtained in much the same way as murine H-2 antigens. Recently, Brij 99, a nonionic detergent, was used (13) in conjunction with papain to solubilize HLA antigens. The detergent extracted a substance which had two subunits, of molecular weight 12,000 and 44,000. When the complex was subjected to papain digestion, the 44,000 molecular weight material was reduced to 34,000 while the 12,000 molecular weight subunit remained unchanged. The association of β_2 microglobulin, a molecule which has homology with a portion of an immunoglobulin, with HLA antigens was made by these and a number of other investigators (14–17) and was recently reviewed (18). Studying partially purified HLA antigens from papain-digested lymphocytes, Thieme (19) used four different alloantisera to demonstrate that four different antigens obtained from a papain digest could be separated from each other; he concluded that the HLA antigens of a single genotype are found on four distinct molecular species.

Since various chemical and physical treatments produced antigens of different molecular weights, several investigators have attempted to isolate a more uniform product of HLA antigens from human plasma or sera or from the culture fluid from lymphoid cells grown in vitro, under the assumption that the cell sheds products into the fluids which bathe it. Pellegrino (20) showed that the membranous materials of several cultured lymphoid cell lines are excellent sources of HLA antigens and are not dependent on cell growth cycle variations. Billing (21,22) was able to isolate HLA antigens from human sera by DEAE sephadex chromatography, concanavalin A sepharose chromatography, and polyacrylamide gel electrophoresis. By this method the isolated antigens were beta globulins containing 10 to 12% carbohydrate and possessing a molecular weight of 130,000. Dawson (23) also used affinity chromatography (lens culinaris hemagglutin bound to sepharose 4B) to remove HLA antigens from deoxycholate-extracted tissue-cultured cells, illustrating that the affinities of carbohydrate moieties of antigens for lectins may be exploited for their isolation.

Isolation of Tumor-Associated Antigens

Since tumor-associated antigens have been demonstrated by transplantation techniques and by serological methods, the extraction and purification of these molecules have become of general importance. In considering current methods for preparing tumor-associated antigens, we must keep several points in mind.

1.   Although antigenic activity in vitro or in vivo does not require solubilization of antigen, chemical characterization does. A "soluble" preparation should be soluble in water or a physiological medium. Detergent extracts, such as those performed with sodium dodecyl sulfate or Non-Idet P40, form semistable micelles with various fragments of the tumor membrane. When an attempt is made to remove the detergents from the preparation by dialysis, precipitation of the antigens often occurs. Alternatively, if one leaves much detergent in the preparation, the materials are toxic to the cells in in vitro assays, unless they are greatly diluted (24).

2.   The antigen should remain soluble through centrifugation at $100,000g$ for at least one hour. Many "soluble" preparations of crude antigens have been made in which the materials have only been centrifuged at $20,000g$ for one-half hour. At this speed ribosomes and plasma membrane remain in the supernatant. Although such materials may contain the antigenic specificity, in this state they are not truly soluble.

3.   Purification of the antigen should take place during the processing. In going from the original tissue through the various steps of the purification,

column chromatography, electrophoresis, etc., greater specific activity per milligram of protein or carbohydrate should be obtained at each step.

4. The assay used for the antigen must be sensitive and applicable. In isolating tumor antigens, most major problems occur with the methodology of the assays and not with the biochemical procedures for isolating putative antigenic fractions. Assays of *tumor transplantation antigen* must measure resistance to transplantation. This requires adequate numbers of animals in both grafted and control groups to make the experiment meaningful. The interval of time between the rejection of the graft by the control and rejection by the antigen-primed animals must be significant. Inhibition assays, such as blocking of in vitro cytotoxicity, must be due to specific antigen and not simple excess of protein. Pellegrino (25) pointed out that a purified histocompatibility antigen should totally inhibit cytotoxic antibody at "zero cytotoxicity" units at a concentration of less than 0.5 microgram of purified antigen per microliter. Many assays which are now being used to measure tumor antigen cannot satisfy this criterion.

Currently, many studies of the isolation of tumor-associated antigens utilize tumor lines in inbred strains of animals. The use of such tumors is much simpler than isolating antigens from human tumors or from tumors in outbred animals, because normal antigens associated with histocompatibility differences are excluded and the only antigenic differences seen are those between normal tissue and tumor. Since this is rarely possible in human tumor systems, great emphasis has been placed on the response of the patient to his own tumor. In allogeneic human tumor systems caution must be exercised to insure that the antigen and the immune response are truly tumor-associated and not the results of histocompatibility differences. As pointed out elsewhere, this problem is even greater when "tumor-specific" antiserum is produced in a foreign species.

TUMOR ANTIGENS: THE ASSAYS AND THE ANTIGENS

At present our capacity to extract and biochemically purify tumor antigens considerably exceeds our capacity to assay the purified materials accurately for specific antigenic activity. This is due in part to the heterogeneity of the antigens themselves and in part to the relative complexity and nonspecificity of some of our biological assays. The tumor cell not only presents a constellation of different antigens, but even any single antigen may be handled quite differently when presented to the immune response as a soluble preparation rather than on the intact cell. This has its counterpart in normal transplantation antigens, where the antigens responsible for serological recognition are distinct from those responsible for graft rejection, although both are under tight genetic control, are closely correlated, and are highly specific for the individual. It is not yet known whether such a dual antigenic system also applies to tumor antigens. However, it is clear that antigenic *recognition* does not necessarily result in an immune response that is detrimental to the tumor; i.e., an antigen preparation that can be recognized is not necessarily one that will induce tumor rejection.

The assays for tumor antigens fall into three general categories: (1) in vivo, (2) in vitro using cellular immunity, and (3) in vitro using antibody.

Cellular Immunity in vivo

Transplant Rejection.   The original assay for tumor antigens, and in some respects the reference for most other assays, is tumor rejection. This was originally developed through the use of intact tumor cells, injected in minute doses which were unable to grow, or in moderate doses which resulted in tumors that were subsequently excised, or in still larger doses of cells inactivated by irradiation (26). Subsequent challenge with graded doses of viable tumor cells showed the immunized animals to be more resistant than untreated controls. Many attempts have been made to induce tumor rejection immunity in vivo with soluble antigen extracts, with only a few successes (27–32). Immunization in vivo with normal transplantation antigen extracts has shown great variability, depending on the antigenic preparation. Moreover, cellular cytotoxicity has been difficult to demonstrate in vitro in these animals.

With respect to soluble antigen preparations from tumors, preimmunization for graft rejection represents a cumbersome assay which is difficult to quantitate. However, the importance of soluble antigenic preparations that induce tumor rejection must not be underestimated, since tumor rejection is the ultimate goal of many studies of tumor immunology. Most assays for tumor antigens currently in use do not measure their capacity to induce tumor rejection, and an important step will be to determine the relationship between those antigens that are measured by other in vitro methods and the capacity of these materials to induce graft rejection. Obviously, studies involving the rejection of viable tumor cells are confined to experimental systems.

Delayed Hypersensitivity by Skin Testing.   Graft rejection is associated with lymphocyte infiltration, and it has long been known that the cellular immune response induced by some antigens in vivo can be detected by a skin reaction to intradermal injections of antigen. The skin reaction of delayed hypersensitivity characteristically appears between 24 and 48 hours after injection and is characterized by infiltration of lymphocytes into the area of the injected antigen. Delayed hypersensitivity, thought to reflect cellular immunity, is a relatively complex reaction in which lymphocytes of the host interact with the antigen and subsequently release soluble factors, which in turn cause inflammatory cells to accumulate in the region where the antigen was injected. The induration and erythema which result may be measured, but precise quantitation of different antigenic materials is obviously difficult.

Extracts of human tumors are usually compared with those from other tumors and preparations from normal tissues. The ideal of testing the extracts in the patient who provided the tumor is frequently not met, raising the possibility that some positive reactions are against normal allogeneic transplantation antigens rather than tumor antigens. Moreover, it has already been shown that some tumor antigens contained in extracts may not elicit positive skin reactions (33). Another problem with in vivo skin testing for delayed hypersensitivity is the incidence of false-positive reactions. The skin is capable of a limited range of responses, and inflammation follows the injection of many materials. The amount of material used to measure delayed hypersensitivity has been shown to be a critical factor, in that the injection of too much protein, even of control material, may provide a false-positive reaction (34).

Assays for delayed cutaneous hypersensitivity against tumor antigen extracts have met with varied success. In the guinea pig, which is the favorite experimental animal for demonstrating delayed hypersensitivity, 3M KCl extracts of ascites tumors and sarcomas have produced positive reactions (35,36). Hollinshead, who probably has utilized this assay for human tumor antigen more than any other investigator, has produced antigens from sonicated extracts of carcinoma of the breast (37,38), squamous cell carcinoma (39), carcinoma of the lung (40), carcinoma of the colon (33), and melanoma (41). Extracts of several solid tumors prepared with 3M KCl have also been shown to contain antigen capable of eliciting delayed cutaneous hypersensitivity (42) as well as in vitro blastogenic responses (43,44).

In order to be the "guinea pig" for an in vivo assay of soluble tumor antigen, the patient must be *able* to respond to the antigen. However, there is now a large body of evidence showing that the general immune capacity of many tumor patients is nonspecifically impaired. This is reflected in their inability to respond with delayed hypersensitivity skin reactions not only to tumor antigen extracts but also to a battery of common skin test antigens including PPD, mumps, streptokinase-streptodornase, DNFB, and candida (45,46). The mechanism of this anergy is not known, but several serum-borne immunosuppressive factors have been identified which may be the cause (47–52).

As with in vivo testing of tumor antigens in experimental systems by the induction of graft rejection, the spectrum of antigens capable of producing delayed hypersensitivity skin reactions is not known. To this end correlative studies between in vitro techniques for detecting tumor antigen and this widely applicable in vivo method are badly needed.

Cellular Immunity in vitro

Cellular Cytotoxicity and Blocking.   Methods developed to demonstrate cellular cytotoxicity in vitro include colony or cell inhibition (53), chromium-51 release (54), and radioactive isotope release (55,56). An extensive review of this subject has been published (57). The objective of much current work in this field is to increase the reliability of these tests for cytotoxicity against human tumor-associated antigens. Of several problems associated with cellular cytotoxicity assays (58) a major one continues to be the nonspecific cytotoxicity of presumably nonimmune lymphocytes from some normal donors in human studies (56,59–61). At present there is no evidence to show whether these "nonspecific" reactions are truly nonspecific or whether they represent some expression of previous exposure of the lymphocyte donor to tumor-related antigens.

The use of radiolabeled cells was introduced as an attempt to provide a more simple and objective method than visual counting for enumerating target cells. Chromium 51 has been useful in allogeneic systems and in some tumor systems but requires that the immunity be relatively strong and the assay of short duration, since the isotope rapidly leaks spontaneously from many tumor cells. Other isotopes localizing in the cytoplasm or the nucleus are more stable, but ^{3}H thymidine must be used with caution, since heavy labeling can damage or kill the target cells. New antigens may be incorporated or develop in the cell membrane upon growth in heterologous serum, as has been demonstrated on cultured human sarcoma cells grown in fetal calf serum (62,63). Normal human serum contains natural antibodies to this antigen, which appear within 24 hours of culture.

In spite of these inherent problems, a massive amount of data has accumulated through the use of cellular cytotoxicity assays (57). Foremost among these is the finding that there are common, cross-reacting antigens on human neoplasms of similar histological type: adenocarcinoma and fibroadenoma of the breast (64), melanoma (58,65–66), and sarcoma (67).

Assays for cellular cytotoxicity do not measure soluble antigen directly, nor do they provide a method for quantitative estimation of cellular antigens. However, they do provide an indirect approach to the qualitative detection of free antigen by its capacity to block cellular immunity. Evidence indicating the presence of factors in tumor-bearing serum which block cellular cytotoxicity is accumulating rapidly (68–75). This is still somewhat presumptive, however, since tumor antigen has not been purified to a high degree from serum and also because other, nonantigen blocking factors have been found in serum. The goal of much ongoing research is the isolation of both purified tumor-associated antigens and purified antitumor antibody, so that the effect of stoichiometrically produced complexes may be studied quantitatively.

The original evidence that blocking factors were associated with IgG came from experiments in which serum from Moloney sarcoma virus (MSV) infected mice with progressively growing tumors blocked colony inhibition (68). The effect was specific, since sera from mice bearing mammary tumors or methylcholanthrene sarcomas were nonblocking for the MSV tumor. When progressor tumor-bearer serum from MSV tumor bearers was fractionated over an Amicon X100 membrane in pH 3.1 glycine buffer, blocking activity was lost in both the fraction retained above and that passing through the membrane. Since the recombined fractions once again demonstrated blocking activity, the factors were assumed to be antigen-antibody complexes (68). Subsequently Ankerst (76) showed that the blocking activity of serum in an adenovirus tumor system was in the IgG fraction recovered from Sephadex G200 and DEA cellulose columns, indicating that the substance associated with the blocking was approximately equal in size and charge to 7s immunoglobulin. Serum blocking factors associated with IgG have been shown recently to be a more general phenomenon in allograft immunity (77–79), and the blocking factors in multiparous mice have been shown to be IgG_2a or IgG_2b (80).

Several other investigators were able to demonstrate blocking factors in the serum of rats bearing hepatomas and sarcomas using the Hellström's assay. Baldwin (70,71) demonstrated that serum from tumor-bearing animals blocked lymphocyte cytotoxicity in a rat hepatoma system. With the addition of membrane proteins to both postexcision serum and tumor-bearer serum he demonstrated variable degrees of blocking activity. This experiment was an initial attempt to make artificial antigen-antibody complexes to block lymphocyte cytotoxicity at the level of the target tumor cell. Addition of membrane antigen to tumor-bearer serum which already contained antigen-antibody complexes produced an excess of antigen, which also blocked cytotoxicity. In a study of the in vivo effect of serum blocking factors, it was demonstrated that when mice who were surgically cured of their tumors, but whose immune response was not fully recovered, were injected with the blocking serum, their recovery was further retarded, since they succumbed more rapidly to a new challenge of the same tumor (8!). In this study the blocking serum was produced in irradiated mice injected with large doses of killed sarcoma cells and was thought to contain free antigen but no antibody or antigen-antibody complexes. Jose (75) has titrated remission serum from patients with neuroblastomas with antigenic material recovered from the media of cultured tumor cells to produce complexes. By culturing neuroblastoma cells and immune lymphocytes in the presence of "synthesized" complexes, he was able to show that complexes in antigen excess showed the greatest blocking, while those in antibody excess showed less. Dauphinee (82) found that another factor, lysozomal enzymes, may enhance blocking activity of antitumor antibody. Antibody against EL-4 lymphoma and P-815 mastocytoma, after incubation with lysozomal enzymes, blocked complement-dependent cytotoxicity more effectively than did antibody alone.

The metabolic requirements for antigen shedding were studied by Fannes and Choi (83), who showed in a DBA/2J mastocytoma system that the shedding of tumor antigens into the medium was an energy-dependent process which required the intact metabolism of the cell at 37°C. Utilizing ^{125}I-labeled isoantibody, purified by absorption and elution on the same population of cells, they found that in 1 hour 20 to 30% of the bound antibody was released and the surface antigen rapidly regenerated. In similar studies two populations of tumor cells were exposed to immune lymphocytes after first being coated with isoantibody and then maintained at 0° or 37° respectively, for 90 minutes. The population which had been incubated at 37° was lysed as if there were no isoantiserum present, indicating that most of the previous coating had been shed. In another experiment indicating that shedding is an energy-dependent process, Leonard (84) used fluorescent staining on line 10 guinea pig ascites tumor to show that tumor cells coated with antitumor antiserum plus a fluoresceinated antiglobulin "capped" at 37° and that the fluorescence pattern disintegrated into patches which were released from the cell surface. Currie and Alexander (85) speculated that it is the shedding phenomenon which immunizes a host to his tumor. By investigating two lines of sarcomas, one of which metastasized rapidly to the lymph nodes and lungs and one which did not, they noticed a striking difference between the two lines in culture: the tumor which metastasized did *not* shed antigen into tissue culture media in vitro.

Lymphocyte Stimulation.   Lymphocyte stimulation is an assay for cell-mediated immunity which does not measure cell-killing capacity but instead measures the ability of a population of immunized lymphocytes, including both T and B lymphocytes, to recognize an antigen and undergo blastogenesis in vitro as monitored by the incorporation of tritiated thymidine. Burk (86) showed that the ability of lymphocytes of methylcholanthrene tumor-bearing mice to undergo blastogenesis in the presence of mitomycin-treated tumor cells was dependent on the size of the growing tumor at the time the lymph node cells were obtained. Blastogenic activity was high during the early tumor-bearing period but decreased markedly as the tumor exceeded one centimeter in size. Stimulation of immune lymphocytes also measured circulating antigen from serum of tumor-bearing animals and has been used to assay for purified tumor antigen (87). Specificity in a lymphocyte-stimulation assay and its correlation with macrophage migration inhibition was first shown with soluble antigens from a guinea pig ascites tumor (35). Lymphocyte blastogenic activity has been studied in conjunction with a chromium release assay to measure responder cells in the spleens and lymph nodes of MSV-infected mice (88) and showed that these two assays measured *different* cellular subpopulations or activities. Lymphocyte blastogenic response has also been measured in patients with acute leukemia (89,90). A positive blastogenic response indicates that the patient is not anergic to his tumor and may be associated with a relatively good prognosis. Law's group has recently demonstrated that lymphocyte blastogenic response correlates with results obtained in in vivo assays, notably graft rejection and Winn assays (91).

Inhibition of Macrophage or Leukocyte Migration.   The exact relationships of these phenomena to lymphocyte stimulation and cellular cytotoxicity are not known, but these two assays appear to reflect the same general arm of the immune response in that they are primarily functions of immune T cells. The macrophage migration inhibition assay, as used by David (92), uses inhibition of normal macrophage migration to measure the release of a soluble inhibiting factor by immune lymphocytes (T cells) in the presence of specific antigen. This assay and its counterpart, in which leukocyte migration inhibition is measured, have been applied to tumor-specific systems (43,93–94). An additional assay based on modification of immune leukocytes—in this case their surface properties—is *inhibition of leukocyte adherence* (95). The adherence of normal peritoneal leukocytes to glass surfaces appears to be measurably reduced when the cells are recovered from animals sensitized to antigenic tumors and soluble antigen is present in the culture.

Antibody Assays

Another correlate of immunity to tumor-associated antigens in both human and animal systems is the antibody response to the tumor. These responses may be visualized by immunofluorescent methods or measured by isotopic-antiglobulin techniques or complement-dependent methods. The use of *fluorescein-labeled antibody,* by the direct or indirect techniques, is difficult to quantitate and is the least sensitive of the humoral assays. However, Baldwin has used this technique well as an indicator for the purification of soluble antigens from a diethylaminoazobenzene-induced rat hepatoma by utilizing the serum from syngeneic rats immunized with irradiated tumor cells (96,97). The same approach was taken in a guinea pig ascites tumor system utilizing serum taken from animals with progressively growing tumors. Antibody was detected at all times during the tumor-bearing period using fluorescein-labeled anti-guinea pig serum (98). In contrast to the fluorescent technique, the use of I^{125}-*labeled antiglobulin* provides an objective method of quantitation of tumor-associated antigens. The antiglobulin technique is much more sensitive than fluorescence and has been used to detect antigens on a Friend virus-induced lymphoma (99) and methylcholanthrene-induced sarcomas (99,100) and indicated weak cross-reactivity between Moloney and Gross virus-induced tumors (101).

A further refinement for cellular localization of antigen is the use of *immunoelectron microscopy* as developed by Aoki (102). This elegant technique has been used to determine the cell surface localization and distribution of normal cellular antigens, tumor antigens, and antigens appearing during virus growth. *Complement fixation* has been used to demonstrate antigens in human sarcoma and melanoma systems (103). The most extensive use of this assay, however, has been for demonstration of the group-specific antigens associated with C-type virus particles found in many tumors and some normal animals (104).

Complement-dependent cytotoxic antibody was first used to detect tumor-specific antigens in murine lymphoma and leukemia systems (105). These virus-induced tumors were noteworthy for their sensitivity to cytotoxic antibody, a factor which distinguished them from solid tumors, in which lysis by antibody and complement was much more difficult to achieve. However, cytotoxic antibody has been used to detect antigens of methylcholanthrene-induced sarcomas in C57BL/10 mice (106). In this study the cytotoxic antibody was found to be IgM and was measured by inhibition of uptake of ^{3}H thymidine by sarcoma cells growing in culture. Using a complement-dependent ^{51}Cr-release assay, Drapkin was unable to detect cytotoxicity against an SV40 tumor or monitor purification of antigens (27). Sera from mice bearing Moloney sarcoma virus (MSV) induced tumors have been studied by a complement-dependent assay to determine the presence of cytotoxic antibodies in their progressor and regressor serum (107).

The use of *xenogeneic antisera* for the detection of tumor-associated antigens requires a special word. Immunization of animals of a different species with tumor, followed by extensive absorption with normal tissues, is an approach that has appealed to many investigators. However, the fact remains that with the single noteworthy exception of the studies of CEA developed by Gold and Freedman (108,109) this approach has not been very fruitful. The reason for numerous failures is not clear, but probably is that the xenogeneic animal "sees" myriads of foreign antigens in the immunizing cells. Very few of these xenoantigens are related to the tumor, and they may be much less immunogenic than the associated normal antigens. Purification of antibody by absorption is always at the expense of some of the specific antibody in question, and extensive absorption with normal tissues may well remove all antibody specific for the tumor in the process.

Radioimmunoassays require either highly purified antigen or highly purified antibody. With respect to tumor-associated antigens, these requirements have been fulfilled on a large scale only in the studies of CEA described elsewhere.

TUMOR ANTIGENS: EXPERIMENTAL SYSTEMS*

After it was shown by Kahan and Reisfeld (110) that hypertonic KCl extracted normal histocompatibility antigens from lymphoid cells, Meltzer (111) used this

---

*Purification of antigens follows the methods which have been already established for the purification of proteins. If the reader wishes to review the theory and practical aspects of techniques, we refer him to the set of volumes *Methods in Enzymology*, published by Academic Press. Volume 22 contains methods by which various organelles may be extracted, solubility separations, chromatographic procedures,

technique to prepare a water-soluble antigen from the lyophilized cells of a diethyl nitrosamine-induced guinea pig hepatoma. The recovered antigen was soluble, as evidenced by the presence of the active fraction in the included volume of a Sephadex G200 column. Intact tumor cells and soluble extracts from two non-cross-reacting tumor lines were tested for delayed cutaneous hypersensitivity reactions in immunized guinea pigs and found to be antigenically distinct. It was the opinion of these investigators that only 15–40% of the antigenic activity present on the original cells was recovered. They speculated that the loss may have been due to destruction of the antigen by the purification procedure or to simple differences in the reactivity of the antigen as it is displayed on the intact cell, compared to its conformation in the soluble form.

Low-frequency sonication (112) has been used to extract tumor transplantation antigens from guinea pig sarcomas. The antigens obtained were active in a test of delayed hypersensitivity (36).

Antigens from the B16 mouse melanoma have been extracted with Non-Idet P40 detergent (113). The materials eluted at column volume from a Sephadex G200 column. By this criterion the authors estimated the molecular weight to be between 150,000 and 200,000. The radio immunoassay used to identify the antigens utilized antiserum made in syngeneic mice by injecting them subcutaneously with irradiated tumor cells, thus avoiding the use of xenogeneic antibody to identify the antigen. It was also found that treatment of the material emerging in the first peak from the column with neuraminidase to remove sialic acid resulted in increased antigenicity.

Probably the most extensive purification of tumor antigens to date from a tumor in inbred animals is the work done by R. W. Baldwin's group on an amino azo dye-induced rat hepatoma (96,97,114). These proteins were extracted from plasma membrane fractions obtained by sucrose gradient centrifugation done in a zonal rotor. The plasma membranes were then digested with papain and the supernatants applied to DEAE cellulose columns and finally to preparative polyacrylamide gel electrophoresis. The resultant active materials had a molecular weight of about 55,000 (97) and were heterogeneous, probably because of the original papain digestion. The technique used to assay for the antigen was inhibition of immunofluorescence of syngeneic antitumor antiserum by the soluble antigen. Baldwin has pointed out the laborious nature and relative insensitivity of this technique (115), which requires the antigenic equivalent of 2×10^8 hepatoma cells per milliliter of serum for significant absorption of tumor-specific antibody. The blocking capacity of artificial antigen-antibody complexes made from the

---

affinity columns, isoelectric focusing procedures, and criteria for homogenicity. Volumes 31 and 32 of this series contain information on biomembranes, while Volume 34 is primarily concerned with affinity techniques. An excellent compendium of the theory and practical aspects of purification of H-2 and HLA antigens is the volume *Transplantation Antigens* by B. D. Kahan and Ralph Reisfeld. This book contains information on proteolytic (Mann) (Sanderson), detergent (Metzgar), hypertonic salt (Reisfeld), sonic (Kahan), and pressure-homogenization (Manson) techniques for extracting antigens.

Additional information about the theoretical and practical aspects of many of the techniques may be obtained from the suppliers: *Sephadex Gel Filtration in Theory and Practice* distributed by Pharmacia or *Isoelectric Focusing in pH Gradients* distributed by LKB Instruments. A concise current review of the theory and general procedures of protein purification, including extraction, fractionation methods, and criteria of purity, may be found in *Proteins: Structure and Function* by Albert Light, published by Prentice-Hall, Inc., 1974.

isolated antigen in a cellular-cytotoxicity assay was demonstrated, confirming the specificity of the prepared antigen (69).

Drapkin (27) isolated antigenic material from an SV40 ascites tumor (m KSA), which induced transplantation resistance when injected into Balb/c mice. The antigens were prepared by papain digestion of tumor membrane obtained from cells by disruption in a Parr bomb. Fifty percent of the activity of the original cell suspension was retained in the crude membrane, but only 5% remained after papain digestion and chromatography on Sephadex G150, as measured by induction of transplantation resistance. Some of the materials with antigenic activity were of approximately 50,000 molecular weight. The size of some of the soluble peptides, however, must have been quite small, since they were retained for almost three column volumes on a Sephadex G150 column.

Extraction by 3M KCl does not guarantee homogeneity of antigenic product. In extracting a line 10 guinea pig hepatoma and utilizing delayed cutaneous hypersensitivity as a test for antigenicity, Leonard (116) discovered that his extracted antigen was nonhomogeneous on both Sephadex G200 and DEAE cellulose and by salting-out criteria.

EMBRYONIC ANTIGENS ASSOCIATED WITH MALIGNANCY

It was postulated years ago that certain normal embryonic properties may be reexpressed in neoplasia and that cancer is a disease of cellular differentiation. As early as 1906 attempts were made to immunize mice with fetal cells in order to prevent tumors (117). The study of embryonic antigens has come of age since it was discovered that such antigens do exist on the cells of many tumors. Attempts are now being made to answer questions about the time of appearance and function of these antigens in embryogenesis, as well as in tumor development, and whether embryonic cells or their extracts are capable of immunizing against tumor growth.

The two best-known and widely studied fetal antigens associated with malignancy are α-fetoprotein (118) and carcinoembryonic antigen (108,109). A number of other embryonic antigens, however, have been found in association with tumors. Various fetal hemoglobins may be found in leukemias (119). Several placental antigens normally do not occur in normal adults (120) but some appear in the serum in pregnancy. Tal (121) described an antigen which he believes to be ceramide lactoside in the serum of pregnant women and many cancer patients. Sulfoglycoprotein, a protein of the fetal alimentary tract, often reappears in gastric cancer (122,123). Recently, the band-V isozyme of 5' nucleotide phosphodiesterase was detected in 88% of a group of hepatoma patients (124). Isoferritins, which cross-react with normal ferritin, are another group of fetal antigens which have been identified in placental tissues and HeLa cells (125). A sensitive test for the Regan isozyme, an alkaline phosphatase found in the serum of cancer patients and normal subjects, has also been developed recently (126).

Studies are now beginning to approach the biochemical identification and functions of various fetal antigens. The fast-moving antigen of Hodgkin's disease has now been shown to be ferritin (127), while the Regan Isozyme is a phosphatase (126). A recent report (128), in which extracts of metastases and primary carcinomas of colon, liver, and pancreas were compared with their normal tissue counterparts, showed that increased carboxylesterase activity resided in the tumor tissue extracts. Perhaps the biological function of CEA is as a carboxylesterase. Murgita (129) has hinted that alpha fetoprotein may be a regulator of immunoglobulin synthesis in the mouse as well as being capable of suppressing the concanavalin A, phytohemagglutin, lipopolysarccharide, and MLC responses of mouse lymphocytes in culture (130). Dattwyler (131) has now established by fluorescence methods that murine α-fetoprotein specifically binds to T cells. A number of conditions other than neoplasia exist in the human in which this material is elevated in the circulation: pregnancy, acute and chronic hepatitis, and ataxia telangiectasia. Tomasi (132) believes that the immunosuppression in each of these conditions may be related to the presence of excess circulating AFP.

α-Fetoprotein

Alpha fetoprotein (AFP), an α-globulin, was first discovered by Abelev (118) in a murine heptatoma (133,134). This discovery was followed shortly by that of Tartarinov (135), who found a similar protein in a human hepatoma. Investigators have subsequently been attempting to develop sensitive assays for detection of AFP and to find it in other types of cancer. AFP is synthesized during gestation by the embryonal liver and yolk sac and is secreted into the fetal serum. This material is of interest because it is diagnostic for two types of cancer: primary liver carcinoma and teratoblastoma. One-third of patients with primary hepatoma have circulating AFP in sufficient quantity to be detectable by simple double diffusion, while a more sensitive radioimmunoassay can detect AFP in the circulation of 85–95% of such patients (136).

Serum α-fetoprotein levels rise in other clinical states, including viral hepatitis (137) and ataxia telangectasia (138). Neonatal levels are also high, 5 mg/100 ml (139). Although the maternal serum level of AFP is not a completely reliable indicator, high levels of AFP in the amniotic fluid before 20 weeks of gestation are predictive of neural tube defects in the fetus: spinal bifida and/or anencephaly (140,141). A rapid rise in AFP level in amniotic fluid after 24 weeks of gestation appears to signal impending fetal death (142).

Since α-fetoprotein is elevated in several human diseases, a number of different assays have been developed to detect its presence in physiological fluids. Sizaret (143) developed a method of electroimmunodiffusion which has been used to detect AFP in hepatocellular carcinoma with 71% accuracy (144). An immunoenzymatic assay for AFP was developed in which horseradish peroxidase-treated sheep antirabbit IgG was developed in conjunction with diaminobenzene to stain immunoprecipitates containing rabbit anti-AFP, the limit of this test being 200–400 nanograms of AFP/ml. For AFP levels as low as 50 nanograms/ml, I^{125}-labeled antibody may be substituted and radioautography used (136).Two other recent radioimmunoassays for AFP have been described which are exquisitely sensitive. One of them detects 2 nanograms of AFP/ml (145), while the other detects 20 nanograms of AFP/ml in as little as 20 microliters of serum (146), making it 500 times as sensitive as the Ouchterlony technique.

Recent studies on developmental changes in the syntheses of AFP and albumin in the fetal mouse (147) indicate that there is a reciprocal relationship between the synthesis of fetoprotein and albumin by the embryonic liver. AFP was found not to be free inside the cell but bound to the membranes and ribosomes. By incorporating radioactive amino acids during protein synthesis and polyacrylamide gel electrophoresis for separating the synthesized proteins, it was demonstrated that the synthesis of $\propto$-fetoprotein decreased from 13 days of gestation to 6 days after birth, while albumin synthesis increased.

Sell's group has isolated and characterized rat fetoprotein from amniotic fluid (148). The protein was purified by a combination of ammonium sulfate precipitation, DEAE cellulose, Pevikon block electrophoresis, Sephadex G200 chromatography, and isoelectric focusing. The isolated protein had an isoelectric point of 4.9, a molecular weight of 70,000, and did not cross-react with human AFP. Utilizing this immunochemically pure AFP, a refined radioimmunoassay was developed which could detect one nanogram of AFP. It was also found that a tenfold increase in sensitivity was obtained by preincubating the goat anti-AFP antiserum with the unlabeled antigen for 20 hours prior to the addition of labeled antigen. This sensitive assay was used to study the synthesis of AFP in fetal hepatocytes in tissue culture; the finding was that the greatest amount of AFP was produced during the logarithmic phase of growth (149).

Several groups have studied the appearance of fetoprotein following treatment of animals with carcinogens. Okita (150) was able to visualize AFP in hyperplastic liver nodules of rats treated with 2-acetylamino-fluorene. Becker (151) noted early elevations of serum AFP in rats treated with N-2-fluorenylacetamide, even though at this point there was no apparent cell damage. The early appearance of AFP was postulated to arise from "a highly selective derepression of protein synthesis" that occurs following the formation of a complex between the metabolite(s) of the carcinogen and specific chromatin.

Carcinoembryonic Antigen (CEA)

Several excellent reviews on the origins, immunology, and chemistry of CEA have been published (152–156). Gold, who first described this fetal antigen in 1965, initially believed that the appearance of CEA in the circulation was specific for adenocarcinoma of the colon (108,109). Subsequently, however, it was found that CEA is not specific for colorectal cancer, is not homogeneous, and is much more complex than previously thought. CEA has been found in a number of other tumors, including carcinoma of the lung (143), breast (157), and bladder (158), sarcomas, and Hodgkin's disease (159), and in several benign diseases —gastrointestinal polyps, alcoholic cirrhosis of the liver, uremia, and inflammatory disease of the bowel (160,161). Since the first radioimmunoassays were developed for the CEA antigens, many refinements have appeared (162–167).

Carcinoembryonic antigen is recovered in good yield from perchloric acid extracts of adenocarcinomas of the colon, their liver metastases, or from fetal tissue of the gastrointestinal tract during the first two trimesters of gestation (168–170). Purification methods have included: Sepharose 4B columns, preparative electrophoresis, Sephadex G200 chromatography, and disruption of immune precipitates. Carcinoembryonic antigens may also be partially purified by affinity column chromatography on a concanavalin A ligand (171–173). It is undoubtedly the carbohydrate content of the antigen which allows the molecule to react with concanavalin A (171), and there is now evidence that CEA contains ABO blood-group substances, including the Lewis antigens (174-176). It has recently been postulated that the protein portion of the molecule of CEA provides the antigenicity and not the carbohydrate portion (177).

It was recently demonstrated that CEA isolated by the perchloric-acid method is not a single homogeneous substance, but in fact has considerable heterogeneity (175,178–180). Since CEA is found not only in adenocarcinoma of the colon but in a variety of other diseases, attempts are being made to identify particular variants or subtypes of CEA with more specific disease states. In order to accomplish this, Rule (179,181) made isoelectric-focusing fingerprints of the CEA derived from normal colon, fetal gut, and primary adenocarcinoma of the gut. These showed marked variability, each fingerprint having different quantities and distribution of isomers at the different isoelectric points tested. Nery (158) looked at the size of CEA fragments appearing in the urine of normal subjects. Differences were obtained in the elution profiles of CEA-like substances when normal and tumor patient's urine specimens were chromatographed on Sepharose 4B, indicating that CEA was shown to be heterogeneous not only on a molecular sieve column but on an affinity column as well. Rogers (173) separated the CEA obtained by perchloric acid extraction of a liver metastasis of a colon carcinoma into two fractions separable by 2% and 10% methyl glucoside on a concanavalin A sepharose column, indicating heterogeneity by still another criterion. David and Reisfeld (172) took advantage of the interaction of concanavalin A and CEA to show that absorption on Sepharose 4B concanavalin A makes an efficient storage method for ^{125}I CEA. Hughes (182) noted pH-dependent changes in the composition of CEA, which he believed to be due to aggregation of a cationic protein and metachromatic material. Coligan also found CEA to be heterogeneous by chromatography on ECTEOLA cellulose and showed that treatment of CEA with neuraminidase altered the electrophoretic migration of the molecules and somewhat decreased their heterogenecity (180).

Reisfeld has reinvestigated the problem of CEA heterogeneity and CEA-like antigens which may contaminate diagnostic reagents as a result of denaturation of the proteins during extraction by perchloric acid. CEA was isolated from several saline extracts of gastrointestinal tumors by virtue of its affinity for concanavalin A sepharose columns (172). The extracts were passed over lectin adsorbants (wheat germ agglutin, soybean agglutin, and maclura pomifera lectin), and thereby the blood group substances A, B, H, and Lea were removed from the preparations (183). These investigators speculate that the heterogeneity of CEA extracts results from the initial treatment with perchloric acid, which may hydrolyze some glycosidic bonds, and from the prolonged dialysis, which may cause denaturation and aggregation of molecules, contaminating the CEA with other proteins containing blood group substances.

Immunology of Fetal Antigens

An excellent review by Coggin and Anderson (184) covers in detail many of the central problems involved in the immunology of fetal antigens. Two of the major questions are whether fetal antigens are distinct from tumor transplantation antigens and whether the fetal antigens play a direct role in tumor rejection. Many investigators have concluded that the contribution of fetal antigens to tumor rejection is small. The major evidence for this comes from transplantation studies of sarcomas induced by chemical carcinogens. In these classic studies it was found that tumors induced by the same chemical carcinogen in animals of highly inbred strains were antigenically different from each other, in that preimmunization with one tumor produced a high degree of resistance against that tumor alone and not against others of the same series. More recently a variety of in vitro studies of the antigenicity of these same tumors have shown evidence of common antigens shared between different tumors of the same series (184). Moreover, these common antigens were frequently found in fetal tissues, and antibody against them appeared in the serum of multiparous females. Taken together, these studies strongly suggest that the highly tumor-specific antigen is responsible for tumor rejection, while the shared antigens, presumably of embryonic origin, are not.

Many virus-induced tumors also appear to have additional embryonic antigens. Ting (185) demonstrated that the fetal antigens of SV40-induced tumors in C3H/HeN mice were indeed distinct from the tumor transplantation antigens. Antisera raised against embryonic cells in males of the same strain were reacted with SV40 tumors, Gross and Rauscher leukemias, EL-4, mammary tumors, and plasma cell tumors. Embryonic tissues and tissues from the various tumors were able to absorb out the antiembryonic activity. The activity of antisera raised against the various tumor types, however, could be removed only by absorption with the specific tumor cell type, and not by absorption with embryonic tissue alone. These same investigators (186) also showed that more than one fetal antigen exists on SV40 tumor cells in mice and that these same antigens may be found on the spleen cells of normal allogeneic mice. Similar observations have been made by Invernizzi (187) in sarcoma of the mouse and by Bowen (188). The separate identities of fetal antigens and TSTA's in amino azo dye-induced and methylcholanthrene fibrosarcomas in rats have been confirmed by Baldwin (189) and Thompson (190).

Coggin (184) has done extensive work on the immunogenicity of fetal antigens expressed on SV40-induced tumors. Vaccines made from fetal tissues from primiparous hamsters were able to prevent SV40 tumors from arising in male hamsters (191). Another striking finding of this work was that the lymph node cells and peritoneal exudate cells of primiparous and multiparous female hamsters were cytotoxic against SV40 tumor cells but not against BHK (baby hamster kidney) cells, indicating that the peritoneal exudate cells and lymph node cells (LNC) were recognizing a familiar cell surface determinant. Similar lymphoid cells from pregnant females had greatly reduced cytotoxicity against SV40 tumor cells during a period in which cytostatic antibody appeared. The conditions of this work (184) should be noted. The times at which the embryos were taken for vaccine preparation were carefully controlled, since the antigens were not expressed throughout the entire gestation periods. It was also necessary for the fetal cells to be viable before irradiation and to be processed by methods which retained the surface antigen (i.e., not trypsinized). The cells were irradiated in order to prevent embryomas from forming. They were obtained from fetal tissues from primiparous females only, since cells from multiparous females were coated with cytostatic antibody which rendered them less immunogenic.

Contrasting results were obtained by another group (192), who implanted normal and immunosuppressed mice with allogeneic and syngeneic fetal tissues. In normal mice which had a previous syngeneic transplant of fetal tissue the second graft grew better. In fact, in those normal mice which had previously been inoculated with fetal tissue an injection of methylcholanthrene produced a tumor more rapidly than in groups of untreated mice. In a recent report (193) irradiated fetal cells from one- to two-week-old embryos did not protect against an SV40 tumor challenge in syngeneic mice, whereas irradiated cells from the SV40 tumor itself did. Rees (94) has demonstrated that immunization with fetal cells reduced the number of tumor nodules appearing in the lungs of mice which were injected intravenously with sarcoma cells.

The phenomenon of reexpression of fetal antigens on tumor cells of different histologic types in various species is being reinvestigated in vitro with the conclusion (195) that the embryonic antigens of colon tumors of rats are expressed in many types of rat embryonic tissue and that these embryonic antigens are immunogenic as tested by cytotoxicity assays utilizing the circulating lymphocytes of multiparous females. Sera from multiparous rats were able to detect embryonic antigens on chemically induced hepatomas, sarcomas, and mammary tumors (189,196–199). Fetal antigens of the rat appear to be at a maximum on the fourteenth and fifteenth day of gestation (198). Sera from multiparous rats were also shown to block the cytotoxicity of LNC from multiparous donors for tumor and fetal cells but did not block the cytotoxic action of immune LNC on the tumor cells (197).

ANTIGENS OF VIRUS-INDUCED TUMORS

A comprehensive review of the antigens of oncogenic viruses and virus-induced tumors is beyond the scope of the present work. The following includes selected aspects of an area which has undergone enormous development in the past few years and cites recent reviews for more details. Virus-induced tumors are characterized by the sharing of common antigens between different tumors induced by the same virus, even in different host species (200,201). This is reasonable when one considers that every cell successfully transformed by a given virus receives essentially the same package of genetic information. It will also be noted below that there is considerable sharing of antigens between related viruses and their respective tumors within larger groups, particularly among the RNA viruses. The sharing of antigens between virus-induced tumors is not necessarily to the exclusion of antigens specific for the individual tumor (202) or of embryonic antigens (184). This is in contradistinction to tumors induced by chemical carcinogens, where individual tumor-specific antigens are the rule but where there is an increasing amount of evidence for common cross-reacting antigens between different tumors, these latter usually of embryonic origin (106).

Virus-tumor systems have two major opportunities for antigen expression: the viruses themselves and new cellular antigens induced by the viruses (203). In both cases the new antigens may be located on the surface or in the interior of the virus or the cell. In the case of the DNA viruses the viral antigens and the cellular antigens have been easily separable by the alternative behavioral pathways seen in these systems. Cells that are "permissive" and produce complete virus particles are lysed in the process and do not undergo malignant transformation. Alternatively, cells that undergo malignant transformation and acquire new tumor-associated antigens carry the virus in a nonreplicating form and rarely produce intact virus. The result is that the viral antigens and new cellular antigens are not present under the same conditions and can be studied separately.

The RNA viruses present a much more complex situation, in that virus production is usually carried out continuously by the infected and transformed cell, so that viral and tumor antigens are present simultaneously. This has made it difficult to distinguish between these two sources of antigens. The problem is made more complicated by the fact that many of the RNA viruses are produced by budding off of the cell surface membranes and can introduce antigenic changes in these membranes during this process. Indeed, the outer membrane of the virus is adapted if not borrowed from the cell membrane in many respects.

Antigens of the DNA Virus-Induced Tumors

The DNA viruses are antigenic, as are the tumors that they induce. These two sources of antigen, virus particle and tumor cell, are separable because of the dichotomy in growth pattern that is characteristic of this group (204). Following infection with an oncogenic DNA virus the cell is usually forced to make a choice between supporting production of more virus, during which process it is eventually lysed, *or* undergoing malignant transformation without the production of intact virus. From cultures of permissive, virus-producing cells one can obtain pure viral materials for antigen study. The corresponding cellular materials are obtained from virus-free cultures of transformed cells. The smaller DNA tumor-inducing viruses, the papova viruses (polyoma and SV40), may represent the simplest model of virus tumor production. The capsid of each of these viruses has its own antigenic specificity or *V antigens,* detected by fluorescent antibody (205, 206).

Of greater importance are the cellular antigens induced by these viruses, none of which appears to have any relationship to structural materials of the virion itself. The *tumor antigen* (T antigen) demonstrated by complement fixation (207) was found to be localized in the nucleus by immunofluorescence (208,209). This antigen appears within 12 to 24 hours of infection with SV40 virus and is found in cells that are to be transformed as well as in cells destined to produce virus (206). In these latter cells it appears before evidence of viral capsid antigen or production of virions. Production of T antigen does not require viral DNA synthesis and therefore appears to be an early function of viral infection. The T antigen induced by SV40 virus in productively infected or transformed cells is antigenically similar even in different species (210). This fact alone establishes quite firmly that the antigen is induced by information coded for by the virus. The T antigen associated with SV40 virus is heat stable and resistant to DNase and RNase but sensitive to trypsin digestion (211). It has an estimated molecular weight of 200,000–250,000 by Sephadex G200 chromatography, but only of 70,000 to 80,000 when assayed by immunoabsorption (212).

A second internal cellular antigen induced by SV40 has been identified (213). The U antigen is found in the perinuclear region and differs from T antigen in being heat stable, but little more is known about it.

Cell Surface Antigens Induced by DNA Viruses (Polyoma and SV40).   The first evidence of cell surface antigen in virus-induced tumors was provided by Sjögren et al. (214) and Habel (215), in which mice and hamsters injected with polyoma virus were rendered resistant to subsequent challenge with viable polyoma tumor cells. Similar antigens were demonstrated by transplantation rejection in the SV40 system (216). These tumor-specific transplantation antigens (TSTA) have no relationship to the V or capsid antigens of the corresponding viruses, since antiviral antibodies have no adverse effect on the tumors. Cells transformed with SV40 can be shown to have TSTA by their capacity to preimmunize hamsters against transplantable SV40 tumor cells or to prevent the development of tumors in animals that were previously inoculated with the virus as newborns (217,218). The TSTA's of SV40-transformed human cells and those of hamster cells appear to be similar (219).

Surface Antigen (S Antigen) of SV40 Cells.   Attempts to demonstrate surface antigens on DNA virus-transformed cells in vitro also were fruitful. Because of the relative ease with which these studies could be carried out compared to immunization and graft rejection, they have been pursued extensively. *S antigen* was first demonstrated on SV40-transformed cells by direct immunofluorescence (220). The antibody gave a ring around the cell surface and was specific for SV40 in that it did not react with normal hamster cells or those transformed with other viruses. The S antigen of SV40-transformed human cells was found to be similar to that of SV40-transformed hamster cells, providing further evidence that this antigen was also induced specifically by the virus (221–223). Cytotoxic antisera has also been used to demonstrate surface antigen on these cells (223,224).

Although TSTA and S antigens are both present on the cell surface, there is evidence that they are *not* the same entity. SV40 cell lines produced by Diamandopoulos et al. (225) and tested by Tevethia et al. (226) were found to be positive for surface antigen but negative for the intranuclear T antigen. They were *not* rejected by immune animals, indicating that they also lacked TSTA. Cytotoxicity studies with hyperimmune mouse serum confirmed these findings (224), and this same cell line has also been found to be lacking SV40 specific messenger RNA (227) and SV40 DNA (228). The presence of the surface antigen in the absence of detectable quantities of SV40 genetic information suggested that expression of the S antigen may not require the viral genome at all. More recent studies have indicated that the S antigen may actually be a normal cellular constituent (229) which is detectable after virus transformation but which may also be revealed after gentle treatment with trypsin (230).

Burkitt Lymphoma and Epstein-Barr Virus.   The antigens associated with Burkitt lymphoma have been widely investigated and well reviewed (231). The first such antigen discovered was a *viral capsid antigen* (VCA) found by indirect immunofluorescence on acetone-fixed smears prepared from cultured lines derived from Burkitt lymphomas (232). The presence of this antigen correlated extremely well with the presence in culture cells of the virus closely associated with this tumor—EBV or Epstein-Barr virus, a member of the Herpes group of viruses (233). Virus-free lines from Burkitt patients did not have this antigen (234). Although the antigen originally described was intracellular, positive sera were able to coat virus particles, and the activity of the antisera could be absorbed out with concentrated virus, indicating that the antigen was a structural component of the virus capsid. It is of interest to note that the Epstein-Barr virus is antigenically very similar to, if not identical with, the agent that is responsible for infectious mononucleosis. Sera from patients with this disease are able to coat the virus and give positive immunofluorescence reactions when tested on Burkitt cells (235).

A second internal cellular antigen was also found by immunofluorescence (236). Because it was found in cells soon after infection with virus it was called *early antigen* (EA) to distinguish it from VCA described above, which appears late in the virus cycle. The production of EA is prevented by inhibitors of protein synthesis but not by inhibitors of DNA synthesis (237). Antibody against EA was present in the serum of Burkitt lymphoma patients more frequently than was anti-VCA, and the titers were high in tumor-bearing patients and low or nonexistent in patients undergoing total regression (238). Continued high titers in the presence of drug-induced regression was associated with a poor prognosis, while long-term survivors had low or nonexistent levels of this antibody.

Cell surface antigens, detected by direct or indirect membrane immunofluorescence, have been found on Burkitt cells, using sera from Burkitt patients. While these antigens are present on the surface of most biopsy specimens of Burkitt lymphoma, they are only found in cell lines that actually produce virus (239). Negative cell lines can be rendered positive for the membrane antigen by infection with EBV (237,240). In cultured cells the membrane antigen appeared 20–24 hours following virus infection and was not influenced by DNA inhibitors. In this sense the membrane antigen is similar to the EA antigen in that both are "early products" of the viral genome and do not require viral DNA synthesis for their expression.

In a competitive blocking assay (241) sera from most patients with Burkitt lymphoma (and nasopharyngeal carcinoma) showed high levels of antibody against the membrane antigen. Normal controls and relatives of Burkitt patients were usually negative (242). Titers of this antibody frequently fell in the course of rapid or extensive tumor growth and rose after successful chemotherapy and tumor regression. In individual patients, recurrence of the tumor following a period of regression was associated with a drop in the level of antibody against the membrane antigen. Whether this decline in antibody level precedes or follows active recurrence of the disease is not known. However, these are important alternatives, because the former situation implies that a loss of immunologic control may be *responsible* for the recurrence. Cells recovered from patients with late tumors have been found to be coated with immunoglobulin that is specific for the membrane antigen and raises the possibility that large amounts of specific antibody are absorbed to the growing tumor cells and that such absorption may contribute to the escape of the tumor through "autoenhancement."

Complement fixation studies using sera from patients and Burkitt cell lines disrupted by freezing and thawing or sonication were first carried out by Armstrong in 1966 (243). Sera positive by complement fixation were usually also positive for immunofluorescence against VCA. Further separation of the complement-fixing antigens resulted in soluble and sedimentable components (244–246). The soluble complement-fixing antigen appeared to be distinct from the VCA, in that it was found in cell lines that were free of EBV by electron microscopy and were negative for VCA by fluorescence. Antibodies against the S antigen could not be absorbed out with EBV-positive or EBV-negative cell lines, and absorption with purified S antigen did not remove antibody directed against VCA. The S antigen could not be localized within the cell by immunofluorescence or on the surface of the cell as a membrane antigen. Instead, it appears to be a cellular rather than a viral antigen, but coded by the viral genome. In this way it resembles the T antigen of other DNA virus systems (246).

Soluble antigen recovered from freeze-thawed and homogenized Burkitt cell lines gave *precipitin reactions* with sera from Burkitt patients (247). The precipitating antigens were found in cells known to produce EBV and which were positive for VCA by immunofluorescence. Antibody against this soluble precipitating antigen fell to low or undetectable levels during tumor regression but reappeared upon recurrence (248). It is felt that this antigen, like the early antigen (EA) detected by immunofluorescence, is probably a cellular antigen representing an early product of viral transformation.

Delayed hypersensitivity skin reactions have been obtained with antigen extracts of Burkitt lymphoma (249). As with other studies of delayed hypersensitivity with tumor antigens, an apparent correlation with prognosis existed.

Carcinoma of the Cervix and Herpes Simplex Type II Virus.   A second virus of the herpes family, Herpes Simplex Type II (HSV-II), has been seriously implicated as the causative agent for carcinoma of the cervix. The initial studies noted the association between infections with genital herpes and cervical dysplasia and cancer (250). Antibody capable of neutralizing HSV-II has been recovered from the circulation of women with cervical neoplasia (251,252). Cellular antigens, not related to the structural material of the virus, were identified using serum extensively absorbed with stable virion antigens (253). Attempts to purify the antigens by low-frequency sonication, centrifugation, and polyacrylamide gel electrophoresis resulted in preparations that gave positive complement fixation reactions with sera from patients with carcinoma of the cervix, carcinoma of the larynx, and other assorted carcinomas of the head and neck (254).

RNA Viruses

RNA viruses are known to be responsible for mammary carcinoma of the mouse and a wide spectrum of leukemias, lymphomas, and sarcomas in experimental animals. They have been implicated in human carcinomas of the breast, acute myelogenous leukemia, transitional cell carcinoma of the urogenital tract, and sarcomas. The C-type RNA tumor viruses are by far the largest single group of oncogenic viruses and one of the best studied so far (255). The members of this complex family of viruses are large, measuring 1,200 to 1,400 Å in diameter, and are assembled by budding off the cell surface or into vacuoles within the cell (256). A complex system of common and shared antigens, both viral and cellular, is found among the tumors induced by these viruses, even in different species, indicating considerable overlap of genetic information carried by the different viruses in the group. The antigens that have been studied fall into two main classes: (1) structural proteins of the virus particles themselves, and (2) cellular antigenic materials induced by viral genetic information. The virus particles have antigens on the envelope of the virus as well as internal antigens. Similarly, the tumor cells have virus-induced antigens on the cell surface and within the cell.

Antigens of the Virus Envelope.   The virus envelope antigens (VEA) fall into at least two different major categories plus two subcategories (257). Sufficient studies have not yet been carried out to determine whether all of the mammalian RNA viruses express all four of these.

Group specific virus envelope antigens (gs-VEA) are common to all of the known murine C-type viruses, regardless of the type of tumor induced. The virus envelope antigens may also include interspecies group specific antigens (interspec. antigens), which are shared between C-type particles responsible for tumors in different mammalian species.

Type specific virus envelope antigens (ts-VEA) are specific for certain tumors within a given species and may even show subtypes for a given tumor. Hence, the murine leukemia virus family shows at least two major serological groups, G (Gross) virus and FMR (Friend, Moloney, Rauscher). In the murine system the original subgroupings of G and FMR on the basis of sera types may be further subdivided into still greater specificity by immunoelectron microscopy (257). Similarly, the feline leukemia viruses have three antigenic subgroups. These antigens appear to be glycoproteins or are carried on glycoprotein molecules, having molecular weights of 40,000 to 60,000 for the smaller species and 70,000 to 93,000 for the larger (258,259). Isolation and characterization of the mammalian virus envelope antigens has not been carried nearly as far as that of the avian viruses.

The envelope antigens, particularly the type specific envelope antigens, may be partially responsible for the specificity of the strains of animals that can be successfully infected with a given virus, presumably through the capacity of the cells to adsorb the virus, although there is now evidence of postpenetration restriction of infection.

Internal Viral Antigens.   The interior of the virus also contains antigenic material, of which two major classes have been identified in mammalian C-type particles. The more inclusive of these is the interspecies group specific antigen (gs-interspec.), which cross-reacts among C-type particles isolated from different mammalian species (260,261). The other is more specific and is the group specific antigen (gs-spec.) for a given species. Both of these appear to be polypeptides of molecular weight approximately 30,000 (262).

It should also be noted that the C-type viruses carry an important enzyme, DNA polymerase or "reverse transcriptase" (263), the function of which is to anticode the RNA information of the virus into DNA for insertion into the genetic apparatus of the cell. Antisera prepared against the reverse transcriptases from different viral species have been compared and have revealed that the antigenic specificity of the enzyme closely correlates with that of the interspecies antigen. The reverse transcriptases of the rodent mammalian viruses appear to be very similar to each other, as do those of the monkey viruses, but these two general categories do not cross-react strongly with each other (264), nor does either of them show antigenic similarity with reverse transcriptase of avian (265) and C-type viruses or the B-type viruses from other species.

Virus-Induced Intracellular Antigens.   Unlike the DNA viruses, where virus production and malignant transformation take place in different cells, the RNA viruses propagate continuously in the transformed cell, a factor which has complicated the search for virus-induced cellular antigens. A trick that has circumvented this problem was the induction of tumors with C-type viruses from heterologous species (i.e., hamster cells transformed with murine sarcoma virus), where the cells undergo transformation but fail to produce infectious virus (266). New antigens of the group specific type were found in these cells (267), but these were later shown to be the internal group specific antigens of the virion (268). The presence of these antigens was indicative of incomplete virus production, since viral-envelope antigens were not found in such cells. At present no truly virus-induced intracellular antigens have been found in the C-type virus mammalian systems. It should be noted that the intracellular gs antigens detected in these nonproducing tumor cells do not correspond to the T antigens which are found in cells transformed by the papova viruses: (1) They are virion antigens and not true cellular antigens. (2) They are localized in the cytoplasm rather than in the nucleus. (3) They are not found in all nonproducing cells and may even disappear from malignant cells; therefore, even this antigenic evidence of abortive virus information is not required for maintenance of malignant cells.

Virus-Induced Cell Surface Antigens.   The surface of the cell transformed with a C-type RNA virus is even more of an antigenic battleground. In addition to new tumor-specific antigens induced by the virus, the virus particles themselves are continuously budding off, expressing their own virion-envelope antigens on the cell surface as they do so. Tumor-specific antigens responsible for graft rejection were first shown for the DNA polyoma virus-induced tumor by Sjögren et al. (214) and Habel (215). Studies in the SV40 system showed conclusively that these tumor-specific transplantation antigens (TSTA) were not structural proteins of the virion. The corresponding TSTA of the RNA virus-induced tumors were first shown by Klein et al. (269) for murine leukemia virus and by Sjögren and Jonsson (270) for Rous sarcoma virus. Because of the ever-presence of the virus it was not clear whether these were truly new cellular antigens or whether they were viral envelope antigens on the cell surface acting as transplantation antigens and responsible for graft rejection. The original demonstration of these antigens was by preimmunization and graft rejection, resulting in their classification as *tumor-specific transplantation antigens* (TSTA). Subsequent studies showed that surface antigens on these cells could be demonstrated in vitro with cytotoxic or fluorescent antibody (105). Because of the ease with which they could be studied, these *tumor-specific surface antigens* (TSSA) have received much more attention. Although it is frequently assumed that TSSA's are the same antigenic specificities as the TSTA's responsible for graft rejection, this has not been proven.

Definitive identification of virus envelope antigens and TSSA as separate identities required the development of antisera with only one specificity. An antiserum against Gross lymphoma cells which had no virus-neutralizing activity was reported by Geering et al. (271). Similarly, absorption of antisera with virus concentrates removed virus-neutralizing capacity but not reactivity with cell surface antigens (272). Antibody has also been produced which is specific for the virion surface and does not bind to the tumor cell surface. Immunoelectron microscopy

(102) demonstrated virus envelope antigen on the cell surface, localized mainly to the sites of virus budding. During this process, when the antigen was still a fixed component of the cell surface, it could easily be the target for cellular cytotoxicity or cytotoxic antibody and thus act as a transplantation-type antigen.

The TSSA is not randomly distributed but rather appears in localized areas on the cell surface. By immunoelectron microscopy it was shown that these areas are devoid of normal histocompatibility antigens (102). Moreover, the expression of TSSA fluctuates throughout the cell cycle, being maximal in the G1 phase (273). Because of difficulties of isolation and characterization of TSSA of RNA virus-induced tumors, little information is available about the biochemical nature of these antigens. A putative viral envelope antigen isolated from murine leukemia cells was a glycoprotein with a molecular weight of about 70,000 (274).

Bauer listed several important conclusions concerning the C-type RNA tumor viruses (255): (1) Failure to detect virion antigen in the cell does not indicate the absence of virus genome. (2) Virion antigens can be present without concomitant production of intact virus particles. Synthesis of virion antigens is not prerequisite to the development or persistence of the malignant state of transformed cells. (3) No antigen has been discovered that is absolutely specific to or required by the malignant cells.

To these may be added the fact that the cell surface represents its most vulnerable point for immune attack, and further characterization of the antigens of virus-induced tumors is greatly needed. The fact that common antigens appear between different tumors induced by the same virus, even in different species, may provide materials for immunotherapy of virus induced tumors. Table 1 summarizes some of the information about tumor viruses.

Table 1   Tumor Viruses

Nucleic Acid	Viral Group	Animal Group	Proposed Human Tumors
RNA	Leukovirus:		
	type B	Murine breast	Breast cancer
	type C	Leukoma, lymphoma, sarcoma	Acute myelogenesis leukemia
			Transitional cell cancer of urogenital tract
			Sarcomas
DNA	Adenovirus	Many	None
	Papovaviruses	SV40, polyoma	Wart, laryngeal papilloma
	Herpes Viruses	Marek's disease, frog	Epstein-Barr-Burkitt lymphoma
		Renal cancer, lymphatic	Nasopharyngeal
		Leukemia in marmosets and owl monkeys	Simplex Type II—cervical cancer
	Pox	Fibromas—rabbits and squirrels	
		Fibromo sarcoma—rabbit	Histocytoma (benign)
		Histocytoma—monkeys	

BIOLOGICAL FUNCTION OF TUMOR-ASSOCIATED ANTIGENS

Tumor-associated antigens appear to be a heterogeneous group of materials. The fetal antigens collectively known as CEA appear to be glycoproteins. Most attempts at purification of tumor-specific antigens have failed to remove all carbohydrate or lipid and therefore provide no conclusive evidence that the antigenic moiety is protein or protein associated with carbohydrate and/or lipid.

Location of Tumor Antigens

Very little is known of the true biological function of tumor antigens. They may be slightly abnormal but relatively unimportant "building blocks" in the cell membrane. An intriguing possibility (186–188) is that some tumor-specific antigens represent altered normal cellular antigens. This is supported by the facts that the isolation procedures that were developed for normal transplantation antigens have been widely applicable to preparation of tumor antigens and that some tumor antigens appear to be biochemically very similar to their normal counterparts. A variation is the possibility that the tumor antigens result from subtle but significant realignments and reorganization of the cell surface membrane, where adjacent configurations express their new relationships as antigenic differences from the original cell (275,276). Finally, some tumor-specific antigens may represent important receptor sites on the surface of the cell or even may have enzymatic activity directly responsible for aggressive malignant behavior.

The concentrations of tumor antigens and normal transplantation antigens on the surface of the cell show an inverse relationship. Those tumors with a high level of tumor antigenicity appear to be the same ones that have a poor representation of normal transplantation antigens, and vice versa (276,277). It is of note that single normal transplantation antigenic specificities do not appear to be completely absent; rather, the representation of all the antigens appears to be deficient. Except in some virus-induced tumors, little is known of the spatial relationship between these two families of antigens. Tumor antigens may be in clusters, replacing clusters of normal antigens, or they may be intermixed with the normal antigens and relatively evenly distributed over the cell surface. The relationship is probably not a simple and direct one, because there is evidence that the genetic determinant for the tumor antigen of an MCA sarcoma is *not* on the same chromosome that carries the H-2 determinants (278).

Like other cell-surface components, tumor-specific antigens appear to undergo fluctuations in their representation on the cell surface that are related to different stages in the cell cycle (273). To the limited extent that this has been studied, antigenic representation appears to be maximal in the G1 phase. However, it is unlikely that this generalization applies to all of the tumor antigens or, perhaps, even to all of the normal transplantation antigens.

All tumor-associated antigens are not necessarily expressed only on the surface of the cell. For obvious reasons those that are on the surface are more easily detected and are in a position to play a more direct role in the interaction between the tumor cell and its environment. However, membrane alterations that are expressed on the surface of the cell may also be present on internal cellular membranes, and some tumor antigens, particularly in virus-induced tumors, are found exclusively within the cell.

Blocking and Enhancement

The shedding of antigen from the surface of tumor cells represents a potential mechanism by which the tumor may escape from immunologic control (279). Such antigens could have free access to the circulation, enabling them to bind to and "neutralize" antibody and immune lymphoid cells in the circulation or in lymphoid organs (280). Production of antigen for "export" may be confined to tumor-specific antigens, in which case it may represent a successful adaptive mechanism to counteract immune control of the tumor. Conversely, release of antigen by the cell may be the result of a high rate of turnover of many cell-membrane materials, including normal and tumor-specific antigens (281). The finding that large amounts of normal HLA antigen can be recovered from the plasma of blood donors suggests that these materials, too, are products of metabolic turnover and release (282). It is not known whether the production and release of normal transplantation antigens are significantly increased in tumor cells.

The first evidence that circulating factors from immunized animals may have an "enhancing" effect on tumor growth came from the use of alloantisera in mouse sarcoma systems (283). Although more difficult to demonstrate, similar enhancement was also obtained with antisera directed against tumor-specific antigens (284). The active component of the sera was thought to be specific antibody. The "blocking" of cellular cytotoxicity by serum from tumor-bearing individuals was proposed as the in vitro counterpart for "enhancement" of tumor growth (285). It was noted that the serum of the immune animal may contain antibody, antigen-antibody complex, or even free antigen, and the emphasis was transferred from antibody to antigen-antibody complexes as the serum factors responsible for blocking (68). The blocking capacity of free antigen has also been strongly implicated by the demonstration that antigen alone, as well as in the form of an immune complex, is bound by immune lymphocytes and "inhibits" their cytotoxic capacity. Also, antibody or complexes may be bound by target cells, in which position they are able to "block" the killing by lymphocytes (286). It should be noted that the presence of free antigen in the circulation of the "tumor immune" individual signifies the saturation of all accessible antigen binding sites, both humoral and cellular, for that antigen. In addition to its capacity to interfere directly with the interaction between immune lymphoid cells and tumor cells, circulating antigen may exert a central depression on the immune response, inducing tolerance.

Disposal of Antigens

Little is known of the mechanism of disposal of antigens that may be released into the circulation by tumors. Oldstone showed that AKR mice, previously thought to be tolerant to Gross leukemia virus, retained large deposits of complexes containing GLV antigen and leukemia cell membranes in their kidneys (287,288). The murine leukemia virus has also been implicated in the complexes found in the glomerular deposits in older NZB mice (289). Other murine tumors showing evidence of such deposits are: the B16 melanoma in C57BL/6 mice (290), the mammary tumor in a Paris R-111 mouse (291), and mice bearing neuroblastomas (292). Analogous deposits have been found in the following human cancers: lymphoma and leukemia (293), colon carcinoma (294), Hodgkin's disease (295), and transitional cell carcinoma (296). However, with the exception of some lymphomas and leukemias, deposition of significant amounts of complexes resulting in impaired renal function is not a common clinical feature, even in advanced malignancy. At least three possibilities may account for this: (1) Antigen-antibody complexes may not be produced in significant amounts. (2) The complexes may be small in size and therefore not fixed to the renal membranes. (3) The antigen component of the complexes may not be sufficiently "foreign" to cause deposition in the membranes. Degradation of complexes in the kidney may permit significant amounts of antigen to be released into the urine, where some studies suggest that it can be found (282,297–298).

Recently a number of procedures have been used to detect immune complexes in serum: polyethylene glycol precipitation (299,300); detection with Clq in agarose (301); precipitation with monoclonal rheumatoid factor (302); detection by uptake by macrophages (303); inhibition of humoral cytotoxicity (304); cytoprecipitation (305); microcomplement consumption (306); and adsorption to the Raji lymphoma cell (307). Of these, only the last has been applied to tumor systems. This method utilizes Raji cells for the immobilization of the complexes to C3b-C3d receptors present on these cells. The lower limit of sensitivity of the test appears to be 200–300 nanograms of immune complex, making it a potential method for detecting complexes in the sera of tumor-bearing individuals. Theofilopoulos has now refined the Raji assay utilizing ^{125}I-radiolabeled antiglobulin in order to make the assay quantitative. Antigen-antibody complexes were measured in the serum of mice with LCM virus, in the serum of rabbits with serum sickness, and in serum of patients with glomerular nephritis, systemic lupus, dengue hemorrhagic fever, vasculitis, subacute sclerosing panencephalitis, and several malignancies, using aggregated human IgG as the standard for quantitation.

An approach to removal of antigen-antibody complexes from serum has been demonstrated with Protein A from *Staphylococcus aureus*. This protein specifically removed IgG and blocking activity from serum (308), as tested with cellular cytotoxicity in polyoma-induced sarcomas and colon carcinoma systems in rats. If the immune response results in continuous production of antibody and the tumor releases significant amounts of antigen, complexes of these two materials may accumulate to quite high levels in the circulation. The separation of such complexes from other serum components would provide starting material from which highly purified antigen and antibody could be isolated.

Uses of Tumor Antigens

A wide range of potential uses exist for purified tumor antigens. For some tumors (i.e., in virus-induced tumors) there may be a direct relationship between the antigen and the cause of the malignancy. The detection of truly specific antigen could provide a reliable diagnostic tool. The presence of free antigen or antigen-antibody complexes in the circulation may be related to the extent of the disease, to the existence of metastasis, and even to the prognosis under various conditions of treatment. Finally, purification of tumor-associated antigen will permit better characterization and identification of the true biological function of these materials, over and above their capacity to stimulate the immune response.

For purposes of specific immunotherapy, soluble antigens offer several advantages over processed tumor cells. They can be freed of viable tumor cells and of residual oncogenic virus, providing a safer material than tumor cells or crude products. Purified antigen would be expected to induce a high level of immunity against a single immunogen and can be stored easily in the frozen state. Tumor antigens solubilized with KCl have been used to immunize animals against syngeneic sarcoma (28,29). In a rigorous set of experiments these investigators showed that immunity against two non-cross-reacting methycholanthrene-induced fibrosarcomas could be obtained with single small doses of soluble antigen. This response was specific, since the mice inoculated with lethal doses of fibrosarcoma C in one flank and fibrosarcoma F in the other flank died from the tumor to which they were not immunized. Surprisingly, the dose of crude KCl extract that protected against tumor challenge was effective only over a very narrow range, since too small a dose simply diminished the rate of growth of the tumor to which the host was immunized while too large a dose gave no protection at all (29). Drapkin (27) was also able to show immunoprotection against SV40 tumors in vivo by papain-solubilized antigen partially purified on a Sephadex G150 column.

Other investigators who have worked with soluble extracts and tumor-membrane preparations to achieve immunoprotection have had little success. Baldwin (71) showed that a membrane suspension given in multiple injections did not immunize rats in vivo or in vitro against the amino azo dye hepatomas from which the crude membranes were made, even when they were admixed with bacterial adjuvants. The sera taken from membrane-immunized animals abrogated cell-mediated cytotoxicity, and the LNC's taken from such animals performed poorly in a colony inhibition assay against plated hepatoma cells (70, 309). In a comparable human study done in vitro with lymphocytes from colon carcinoma patients, soluble, papain-digested colon tumor membrane inhibited cytotoxicity, but extracts of melanoma or normal colon did not (310). Mice injected with 500 μg of 3M KCl extract of the EL4 lymphoma (311) showed impaired cellular cytotoxicity in their spleen cells against ^{51}Cr-labeled EL-4 cells. Their serum lacked complement-dependent cytotoxic antibodies, in contrast to the serum of mice which had received irradiated cells for immunization.

Induction of cell-mediated immunity in vitro against *normal* alloantigens has been accomplished by a number of investigators. However, the response to cell-bound alloantigen has been quite predictable, in contrast to the conflicting results obtained with subcellular and soluble preparations of alloantigen. In some studies exposure of immunocompetent murine lymphocytes in vitro to alloantigen not only produced a proliferative response but also stimulated the maturation of cytotoxic lymphocytes (312–314). Koldovsky (313) observed that C57BL/6 spleen and lymph-node cells when mixed with a crude membrane extract of BALB/c origin for 4–5 hours and then allowed to mature for 4–5 days in diffusion chambers implanted in the peritoneal cavity of Swiss mice or in petri dishes with a monolayer of C57 embryo fibroblasts become cytotoxic toward BALB/c fibroblasts. Similarly, Wagner (314) found that CBA thymocytes exposed in vitro for 6 days to a membrane preparation of alloantigenic mastocytoma cells (P815-X-Z) or lymphoma cells (EL-4) became specifically cytotoxic toward whole tumor cells in a Cr^{51}-release assay. More recently Corley (312) reported that normal human peripheral blood lymphocytes that were incubated in vitro with a membrane preparation of PHA-stimulated IM-1 lymphoblasts underwent proliferation as well as a cytotoxic response. In contrast to these studies, which imply that subcellular antigen preparations are good immunogens, Bonavida (315) observed in an allogeneic murine system that 3M KCl-extracted antigen *inhibited* the cytotoxicity of immune lymphocytes if preincubated with them prior to their use in a Cr^{51}-release assay.

Attempts to immunize lymphoid cells with soluble cellular antigen in vitro have frequently met with failure to induce demonstrable cellular cytotoxicity. Our laboratory has investigated the ability of a 3M KCl extract of an MCA sarcoma to induce a secondary immune response in vitro. We observed that C3H/HeJ spleen cells resected from mice 8–12 weeks after amputation of a progressively growing sarcoma were not cytotoxic in a microcytotoxicity assay, but they could generate a cytotoxic population of cells if incubated with whole, live, isologous mitomycin-treated tumor cells for 72 hours or longer. In contrast, a 3M KCl extract of isologous tumor cells that was capable of stimulating a *proliferative response* (i.e., lymphocyte stimulation) did *not* consistently induce maturation of cytotoxic lymphocytes in vitro in the same population of immune lymphocytes that responded to the intact tumor cells. The form in which the antigen is presented to the immune system and the mechanism by which it is handled are undoubtedly important factors in determining the nature and extent of the immune response.

REFERENCES

1. Nathenson, S. G., *Ann. Rev. Genetics* **4,** 69–90 (1970).
2. Nathenson, S. G., and Cullen, S. E., *Biochem. et Biophys. Acta* **344,** 1–25 (1974).
3. Mann, D. L., and Fahey, J. L., *Ann. Rev. Micro.* **25,** 679–710 (1971).
4. Kahan, B. D., and Reisfeld, R. A., eds., *Transplantation Antigens: Markers of Biological Individuality*, Academic Press, New York, 1972.
5. Shreffler, D. C., and David, C. S., *Adv. in Immunol.* **20,** 125–195 (1975).
6. Yamane, K., and Nathenson, S. G., *Biochem.* **9,** 4743–4750 (1970).
7. Schwartz, B. D., and Nathenson, S. G., *J. Immunol.* **107,** 1363–1367 (1971).
8. Nathenson, S. G., Schwartz, B. D., and Cullen, S. E., in *Membranes and Viruses in Immunopathology* (R. A. Good and Stacey Day, eds.), Academic Press, New York, 1972, pp. 117–129.
9. Cullen, S. E., and Nathenson, S. G., *J. Immunol.* **107,** 563–570 (1971).
10. Cullen, S. E., David, C. S., Shreffler, D. C., and Nathenson, S. G., *Proc. Natl. Acad. Sci. USA* **71,** 648–652 (1974).
11. Von Hippel, P. H., and Schleich, T., in *Structure and Stability of Biological Macromolecules* (Serge Timasheff and Gerald D. Fasman, eds.), Marcel Dekker, Inc., 1969, pp. 417–574.
12. Mann, D. L., *Transplan.,* **14,** 398–401 (1972).
13. Springer, T. A., Strominger, J. L., and Mann, D., *Proc. Natl. Acad. Sci. USA* **71,** 1539–1543 (1974).

14. Nakamuro, K., Tanigaki, N., and Pressman, D., *Proc. Natl. Acad. Sci. USA* **70**, 2863–2865 (1973).

15. Cresswell, P., Springer, T., Strominger, J. L., Turner, M. J., Grey, H. M., and Kubo, R. T., *Proc. Natl. Acad. Sci. USA* **71**, 2123–2127 (1974).

16. Peterson, P. A., Rask, L., and Lindblom, J. B., *Proc. Natl. Acad. Sci. USA* **71**, 35–39 (1974).

17. Vitetta, E. S., Uhr, J. W., and Boyse, E. A., *J. Immunol.* **114**, 252–254 (1975).

18. "β₂-Microglobulin and HL-A Antigen," Moller, G., ed., *Transplan. Rev.* **21**, 3–143, Munksgaard Copenhagen, 1974.

19. Thieme, T. R., Raley, R. A., and Fahey, J. L., *J. Immunol.* **113**, 323–328 (1974).

20. Pellegrino, M. A., Pellegrino, A., Ferrone, S., Kahan, B. D., and Reisfeld, R. A., *J. Immunol.* **111**, 783–788 (1973).

21. Billing, R. J., Mittal, K. K., and Terasaki, P. I., *Tissue Antigens* **3**, 251–256 (1973).

22. Billing, R. J., and Terasaki, P. J., *J. Immunol.* **112**, 1124–1130 (1974).

23. Dawson, J. R., Silver, J., and Sheppard, L. B., et al., *J. Immunol.* **112**, 1190–1193 (1974).

24. Dawson, J. R., Shasby, S. S., and Amos, D. B., *J. Immunol.* **111**, 281–283 (1973).

25. Pellegrino, M. A., Ferrone, S., and Pellegrino, A., in *Transplantation Antigens: Markers of Biological Individuality* (Barry Kahan and Ralph Reisfeld, eds.), Chap. 21, "Serologic Detection of Soluble HLA Antigens," pp. 433–452, Academic Press, New York, 1972.

26. Klein, G., Sjögren, H. O., Klein, E., and Hellström, K. E., *Cancer Res.* **20**, 1561–1572 (1960).

27. Drapkin, M. S., Appella, E., and Law, L. W., *J. Natl. Cancer Inst.* **52**, 259–264 (1974).

28. Pellis, N. R., Tom, B. H., and Kahan, B. D., *J. Immunol.* **113**, 708–711 (1974).

29. Pellis, N. R., and Kahan, B. D., *J. Immunol.* **115**, 1717–1722 (1975).

30. Kahan, B. D., and Pellis, N. R., at the Eighth Annual Meeting of the Assoc. for Academic Surgery, Los Angeles, Nov. 7–9 (1975) (in press).

31. Meltzer, M. S., Leonard, E. J., Hardy, A. S., and Rapp, H. J., *J.N.C.I.* **54**, 1349–1354 (1975).

32. Law, L. W., Henriksen, O., and Appella, E., *Nature* **257**, 234–235 (1975).

33. Hollinshead, A. C., McWright, C. G., Alford, T. C., Glew, D. H., et al., *Science* **177**, 887–889 (1972).

34. Oren, M. E., and Herberman, R. B., *Clin. Exp. Immunol.* **9**, 45–56 (1971).

35. Meltzer, M. S., Oppenheim, J. J., Littman, B. H., Leonard, E. J., and Rapp, H. J., *J.N.C.I.* **49**, 727–734 (1972).

36. Holmes, E. C., Reisfeld, R. A., and Morton, D. L., *Cancer Res.* **33**, 199–202 (1973).

37. Hollinshead, A. C., Jaffurs, W. T., Alpert, L. K., Harris, J. E., and Herberman, R. B., *Cancer Res.* **34**, 2961–2968 (1974).

38. Alford, C., and Hollinshead, A. C., *Ann. Surgery* **178**, 20–24 (1973).

39. Hollinshead, A., Tarro, G., Foster, W. A., Jr., Seigel, L. J., and Jaffurs, W., *Cancer Res.* **34**, 1122–1125 (1974).

40. Hollinshead, A. C., Stewart, T. H., and Herberman, R. B., *J.N.C.I.* **52**, 327–338 (1974).

41. Hollinshead, A. C., *Fed. Proc.* **34**, 1042 (1975).

42. Roth, J., Slocum, H. A., Pellegrino, M., Holmes, E. C., and Reisfeld, R. A., *Cancer Res.* (1976) (in press).

43. McCoy, J. L., Jerome, L. F., Dean, J. H., et al., *J.N.C.I.* **53**, 11–17 (1974).

44. Mavligit, G. M., Ambus, U., Gutterman, J. U., Hersh, E. M., and McBride, C. M., *Nat. New Biol.* **243**, 188–190 (1973).

45. Eilber, F. R., Morton, D. L., and Ketcham, A. S., *Amer. J. Surgery* **128**, 534–538 (1974).

46. Pinsky, C. M., Domeiri, A., Caron, A. S., Knapper, W. H., and Oettgen, H. F., "Delayed-Hypersensitivity Reactions in Patients with Cancer," *Recent Results in Cancer Research*, Vol. 47 (G. Mathe and R. Weiner, eds.), Springer-Verlag, Berlin, New York, 1974.

47. Occhino, J. C., Glasgow, A. H., Cooperband, S., Mannick, J. A., and Schmid, K., *J. Immunol.* **110**, 685–694 (1973).

48. Glaser, M., and Herberman, R. B., *J.N.C.I.* **53**, 1767–1769 (1974).

49. Frost, P., and Lance, E. M., *Nature* **246,** 101–103 (1973).

50. Nelken, D., *J. Immunol.* **110,** 1161–1162 (1973).

51. Veit, B., and Michael, J. G., *J. Immunol.* **111,** 341–351 (1973).

52. Bernstein, I. D., Zbar, B., and Rapp, H. J., *J.N.C.I.* **49,** 1641–1647 (1972).

53. Hellström, I., *Int. J. Cancer* **2,** 65–68 (1967).

54. Brunner, K. T., Manuel, J., Cerottini, J. C., and Chapuis, B., *Immunol.* **14,** 181–196 (1968).

55. Jagarlamoody, S. M., Aust, J. C., Tew, R. H., and McKhann, C. F., *Proc. Natl. Acad. Sci. USA* **68,** 1346–1350 (1971).

56. Bean, M. A., Pees, H., Fogh, J. E., Grabstald, H., and Oettgen, H. F., *Int. J. Cancer* **14,** 186–197 (1974).

57. Hellström, K. E., and Hellström, I., *Adv. Immunol.* **18,** 209–277 (1974).

58. McKhann, C. F., Cleveland, P. H., and Burk, M. W., *Natl. Cancer Inst. Monogr.* **37,** 37–39 (1973).

59. Takasugi, M., Mickey, M. R., and Terasaki, P. I., *Cancer Res.* **33,** 2898–2902 (1973).

60. Pierce, G. E., and DeVald, B. L., *Cancer Res.* **35,** 1830–1839 (1975).

61. Heppner, G., Henry, E., Stolbach, L., Cummings, F., McDonough, E., and Calabresi, P., *Cancer Res.* **35,** 1931–1937 (1975).

62. Irie, R. F., Irie, K., and Morton, D. L., *J.N.C.I.* **52,** 1051–1058 (1974).

63. Irie, R. F., Irie, K., and Morton, D. L., *J.N.C.I.* **53,** 1545–1551 (1974).

64. Avis, F., Mosonov, I., and Haughton, G., *J.N.C.I.* **52,** 1041–1049 (1974).

65. Hellström, I., Warner, G. A. Hellström, K. E., and Sjögren, H. O., *Int. J. Cancer* **11,** 280–292 (1973).

66. Heppner, G. H., Stolbach, L., Byrne, M., Cummings, F. J., McDonough, E., and Calabresi, P., *Int. J. Cancer* **11,** 245–260 (1973).

67. Wood, W. C., and Morton, D. L., *Science* **170,** 1318–1320 (1970).

68. Sjögren, H. O., Hellström, I., Bansal, S. C., and Hellström, K. E., *Proc. Natl. Acad. Sci.* **68,** 1372–1375 (1971).

69. Baldwin, R. W., Price, M. R., and Robins, R. A., *Nat. New Biol.* **238,** 185–186 (1972).

70. Baldwin, R. W., Embleton, M. J., and Robins, R. A., *Int. J. Cancer* **11,** 1–10 (1973).

71. Baldwin, R. W., Embleton, M. J., and Moore, M., *Br. J. Cancer* **28,** 389–399 (1973).

72. Thomson, D. M., Eccles, S., and Alexander, P., *Br. J. Cancer* **28,** 6–15 (1973).

73. Thomson, D. M., Steele, K., and Alexander, P., *Br. J. Cancer* **27,** 27–34 (1973).

74. Kolb, J. P., Poupon, M. F., and Lespinats, G., *J.N.C.I.* **52,** 723–727 (1974).

75. Jose, D. G., and Seshadri, R., *Int. J. Cancer* **13,** 824–838 (1974).

76. Ankerst, J., *Cancer Res.* **31,** 997–1003 (1971).

77. Wright, P., Hargreaves, R. E., Bansal, S. C., Bernstein, I., and Hellström, K. E., *Proc. Natl. Acad. Sci.* **70,** 2539–2543 (1973).

78. Bansal, S. C., and Sjögren, H. O., *Int. J. Cancer* **12,** 179–193 (1973).

79. Wright, P. W., Hargreaves, R. E., Bernstein, I. D., and Hellström, I., *J. Immunol.* **112,** 1267–1270 (1974).

80. Tamerius, J., Hellström, I., and Hellström, K. E., *Int. J. Cancer* **16,** 456–464 (1975).

81. Vaage, J., *Cancer Res.* **34,** 2979–2983 (1974).

82. Dauphinee, M. J., Talal, N., and Witz, I. P., *J. Immunol.* **113,** 948–953 (1974).

83. Faanes, R. B., and Choi, Y. S., *J. Immunol.* **113,** 279–288 (1974).

84. Leonard, E. J., *J. Immunol.* **110,** 1167–1169 (1973).

85. Currie, G. A., and Alexander, P., *Br. J. Cancer* **29,** 72–75 (1974).

86. Burk, M. W., Yu, S., Ristow, S. S., and McKhann, C. F., *Int. J. Cancer* **15,** 99–108 (1975).

87. Burk, M. W., Ristow, S. S., and Yu, S., *Fed. Proc.* **34,** 1042 (1975).

88. Senik, A., Gomard, E., Plata, F., and Levy, J. P., *Int. J. Cancer* **12,** 233–241 (1973).

89. Gutterman, J. U., Mavligit, G., McCredie, K. B., Freireich, E. J., and Hersh, E. M., *Int. J. Cancer* **11,** 521–526 (1973).

90. Gutterman, J. U., Rossen, R. D., Butter, W. T., McCredie, K. B., Bodey, G. P., Freireich, E. J., and Hersh, E. M., *N. Eng. J. Med.* **288,** 169–175 (1973).

91. Dean, J. H., McCoy, J. L., Lewis, D., Appello, E., and Law, L. W., *Int. J. Cancer* **16,** 465–475 (1975).

92. David, J. R., *Proc. Natl. Acad. Sci. USA* **56,** 72–77 (1966).

93. Bloom, B. R., Bennett, B., Oettgen, H. F., McLean, E. P., and Old, L. J., *Proc. Natl. Acad. Sci. USA* **64,** 1176–1180 (1969).

94. Churchill, W. H., Zbar, B., Belli, J. A., and David, J. R., *J.N.C.I.* **48,** 541–549 (1972).

95. Halliday, W. J., and Miller, S., *Int. J. Cancer* **9,** 477–483 (1972).

96. Baldwin, R. W., and Glaves, D., *Clin. Exp. Immunol.* **11,** 51–56 (1972).

97. Baldwin, R. W., Harris, J. R., and Price, M. R., *Int. J. Cancer* **11,** 385–397 (1973).

98. Smith, P. J., Robinson, C. M., and Reif, A. E., *Cancer Res.* **34,** 169–175 (1974).

99. Harder, F. H., and McKhann, C. F., *J.N.C.I.* **40,** 231–241 (1968).

100. Burdick, J. F., Cohen, A. M., and Wells, S. A., *J.N.C.I.* **50,** 285–289 (1973).

101. Burdick, J. F., and Wells, S. A., Jr., *J.N.C.I.* **51,** 1149–1156 (1973).

102. Aoki, T., Boyse, E. A., Old, L. J., deHarven, E., Hammerling, U., and Wood, H. A., *Proc. Natl. Acad. Sci. USA* **65,** 569–576 (1970).

103. Eilber, F. R., and Morton, D. L., *J.N.C.I.* **44,** 651–656 (1970).

104. Huebner, R. J., and Todaro, G. J., *Proc. Natl. Acad. Sci. USA* **64,** 1087–1094 (1969).

105. Wahren, B., *J.N.C.I.* **31,** 411–423 (1963).

106. Cleveland, P. H., McKhann, C. F., Johnson, K., and Nelson, S., *Int. J. Cancer* **14,** 417–426 (1974).

107. Tamerius, J. D., and Hellström, I., *J. Immunol.* **112,** 1987–1996 (1974).

108. Gold, P., and Freedman, S. O., *J. Exp. Med.* **121,** 439–462 (1965).

109. Gold, P., and Freedman, S. O., *J. Exp. Med.* **122,** 467–481 (1965).

110. Reisfeld, R. A., Pellegrino, M. A., and Kahan, B. D., *Science* **172,** 1134–1136 (1971).

111. Meltzer, M. S., Leonard, E. J., Rapp, H. J., and Borsos, T., *J.N.C.I.* **47,** 703–709 (1971).

112. Holmes, E. C., Kahan, B. D., and Morton, D. L., *Cancer* **25,** 373–379 (1970).

113. Bystryn, J. C., Schenkein, I., Baur, S., and Uhr. J. W., *J.N.C.I.* **52,** 1263–1269 (1974).

114. Price, M. R., and Baldwin, R. W., *Br. J. Cancer* **30,** 382–393 (1974).

115. Baldwin, R. W., and Barker, C. R., *Br. J. Cancer* **21,** 793–800 (1967).

116. Leonard, E. J., Richardson, A. K., Hardy, A. S., and Rapp, H. J., **55,** 73–78 (1975).

117. Schone, G., *Muenchen, Med. Wochenschr.* **53,** 2517–2519 (1906).

118. Abelev, G. I., Perova, S. D., Khramkova, N. I., Postnikova, Z. A., and Irlin, I. S., *Transplan.* **1,** 174–180 (1963).

119. Miller, D. R., *Br. J. Haemat.* **17,** 103–112 (1969).

120. Hoffman, R., Friemel, H., and Brock, J., *Arch. Gynak.* **208,** 187–195 (1969).

121. Tal, C., in *Embryonic and Fetal Antigens in Cancer* (N. G. Anderson and J. H. Coggin, Jr., eds.) Vol. II, USAEC Division of Technical Information, Springfield, Va., 1972, p. 53.

122. Hakkinen, I. P., *Transplan. Rev.* **20,** 61–76 (1974).

123. Hakkinen, I. P., and Viikari, S., *Ann. Surg.* **169,** 277–281 (1969).

124. Tsou, K. C., McCoy, M. G., and Lo, K. W., *Cancer Res.* **34,** 2459–2463 (1974).

125. Drysdale, J. W., and Singer, R. M., *Cancer Res.* **34,** 3352–3354 (1974).

126. Usategui-Gomez, M., Yeager, F. M., and Fernandez de Castro, A., *Cancer Res.* **34,** 2544–2545 (1974).

127. Eshhar, Z., Order, S. E., and Katz, D. H., *Proc. Natl. Acad. Sci. USA* **71,** 3956–3960 (1974).

128. Munjal, D., Zamcheck, N., Kupchik, H. Z., and Saravis, C. A., *Cancer Res.* **34,** 2936–2939 (1974).

129. Murgita, R. A., and Tomasi, T. B., Jr., *J. Exp. Med.* **141,** 269–286 (1975).

130. Murgita, R. A., and Tomasi, T. B., Jr., *J. Exp. Med.* **141,** 440–452 (1975).

131. Dattwyler, R. J., Murgita, R. A., and Tomasi, T. B., Jr., *Nature* **256,** 656–657 (1975).

132. Tomasi, T. B., Jr., Dattwyler, R. J., Murgita, R. A., and Keller, R. H., *Trans. Assoc. Amer. Physicians* (1975) (in press).

133. Abelev, G. I., *Transplan. Rev.* **20**, 3–37 (1974).

134. Ruoslahti, E., Pihko, H., and Seppälä, M., *Transplan. Rev.* **20**, 38–60 (1974).

135. Tartarinov, I. S., *Vop. Med. Khim.* **10**, 90–91 (1964).

136. Alpert, E., Coston, R., and Perrotto, J., *Lancet* **1**, 626 (1974).

137. Silver, H. K., Deneault, J., Gold, P., et al., *Cancer Res.* **34**, 244–247 (1974).

158. Waldmann, T. A., and McIntire, K. R., *Lancet* **2**, 1112–1115 (1972).

139. Alpert, E., *Natl. Cancer Inst. Monogr.* **35**, 415–420 (1972).

140. Allan, L. D., Ferguson-Smith, M. A., Donald, I., et al., *Lancet* **2**, 522–525 (1973).

141. Harris, R., Jennison, R. F., Barson, A. J., et al., *Lancet* **1**, 428–429 (1974).

142. Guibaud, S., Bonnet, M., Thoulon, J. M., and Dumont, M., *Lancet* **1**, 1261 (1973).

143. Sizaret, P., and Martin, F., *J.N.C.I.* **50**, 807–810 (1973).

144. McIntire, K. R., Vogel, C. L., Princler, G. L., and Patel, I. R., *Cancer Res.* **32**, 1941–1946 (1972).

145. Chayvialle, J. A., and Ganguli, P. C., *Lancet* **1**, 1355–1357 (1973).

146. Silver, H. K., Gold, P., Feder, S., Freedman, S., and Shuster, J., *Proc. Natl. Acad. Sci. USA* **70**, 526–530 (1973).

147. Tamaoki, T., Thomas, K., and Schindler, I., *Nature* **249**, 269–271 (1974).

148. Sell, S., Jalowayski, I., Bellone, C., and Wepsic, H. T., *Cancer Res.* **32**, 1184–1189 (1972).

149. Leffert, H. L., and Sell, S., *J. Cell. Biol.* **61**, 823–829 (1974).

150. Okita, K., Gruenstein, M., Klaiber, M., and Farber, E., *Cancer Res.* **34**, 2758–2763 (1974).

151. Becker, F. F., and Sell, S., *Cancer Res.* **34**, 2489–2494 (1974).

152. Zamcheck, N., *Adv. Intern. Med.* **19**, 413–433 (1974).

153. Kupchik, H. Z., Zamcheck, N., and Saravis, C. A., *J.N.C.I.* **51**, 1741–1749 (1973).

154. Neville, A. M., and Laurence, D. J. R., *Int. J. Cancer* **14**, 1–18 (1974).

155. Fuks, A., Banjo, C., Shuster, J., Freedman, S. O., and Gold, P., *Biochem. et Biophys. Acta* **417**, 123 (1975).

156. Terry, W. D., Henkart, P. A., Coligan, J. E., and Todd, C. W., *Transplan. Rev.* **20**, 100–129 (1974).

157. Steward, A. M., Nixon, D., Zamcheck, N., and Aisenberg, A., *Cancer* **33**, 1246–1252 (1974).

158. Nery, R., James, R., Barsoum, A. L., and Bullman, H., *Br. J. Cancer* **29**, 413–424 (1974).

159. Khoo, S. K., Warner, N. L., Lie, J. T., and Mackay, I. R., *Int. J. Cancer* **11**, 681–687 (1973).

160. Moore, T. L., Kupchik, H. Z., Marcon, N., and Zamcheck, N., *Am. J. Dig. Dis.* **16**, 1–7 (1971).

161. Laurence, D. J., Stevens, U., Bettelheim, R., et al., *Br. Med. J.* **3**, 605–609 (1972).

162. Egan, M. L., Lautenschleger, J. T., Coligan, J. E., and Todd, C. W., *Immunochem.* **9**, 289–299 (1972).

163. Egan, M. L., Coligan, J. E., and Todd, C. W., *Cancer* **34**, 1504–1509 (1974).

164. Wu, J. T., Madsen, A., and Bray, P. F., *J.N.C.I.* **53**, 1589–1595 (1974).

165. Coller, J. A., Crichlow, R. W., and Yin, L. K., *Cancer Res.* **33**, 1684–1688 (1973).

166. MacSween, J. M., Warner, N. L., and Mackay, I. R., *Clin. Immunol. Immunopathol.* **1**, 330–345 (1973).

167. Coligan, J. E., Egan, M. L., and Todd, C. W., *Natl. Cancer Inst. Mongr.* **35**, 427–432 (1972).

168. Krupey, J., Wilson, T., Freedman, S. O., and Gold, P., *Immunochem.* **9**, 617–622 (1972).

169. Coligan, J. E., Lautenschleger, J. T., Egan, M. L., and Todd, C. W., *Immunochem.* **9**, 377–386 (1972).

170. Reif, A. E., and Robinson, C. M., *Immunol. Commun.* **1**, 351–365 (1972).

171. Chu, T. M., Holyoke, E. D., and Murphy, G. P., *Cancer Res.* **34**, 212–214 (1974).

172. David, G. S., and Reisfeld, R. A., *J.N.C.I.* **53**, 1005–1010 (1974).

173. Rogers, G. T., Searle, F., and Bagshawe, K. D., *Nature* **251**, 519–521 (1974).

174. Holburn, A. M., Mach, J. P., MacDonald, D., and Newlands, M., *Immunol.* **26,** 831–843 (1974).

175. Gold, J. M., Banjo, C., Freedman, S. O., and Gold, P., *J. Immunol.* **111,** 1872–1879 (1973).

176. Simmons, D. A. R., and Perlmann, P., *Cancer Res.* **33,** 313–322 (1973).

177. Morris, J. E., Egan, M. L., and Todd, C. W., *Cancer Res.* **35,** 1804 (1975).

178. Banjo, C., Gold, P., Freedman, S. O., and Krupey, J., Nat. New Biol. **238,** 183–185 (1972).

179. Rule, A. H., and Goleski-Reilly, C., *Br. J. Cancer* **28,** 464–468 (1973).

180. Coligan, J. E., Henkart, P. A., Todd, C. W., and Terry, W. D., *Immunochem.,* **10,** 591–599 (1973).

181. Rule, A. H., and Goleski-Reilly, C., *Immunol. Commun.* **2,** 213–226 (1973).

182. Hughes, N. R., *Nature* **243,** 523–526 (1973).

183. Reisfeld, R. A., David, G. S., Wang, R., Chino, T., and Sevier, E. D., *Proceedings of the 28th Annual Symposium on Fundamental Cancer Research,* Houston, Texas (1975) (in press).

184. Coggin, J. H., Jr., and Anderson, N. G., *Adv. Cancer Res.* **19,** 105–165 (1974).

185. Ting, C. C., Lavrin, D. H., Shiu, G., et al., *Proc. Natl. Acad. Sci. USA* **69,** 1664–1668 (1972).

186. Ting, C. C., Ortaldo, J. R., and Herberman, R. B., *Int. J. Cancer* **12,** 511–518 (1973).

187. Invernizzi, G., and Parmiani, G., *Nature* **254,** 713 (1975).

188. Bowen, J. G., and Baldwin, R. W., *Nature* **258,** 75–76 (1975).

189. Baldwin, R. W., Glaves, D., Pimm, M. V., and Vose, B. M., *Ann. Inst. Pasteur* **122,** 715 (1972).

190. Thomson, D. M., and Alexander, P., *Br. J. Cancer* **27,** 35–47 (1973).

191. Girardi, A., Reppucci, P., Dierlam, P., Rutala, W., and Coggin, J. H., *Proc. Natl. Acad. Sci. USA* **70,** 183–186 (1973).

192. Castro, J. G., Lance, E. M., Medawar, P. B., Zanelli, J., and Hunt, R., *Nature* **243,** 225–226 (1973).

193. Ting, C. C., Rodrigues, D., and Herberman, R. B., *Int. J. Cancer* **12,** 519–523 (1973).

194. Rees, R. C., Shah, L. P., and Baldwin, R. W., *Nature* **255,** 329–330 (1975).

195. Steele, G., Jr., and Sjögren, H. O., *Int. J. Cancer* **14,** 435–444 (1974).

196. Baldwin, R. W., Glaves, D., and Vose, B. M., *Int. J. Cancer* **10,** 233–243 (1972).

197. Baldwin, R. W., Glaves, D., and Vose, B. M., *Br. J. Cancer* **29,** 1–10 (1974).

198. Baldwin, R. W., and Vose, B. M., *Transplan.* **18,** 525–530 (1974).

199. Baldwin, R. W., and Vose, B. M., *Br. J. Cancer* **30,** 209–214 (1974).

200. Hellström, I., Sjögren, H. O., *J. Exp. Med.* **125,** 1105–1118 (1967).

201. Klein, E., Klein, G., Nadkarni, J. S., Nadkarni, J. J., Wigzell, H., and Clifford, P., *Cancer Res.* **28,** 1300–1310 (1968).

202. Heppner, G. H., and Pierce, G., *Int. J. Cancer* **4,** 212–218 (1969).

203. Allen, D. W., and Cole, P., *N. Eng. J. Med.* **286,** 70–82 (1972).

204. Butel, J. S., Tevethia, S. S., and Melnick, J. L., *Adv. Cancer Res.* **15,** 1–55 (1972).

205. Mayor, H. D., Stinebaugh, S. E., Jamison, R. M., Jordon, L. E., and Melnick, J. L., *Exp. Molec. Path.* **1,** 397–416 (1962).

206. Rapp, F., Butel, J. S., Feldman, L. A., Kitahara, T., and Melnick, J. L., *J. Exp. Med.* **121,** 935–944 (1965).

207. Huebner, R. J., Rowe, W. P., Turner, H. C., and Lane, W. T., *Proc. Natl. Acad. Sci.* **50,** 379–389 (1963).

208. Rapp, F., Butel, J. S., and Melnick, J. L., *Proc. Soc. Exp. Biol. Med.* **116,** 1131–1135 (1964).

209. Pope, J. H., and Rowe, W. P., *J. Exp. Med.* **120,** 121–128 (1964).

210. Rapp, F., Kitahara, T., Butel, J. S., and Melnick, J. L., *Proc. Natl. Acad. Sci. USA* **52,** 1138–1142 (1964).

211. Gilden, R. V., Carp, R. I., Taguchi, F., and Defendi, V., *Proc. Natl. Acad. Sci.* **53,** 684–692 (1965).

212. Del Villano, B., and Defendi, V., *Bacteriolog. Proc.,* p. 188 (1970).

213. Lewis, A. M., Jr., Levin, M. J., Wiese, W. H., Crumpacker, C. S., and Henry, P. H., *Proc. Natl. Acad. Sci. USA* **63,** 1128–1135 (1969).

214. Sjögren, H. O., Hellström, I., and Klein, G., *Exp. Cell. Res.* **23,** 204–208 (1961).

215. Habel, K., *Proc. Soc. Exp. Biol. and Med.* **106,** 722–725 (1961).

216. Khera, K. S., Ashkenazi, A., Rapp, F., and Melnick, J. L., *J. Immunol.* **91,** 604–613 (1963).

217. Girardi, A. J., *Proc. Natl. Acad. Sci. USA* **54,** 445–451 (1965).

218. Lausch, R. N., Tevethia, S. S., and Rapp, F., *J. Immunol.* **101,** 645–649 (1968).

219. Jensen, F., and Defendi, V., *J. Virol.* **2,** 173–177 (1968).

220. Tevethia, S. S., Katz, M., and Rapp, F., *Proc. Soc. Exp. Biol. Med.* **119,** 896–901 (1965).

221. Hayry, P., and Defendi, V., *Virol.* **36,** 317–321 (1968).

222. Metzgar, R. S., and Oleinick, S. R., *Cancer Res.* **28,** 1366–1371 (1968).

223. Tevethia, S. S., Crouch, N. A., Melnick, J. L., and Rapp, F., *Int. J. Cancer* **5,** 176–184 (1970).

224. Wright, P. W., and Law, L. W., *Proc. Natl. Acad. Sci. USA* **68,** 973–976 (1971).

225. Diamandopoulos, G. T., Tevethia, S. S., Rapp, F., and Enders, J. F., *Virol.* **34,** 331–336 (1968).

226. Tevethia, S. S., Diamandopoulos, G. T., Rapp, F., and Enders, J. F., *J. Immunol.* **101,** 1192–1198 (1968).

227. Levin, M. J., Oxman, M. N., Diamandopoulos, G. T., Levine, A. S., Henry, P. H., and Enders, J. F., *Proc. Natl. Acad. Sci. USA* **62,** 589–596 (1969).

228. Levine, A. S., Oxman, M. N., Henry, P. H., Levin, M. J., Diamandopoulos, G. T., and Enders, J. F., *J. Virol.* **6,** 199–207 (1970).

229. Hayry, P., and Defendi, V., *Virol.* **41,** 22–29 (1970).

230. Burger, M. M., *Proc. Natl. Acad. Sci. USA* **62,** 994–1001 (1969).

231. Klein, G., *Adv. Immunol.* **14,** 187–250 (1971).

232. Henle, G., and Henle, W., *Bacteriology* **91,** 1248–1256 (1966).

233. Epstein, M. A., Achong, B. G., and Barr, Y. M., *Lancet* **1,** 702–703 (1964).

234. Epstein, M. A., Achong, B. G., Barr, Y. M., Zajac, B., Henle, G., and Henle, W., *J.N.C.I* **37,** 547–559 (1966).

235. Henle, W., and Henle, G., *Epstein-Barr Virus: The Cause of Infectious Mononucleosis—A Review, Oncogenesis and Herpes Viruses* (G. de The, P. M. Biggs, and L. N. Payne, IARC Scientific Publications, Lyons, France, pp. 269–274 (1972).

236. Henle, W., Henle, G., Zajac, B. A., Pearson, G., Waubke, R., and Scriba, M., *Science* **169,** 188–190 (1970).

237. Gergely, L., Klein, G., and Ernberg, I., *Virol.* **45,** 22–29 (1971).

238. Henle, G., Henle, W., Klein, G., Gunven, P., Clifford, P., Morrow, R. H., and Ziegler, J. L., *J.N.C.I.* **44,** 225 (1970).

239. Klein, G., *Cancer Res.* **28,** 625–635 (1968).

240. Henle, W., and Henle, G., in *Comparative Leukemia Research* (R. M. Dutcher, ed.), Karger, Basel, 1970, p. 706.

241. Goldstein, G., Klein, G., Pearson, G., and Clifford, P., *Cancer Res.* **29,** 749–752 (1969).

242. Gunven, P., Klein, G., Henle, G., Henle, W., and Clifford, P., *Nature* (London) **228,** 1053–1056 (1970).

243. Armstrong, D., Henle, G., and Henle, W., *J. Bacteriol.* **91,** 1257–1262 (1966).

244. Gerber, P., and Deal, D. R., *Proc. Soc. Exp. Biol. Med.* **134,** 748–751 (1970).

245. Pope, J. H., Horne, M. K., and Scott, W., *Int. J. Cancer* **4,** 255–260 (1969).

246. Vonka, V., Benyesh-Melnick, M. D., and McCombs, R. M., *J.N.C.I.* **44,** 865–872 (1970).

247. Old, L. J., Boyse, E. A., Oettgen, H. F., deHarven, E., Geering, G., Williamson, B., and Clifford, P., *Proc. Natl. Acad. Sci. USA* **56,** 1699–1704 (1966).

248. Klein, G., Clifford, P., Henle, G., Henle, W., Old, L. J., and Geering, L., *Int. J. Cancer* **4,** 416–421 (1969).

249. Fass, L., Herberman, R. B., and Ziegler, J., *N. Eng. J. Med.* **282,** 776–780 (1970).

250. Naib, Z. M., Nahmias, A. J., and Josey, W. E., *Cancer* **19,** 1026–1031 (1966).

251. Rawls, W. E., Tompkins, W. A. F., and Melnick, L. J., *Am. J. Epidem.* **89,** 547–554 (1969).

252. Nahmias, A. J., Josey, W. E., and Naib, Z. M., et al., *Am. J. Epidem.* **91,** 547–552 (1970).

253. Tarro, G., and Sabin, A. B., *Proc. Natl. Acad. Sci. USA* **65,** 753–760 (1970).

254. Hollinshead, A. C., Lee, O., Chretien, P. B., Tarpley, J. L., Rawls, W. E., and Adam, E., *Science* **182,** 713–715 (1973).

255. Bauer, H., *Adv. Cancer Res.* **20,** 275–341 (1974).

256. Haguenau, F., and Beard, J. W., in *Tumors Induced by Viruses: Ultrastructural Studies* (A. J. Dalton and F. Haguenau, eds.), Vol. 1, Academic Press, New York, 1962, pp. 1–59.

257. Aoki, T., Huebner, R. J., Chang, K. S., Sturm, M. M., and Lui, M., *J.N.C.I.* **52,** 1189–1197 (1974).

258. Duesberg, P. H., Martin, G. S., and Vogt, P. K., *Virol.* **41,** 631–646 (1970).

259. Oroszlan, S., Huebner, R. J., and Giden, R. V., *Proc. Natl. Acad. Sci. USA* **68,** 901–904 (1971).

260. Geering, G., Aoki, T., and Old, L. J., *Nature* (London) **226,** 265–266 (1970).

261. Schafer, W., Lange, J., Pister, L., Seifert, E., de Noronha, F., and Schmidt, F. W., *Z. Naturforsch. (B.)* **25,** 1029–1036 (1970).

262. Gilden, R. V., Oroszlan, S., and Huebner, R. J., *Nat. New Biol.* (London) **231,** 107–108 (1971).

263. Baltimore, D., *Nature* (London) **226,** 1209–1211 (1970).

264. Aaronson, S. A., Parks, W. P., Scolnick, E. M., and Todaro, G. J., *Proc. Natl. Acad. Sci. USA* **68,** 920–924 (1971).

265. Scolnick, E. M., Parks, W. P., Todaro, G. J., and Aaronson, S. A., *Nat. New Biol.* (London) **235,** 35–40 (1972).

266. Gelderblom, H., Bauer, H., and Frank, H., *J. Gen. Virol.* **7,** 33–45 (1970).

267. Huebner, R. J., Armstrong, D., Okuyan, M., Sarma, P. S., and Turner, H. C., *Proc. Natl. Acad. Sci. USA* **51,** 742–750 (1964).

268. Bauer, H., and Schafer, W., *Virol.* **29,** 494–497 (1966).

269. Klein, G., Sjögren, H. O., and Klein, E., *Cancer Res.* **22,** 955–961 (1962).

270. Sjögren, H. O., and Jonsson, N., *Exp. Cell. Res.* **32,** 618–621 (1963).

271. Geering, G., Old, L. J., and Boyse, E. A., *J. Exp. Med.* **124,** 753–772 (1966).

272. Steeves, R. A., *Cancer Res.* **28,** 338–342 (1968).

273. Cikes, M., and Friberg, S., *Proc. Natl. Acad. Sci. USA* **68,** 566–569 (1971).

274. Kennel, S. J., Del Villano, B. C., Levy, R. L., and Lerner, R. A., *Virol.* **55,** 464–475 (1973).

275. Boyse, E. A., in *Immune Surveillance* (R. T. Smith and M. Landy, eds.), Academic Press, New York, 1970, p. 3.

276. Haywood, G. R., and McKhann, C. F., *J. Exp. Med.* **133,** 1171–1187 (1971).

277. Ting, C. C., and Herberman, R. B., *Nat. New Biol.* **232,** 118–120 (1971).

278. Klein, G., and Klein, E., *Int. J. Cancer* **15,** 879–887 (1975).

279. McKhann, C. F., in *Frontiers in Radiation Therapy and Oncology* (J. M. Vaeth, ed.), S. Karger, Basel, 1972, p. 16.

280. Thomson, D. M. P., *Int. J. Cancer* **15,** 1016–1029 (1975).

281. Fujimoto, S., Chen, C. H., Sabbadini, E., and Sehon, A. H., *J. Immunol.* **111,** 1093–1100 (1973).

282. Reisfeld, R. A., Allison, J. P., Ferrone, S., Pellegrino, M. A., Poulik, M. D., *Transplan. Proc.* (1976) (in press).

283. Kaliss, N., *Cancer Res.* **18,** 992–1003 (1958).

284. Moller, G., *Nature* (London) **204,** 846–847 (1964).

285. Hellström, I., Evans, C. A., and Hellström, K. E., *Int. J. Cancer* **4,** 601–607 (1969).

286. Robins, R. A., and Baldwin, R. W., *Int. J. Cancer* **14,** 589–597 (1974).

287. Oldstone, M. B. A., Tishon, A., Tonietti, G., and Dixon, F. J., *Clin. Immunol. Immunopath.* **1,** 6–14 (1972).

288. Oldstone, M. B., Aoki, T., and Dixon, F. J., *Proc. Natl. Acad. Sci. USA* **69,** 134–138 (1972).

289. Yoshki, T., Mellors, R. C., Strand, M., and August, J. T., *J. Exp. Med.* **140,** 1011–1027 (1974).

290. Poskitt, P. K., Poskitt, T. R., and Wallace, J. H., *J. Exp. Med.* **140,** 410–425 (1974).

291. Pascal, R. R., Rollwagen, F. M., Harding, T. A., and Schiavone, W. A., *Cancer Res.* **35,** 302–304 (1975).

292. Oldstone, M. B. A., *J.N.C.I.* **54**, 223–228 (1975).

293. Sutherland, J. C., and Mardiney, M. R., Jr., *J.N.C.I.* **50**, 633–644 (1973).

294. Costanza, M. E., Pinn, V., Schwartz, R. S., and Nathanson, L., *N. Eng. J. Med.* **289**, 520–522 (1973).

295. Sutherland, J. C., Markham, R. V., Jr., Ramsey, H. E., and Mardiney, M. R., *Cancer Res.* **34**, 1179–1181 (1974).

296. Jones, L. W., Levin, A., and Fudenberg, H. H., *Surg. Gynecol. Obstet.* **140**, 896–898 (1975).

297. Anderson, N. G., Holladay, D. W., Caton, J. E., Candler, E. L., Dierlam, P. J., et al., *Cancer Res.* **34**, 2066–2076 (1974).

298. Anderson, N. G., Willis, D., Holladay, D. W., Caton, J. E., Holleman, J. W., Eveleigh, J. W., Attrill, J. E., Ball, F. L., and Anderson, N. L., *Ann. Biochem.* **66**, 159–174 (1975).

299. Creighton, W. D., Lambert, P. H., and Miescher, P. A., *J. Immunol.* **111**, 1219–1227 (1973).

300. Nydegger, U. E., Lambert, P. H., Gerber, H., and Miescher, P. A., *J. Clin. Invest.* **54**, 297–309 (1974).

301. Agnello, V., Winchester, R. J., and Kunkel, H. G., *Immunol.* **19**, 909–919 (1970).

302. Winchester, R. J., Kunkel, H. G., and Agnello, V., *J. Exp. Med.* **134**, 286s–295s (1971).

303. Onyewotu, I. I., Holborow, E. J., and Johnson, G. D., *Nat. New Biol.* **248**, 156–159 (1974).

304. Jewell, D. P., and MacLennan, I. C., *Clin. Exp. Immunol.* **14**, 219–226 (1973).

305. Brouet, J. C., Clavel, J. P., Danon, F., Klein, M., and Seligmann, M., *Am. J. Med.* **57**, 775–788 (1974).

306. Mowbray, J. F., Hoffbrand, A. V., Holborow, E. J., Seah, P. P., and Fry, L., *Lancet* **1**, 400–402 (1973).

307. Theofilopoulos, A. N., Wilson, C. B., and Dixon, F. B., *J. Clin. Invest.* **57**, 169–182 (1976).

308. Steele, G., Jr., Ankerst, J., and Sjögren, H. O., *Int. J. Cancer* **14**, 83–92 (1974).

309. Baldwin, R. W., Price, M. R., and Robins, R. A., *Int. J. Cancer* **11**, 527–535 (1973).

310. Baldwin, R. W., Embleton, M. J., and Price, M. R., *Int. J. Cancer* **12**, 84–92 (1973).

311. Zighelboim, J., Bonavida, B., Rao, V. S., and Fahey, J. L., *J. Immunol.* **112**, 433–435 (1974).

312. Corley, R. B., Dawson, J. R., and Amos, D. B., *Cell. Immunol.* **16**, 92–105 (1975).

313. Koldovsky, P., Turano, A., and Fadda, G., *J. Cell. Physiol.* **74**, 31–36 (1969).

314. Wagner, H., and Boyle, W., *Nat. New Biol.* **240**, 92–94 (1972).

315. Bonavida, B., *J. Immunol.* **112**, 926–934 (1974).

Chapter Six

Immunologic Enhancement of Tumor Growth

KARL ERIK HELLSTRÖM AND INGEGERD HELLSTRÖM

Division of Immunology, Fred Hutchinson Cancer Research Center, Seattle, Washington, and Departments of Pathology and Microbiology & Immunology, University of Washington Medical School, Seattle, Washington

The preceding chapters of this volume have described ways in which the immune system can serve as a means of host defense against tumor growth. The wide prevalence of clinical neoplastic disease is evidence that these defenses are not always effective. In this chapter we will focus attention on mechanisms of immunologic enhancement that allow tumors to escape from immunologic control.

Immunologic enhancement has been defined as a mechanism by which antibody can facilitate the growth of a transplant, usually of neoplastic origin, which would otherwise be rejected (1,2). It can be detected as an active enhancement in animals forming antibodies upon immunization with cells or cell extracts containing foreign histocompatibility antigens and challenged with tumor cells containing the same foreign antigens. It can also be seen as a passive enhancement in animals inoculated with antibodies to foreign alloantigens and then grafted with cells carrying these antigens.

Depending on where the enhancing antibodies are believed to act, one may contrast three forms of enhancement (1,2): *afferent* enhancement, in which the antibodies combine with antigens present on the transplant, preventing them from immunizing the host; *efferent* enhancement, in which they bind to antigens in such a way that they are "masked" and not detected by the host's immune cells; and *central* enhancement, in which they act directly on host lymphoid cells and prevent these from mediating graft rejection.

The work of the authors has been supported by the following grants and contracts: CA 19148, CA 19149, and SO 7 RRO 5520 from the National Institutes of Health, by IM-43G from the American Cancer Society, by contract NO1 CB 64018 from the National Cancer Institute, and by contract NO1 CP 53570 within the Virus Cancer Program of the National Cancer Institute NIH, PHS.

Immunologic enhancement has traditionally been distinguished from immunologic tolerance, in which the host is rendered specifically incapable of mounting an immune response against the antigens of the tolerated graft (1–3). Tolerance is generally ascribed to central inhibition, resulting from either a depletion of specific lymphocyte clones or a long-lasting suppression of their functions. This depletion (or suppression) is most likely the result of contact between appropriate lymphoid cells and tolerizing antigen (4).

Studies performed during the last few years have blurred the distinction between enhancement and tolerance (5). Evidence suggesting that enhancement may occur by central inhibition has come from work demonstrating that "enhancing" antibodies, present in hyperimmune sera, bind to antigens on the enhanced tissue and release substances, probably antigen-antibody complexes. These substances interact with immunologically competent cells and prevent them from destroying the graft (6,7). Other studies have shown that some forms of allograft tolerance may, at least partially, result from inhibition of an ongoing immune response by circulating serum factors (3). Mice and rats rendered "operationally tolerant" to allogeneic skin grafts (i.e., able to retain their grafts for at least 100 days) often possess lymphocytes capable of destroying cultivated cells carrying the tolerated antigens, as well as serum factors which specifically block (inhibit) the cytotoxic activity of the "tolerant" lymphocytes (3). These serum factors are probably complexes of the tolerated antigens and their IgG antibodies (9,10). They can block lymphocyte reactivity when added to either the lymphocytes or the target cells in vitro.

The early work on immunologic enhancement of tumor growth, though performed with H-2 incompatible, allografted tumor cells (1,2), suggested that an enhancement mechanism might provide a route of escape from immunologic destruction of antigenic tumors in the autochthonous or syngeneic host. The first experimental support for this view came in 1964, when Möller demonstrated that inoculation of hyperimmune serum, containing antibodies to tumor-specific transplantation antigens of chemically induced mouse sarcomas, could facilitate tumor growth in syngeneic hosts (11). This implied that antibodies to tumor-specific antigens can, indeed, act as enhancing antibodies.

Hellström et al., working with an in vitro assay system of cellular immunity to antigenic tumors, reported in 1969 that sera from mice with primary Moloney sarcomas, as well as from mice with spontaneous mammary carcinomas and rabbits with Shope virus-induced papillomas, could block specific cell-mediated destruction of cells carrying the tumor-specific antigens of the respective neoplasms (12). They postulated that a phenomenon akin to immunologic enhancement was involved and that this phenomenon might provide a mechanism of escape from immunologic control for tumors in the autochthonous host. The in vitro studies on which this view has, to a large extent, been based have been confirmed and extended to a variety of systems (3). There are also data from in vivo studies indicating that antigen-antibody complexes, and free tumor antigens, can enhance the growth of autochthonous and syngeneic neoplasms (3). The latter data are, however, still not conclusive.

In this article we will discuss evidence that "blocking" serum factors are present in animals and human patients with tumors and that they may permit neoplastic cells to escape from immunologic control in a way akin to immunologic enhancement. We will also discuss the nature of the blocking factors, as well as their significance for diagnosis and therapy of tumors. The present state of knowledge will be described; for a more complete literature review of earlier work in this area, the reader is referred to five fairly recent articles (3,5,13–15).

DETECTION OF BLOCKING FACTORS TO TUMOR ANTIGENS IN VARIOUS SYSTEMS

Microcytotoxicity Assays of Blocking Serum Effects

The microcytotoxicity assay (16), as well as radioisotope assays measuring tumor cell destruction over a 20–40 hour period (17), have been used for most work on blocking effects with tumor bearer sera, while such effects are more rarely seen with short-term (4–6 hour) assays. Abrogation of specific lymphocyte-mediated destruction of plated tumor cells has been observed, when either the target cells or the lymphocytes have been preincubated with serum from individuals bearing a tumor with the same antigens as the target cells. The possibility that inhibition of the lymphocyte reactivity resulted from the presence of free serum factors is ruled out by the fact that the incubated cells were washed before testing.

"Blocking" versus "Inhibition"

Some authors refer to the ability of serum to abrogate lymphocyte reactivity as "inhibition" and the effect on the target cells as "blocking." Since the inhibitory effects of tumor bearer serum on the lymphocytes and the target cells were originally both referred to as "blocking" (18), we will continue to use that term, for simplicity. The blocking effect seen on lymphocytes is probably the more important one (3,18), but one must acknowledge a significant role, in certain instances, for true efferent enhancement by blocking factors present in sera from tumor bearers as well as in some hyperimmune sera.

Tumor Systems in Which a Blocking Effect of Tumor Bearers' Serum Has Been Detected by Microcytotoxicity Assays

The original demonstration that sera from mice with primary Moloney sarcomas (12,19) or spontaneous mammary carcinomas (12,20), and from rabbits with Shope papillomas (12,21), can specifically abrogate cell-mediated destruction of plated neoplastic cells carrying the respective antigens, has been extended to a variety of systems (3,13).

Sjögren and Borum reported that sera from rats with polyoma virus-induced sarcomas could specifically abrogate cell-mediated destruction of polyoma tumor cells (22), and Sjögren and Bansal extended these observations to a larger number of polyoma tumors (23,24). Hellström et al. showed that sera from mice with primary methylcholanthrene (MCA)-induced sarcomas, and from mice and rats with transplanted MCA sarcomas, had blocking activity which was specific with respect to the unique antigens of each sarcoma (25). Baldwin et al. found a specific blocking effect of sera from rats with transplanted, chemically induced hepatomas (13,26–29). Gorczynski and Knight observed blocking activity in sera from mice with primary Moloney sarcomas using an isotope-release assay (30), essentially confirming microcytotoxicity studies by Hellström and Hellström (19). Steele et al. demonstrated that sera from rats with primary or transplanted chemically induced carcinomas of the colon could specifically abrogate lymphocyte-mediated reactivity against antigens common to these tumors and absent from control neoplasms, including polyoma-induced sarcomas and chemically and virally induced breast carcinomas (31,32). Stolfi et al. found blocking factors in sera of mice with growing, transplanted mammary carcinomas (33).

Blocking factors with specificity for common, presumably embryonic antigens present in chemically induced murine sarcomas and hepatomas have been detected in sera from tumor-bearing and from multiparous syngeneic animals (34–38). Such blocking factors have been also detected in sera of tumor-free mice which have been immunized with either embryonic cells or tumor cells, and there is evidence suggesting that the putatively embryonic antigens are more prone to elicit the formation of blocking serum factors than are the individually unique antigens of each chemically induced neoplasm (37,38).

Studies with human tumors also show blocking factors in sera from patients with a variety of neoplasms, including carcinomas of the lung, colon, breast, various sarcomas, and melanoma (39–41). Hellström et al. reported that these blocking factors have the same tissue-type specificity as the patients' lymphocytes, when tested against cultivated neoplastic cells (39). Baldwin et al. obtained similar findings in patients with breast carcinomas and colonic carcinomas (42), as did Avis et al., studying patients with breast carcinomas (43).

Detection of Blocking Effects with Assays Measuring Macrophage Migration Inhibition, Leukocyte Adherence Inhibition, and Lymphocyte Proliferation

When in vitro techniques other than the microcytotoxicity assay have been used, essentially similar findings have been obtained. Halliday showed that sera from mice with growing chemically induced sarcomas contain blocking factors which can be demonstrated with the macrophage migration inhibition assay; specific macrophage migration inhibition was detected in the presence of control sera, whereas sera from mice bearing the respective neoplasms could abrogate this inhibition (44,45). Poupon et al. obtained essentially similar findings, studying mice with growing carcinomas (46). Halliday et al. (47), using the leukocyte adherence inhibition technique, showed that sera from animals with chemically induced sarcomas could specifically prevent the in vitro expression of cell-mediated reactivity against the given sarcomas. They have recently described analogous findings on human patients with a variety of tumors, particularly melanoma (48,49).

Vanky et al. detected blocking serum effects in human patients with sarcomas, measuring DNA synthesis in lymphocytes exposed to putative tumor antigen (50). Sera from patients with growing sarcomas were found to prevent their own lymphocytes from transforming to lymphoblasts in the presence of the appropriate tumor antigens, while sera from tumor-free patients had no detectable blocking activity.

Exceptions to the Detection of Blocking Factors in Sera from Tumor-Bearing Individuals

In a few systems no blocking effect by tumor bearer sera has been observed. Wright and Bernstein did not detect any specific blocking-serum activity when investigating lymphocyte-mediated tumor cell destruction in rats with Gross virus-induced lymphomas (51), although Knight et al. have found that circulating viral antigen P30 may act as a blocking factor in rats with the same tumor (52). Deckers et al. found no blocking effect of sera from C57BL mice bearing a chemically induced sarcoma (53). Gutterman et al. used an assay for antigen-induced lymphocyte proliferation in human patients with leukemia and found that the presence of blocking activity in these sera was associated with improved prognosis (54).

It is difficult to conclude whether failures to find blocking serum factors in animals and patients with growing tumors have a technical explanation, or whether the blocking phenomenon just plays a minor part (or no part at all) in facilitating the growth of some tumors. The latter explanation cannot be dismissed. One should also realize, however, that the different techniques used to measure blocking serum activity may give different results. There is evidence from studies on allograft tolerance in rats that proliferation assays may be easily blocked by antibodies, but not regularly by complexes or free antigens (55); cytotoxicity assays, on the other hand, are commonly blocked by complexes and free antigens but not by antibodies (55). Similarly, techniques measuring the ability of sera to inhibit lymphocyte proliferation upon exposure to tumor antigens may measure something different from techniques measuring blockade of cell-mediated cytotoxicity.

Blocking Factors Eluted from Lymphoid Cells

Blocking factors not only are present in serum but also appear to be bound to lymphoid cells from animals and human patients with tumors. Hattler and Soehnlen (56) showed that blood lymphocytes from tumor patients had some material bound to their surface, which could be eluted at low pH and which could block the in vitro transformation of the patients' lymphocytes to lymphoblasts upon contact with autologous tumor extracts. The material responsible for this blockade appeared to consist of antigen-antibody complexes; neither presumptive antigen nor antibody isolated from lymphocyte eluates was blocking when tested alone.

Recent studies have extended these findings by indicating that lymph node and spleen cells from mice with growing methylcholanthrene-induced sarcomas carry blocking factors, which can be eluted at low pH (57). These factors specifically inhibited the cytotoxic effect on tumor target cells of lymphocytes from tumor-bearing mice. Repeated washing of the lymphocytes in culture medium did not remove the blocking factors. The nature of the lymphoid cells from which the blocking factors were eluted is not known.

The finding that some lymphoid cells from tumor-bearing individuals have blocking factors bound to their surfaces may explain why incubation of lymphocytes in vitro prior to assay for specific tumor cell cytotoxicity sometimes increases their reactivity (58,59), and why treatment of lymphocytes from tumor-bearing animals with papain can have similar effects (60). It may also explain the "eclipse" in antitumor reactivity, which has been detected in some animals with large tumors by using the microcytotoxicity test (61–63), the macrophage migration inhibition assay (60), an assay for delayed hypersensitivity to tumor antigens in vivo (64), tests for neutralization of tumor outgrowth by admixed lymphocytes (65), or tests for tumor-specific transplantation immunity (66). Reactivity to tumor antigens in delayed hypersensitivity assays decreased (67), as did tumor-specific transplantation resistance (68), following inoculation of previously immune hosts with cells (or cell-free material) containing the specific tumor antigens. Tumor bearer lymphocytes regained reactivity following transplantation to sublethally irradiated syngeneic hosts also challenged with the given tumor antigens (69). Altogether these results suggest that tumor antigens (existing in free form and/or as complexes) may be responsible for the lower reactivity seen in many individuals with growing tumors. Presumably many lymphocytes would be capable of reacting in vivo, were they not prevented from doing so by blocking factors bound to them.

None of the findings mentioned excludes the possibility that additional mechanisms contribute to the frequent failure of tumor bearer lymphocytes to show antitumor reactivity in vivo. Certain essential lymphocyte clones may be missing (5), e.g., as a result of prolonged contact with antigens (and/or immune complexes). This is not at all excluded by the demonstration of reactivity in microcytotoxicity tests, since different lymphocyte functions may be measured in vitro than those most relevant in vivo, and different antigens may be involved as targets (5). Specific and nonspecific mechanisms not necessarily mediated by antigens or complexes may be involved as well. For example, various substances formed by the tumor may, by acting in a nonspecific way, decrease the ability of the host to mount an effective immune reaction against the tumor, or prevent destruction of tumor cells by lymphocytes and macrophages (70,71).

Conclusions

There is evidence that suppressive factors exist in the sera of tumor-bearing individuals but also bound to lymphoid cells and that they can specifically abrogate certain aspects of cell-mediated immune responses to tumors. The possible role of such factors in vivo will be discussed next.

RELATIONSHIP BETWEEN BLOCKING SERUM FACTORS DETECTED IN VITRO AND TUMOR ENHANCEMENT IN VIVO

Blocking Factors in Sera from Tumor-Bearing But Not Tumor-Free Individuals

Early studies showed that sera from animals with growing neoplasms can block specific cell-mediated antitumor reactivity, while sera from animals whose tumors have regressed (12,19,72) or have been removed (25) generally do not block.

In most systems the distinction between tumor-bearing and tumor-free animals with respect to detection of blocking serum activity has been rather sharp (3,13,23). Thus, blocking factors in mice with methylcholanthrene-induced sarcomas (25), in mice with transplanted mammary carcinomas (33), in rats with polyoma tumors (23,24), in rats with chemically induced hepatomas (13,26), and in rats with chemically induced colonic carcinomas (32) generally have been found to disappear within 6–15 days following tumor removal. Sera from tumor-bearing and tumor-free animals have been titrated in several of these systems, no blocking activity being detected at any of the serum dilutions tested when the animals have been tumor free. It has, likewise, been demonstrated that human patients who, following primary surgery, are clinically tumor free only rarely have sera which block specific cell-mediated tumor destruction in vitro (39,41,73).

The fact that blocking serum activity generally disappears in animals whose neoplasms have been removed is interesting in view of the finding that such animals often have higher tumor-specific transplantation resistance to subsequent challenge with the same tumor than do animals carrying tumors, as shown by Stjernswärd in mice with primary chemically induced sarcomas (74). Bansal and Sjögren (24) demonstrated that rats with growing polyoma-induced sarcomas (whose sera blocked in vitro) accepted a smaller test graft of polyoma tumor cells than did rats whose polyoma tumors had been removed (and whose sera did not block). The correlation between in vivo and in vitro data suggests that the blocking serum activity detected in vitro may facilitate tumor growth in vivo. It does, however, not suffice as proof for an in vivo role of the blocking serum factors.

Work by Skurzak et al. (74) challenged the notion that there is a clear distinction between blocking factors being seen in sera from tumor-bearing but not from tumor-free individuals. Skurzak et al. found that some dilutions of sera from mice whose Moloney sarcomas had regressed could block lymphocyte-mediated reactivity, while other dilutions of sera could not, and that there was no sharp distinction between sera from regressor animals and sera from animals with growing tumors. The finding that sera from many tumor-bearing, as well as tumor-free, animals contain lymphocyte-dependent antibodies with specificity for tumor antigens (75) may contribute to Skurzak's findings: at some serum dilutions blocking effects may be seen, while at other dilutions one may rather see increased cytotoxicity due to the lymphocyte-dependent antibodies.

Findings by Hayami et al. on Japanese quail with Rous sarcomas agreed with Skurzak's observations, to the extent that sera from some of the quail whose sarcomas had regressed were blocking (76,77). However, the titer of the blocking serum activity in "regressor" quail was lower than in quail with growing tumors. Furthermore, it could be shown, as further discussed below, that the blocking effect of the regressor sera was probably due to the release of immunosuppressive factors (perhaps antigen-antibody complexes) upon contact of the sera with the tumor target cells (77).

Enhancement in vivo with Hyperimmune and with Tumor Bearer Sera

Sera from mice hyperimmune to tumor antigens can enhance tumor growth in vivo (11). Whether they do so by mediating an afferent, an efferent, or a central form of enhancement has not been determined; conceivably, all of these mechanisms may be involved.

The evidence that tumor bearer sera will enhance tumor growth in vivo is less clear cut. Pierce showed in 1971 that sera from mice with growing Moloney sarcomas could facilitate the growth of such tumors in vivo (78), and analogous findings were reported by Bansal et al., who studied rats with polyoma-induced sarcomas (24,79). The latter investigators prepared a pool of serum from rats with growing polyoma tumors and established that it could block specific lymphocyte-mediated destruction of polyoma tumor cells in vitro. They then inoculated serum from this pool into untreated rats and subsequently challenged them with syngeneic polyoma tumor cells. The rats were bled and tested at various time points. They were found to have developed detectable levels of blocking serum activity as a result of their inoculation with serum. The growth of polyoma tumors in rats with blocking sera was, indeed, enhanced, as compared to that in rats which had been inoculated with control sera and whose own sera did not block. However, the number of animals studies by Bansal et al. (79) was relatively small, and full controls for antigenic specificity were not included. This is, then, clearly an area in which more work is needed.

Failure to Detect Enhancement with Tumor Bearers' Sera

The conclusion that sera from tumor-bearing animals can enhance tumor growth in vivo has been challenged. Vaage found no enhancement in mice receiving tumor bearer serum but rather, in some cases, an inhibition of tumor growth (80). Proctor et al. (81) and Howell et al.(65) also failed to show any enhancing effect in mice inoculated with tumor bearer sera. However, none of these investigators determined whether the experimental animals had received serum in sufficient doses and at sufficiently short intervals to assure a constant blocking serum activity. In the absence of such tests it is difficult to evaluate why no enhancement was observed. Conceivably, serum factors which block in higher concentrations may, when more diluted, act as (or exist together with) lymphocyte-dependent antibodies, counteracting tumor growth.

On the other hand, Vaage (68) found that when mice whose tumors had been removed were inoculated with antigenic tumor extracts or irradiated tumor cells and then challenged with tumor cells having the same antigenic specificity, they had a decreased transplantation resistance to the challenge. This shows that material, namely tumor antigen, which we know can block lymphocyte-mediated cytotoxicity in vitro, can facilitate tumor growth when inoculated in vivo, perhaps by mediating an active form of enhancement.

A possible explanation as to why antigen may give more consistent enhancement of tumor growth in vivo than does whole tumor bearer serum is that antigens may be eliminated less quickly upon inoculation than are antigen-antibody complexes in tumor bearer sera. The antigen could block by itself, but it could also stimulate the host to synthesize antibodies which combine with the antigen to form immune complexes. Furthermore, the amount of circulating antigen and complexes in tumor bearer sera may be much less than the amount present in cells or extracts enhancing tumor growth.

Conclusions

Inoculation of certain hyperimmune sera or of certain antigen preparations from tumors can facilitate tumor growth in vivo. Whether this facilitation is due to a blocking mechanism akin to immunological enhancement, or has some other explanation, has not been clarified. More critical work is needed to establish the extent to which serum blocking factors detected in vitro play a role in vivo. It is unfortunate that only one relatively small study (79) has been carried out which tested both for the presence of detectable serum blocking activity in animals following inoculation with tumor bearer sera and for subsequent enhancement of the growth of a tumor challenge.

THE NATURE OF THE BLOCKING SERUM FACTORS AND THEIR MODE OF ACTION

Evidence Suggesting That Blocking Factors Contain Both Antigens and Antibodies

The fact that serum blocking activity generally disappears shortly after tumor removal or regression (3) suggests that the tumor contributes some important component of blocking factors, probably a tumor antigen. The finding that blocking activity can generally be removed from serum by absorption with appropriate tumor cells (19) indicates that another component of blocking factors may be antibodies; this is true also when the blocking effect is tested by preincubating the effector cells with serum and then washing them prior to the assay (76). The simplest way to cope with these findings would be to postulate that the blocking factors are often antigen-antibody complexes (82). This postulate has been supported by experimental data.

The first experimental evidence suggesting that free tumor antigens, as well as antigen-antibody complexes, can act as blocking factors was published in 1971 (18). Sera from mice bearing either a methylcholanthrene-induced sarcoma or a Moloney sarcoma were separated into two components by ultrafiltration at pH 3.1. One serum component was present in a fraction with a molecular weight between 10,000 and 100,000, while the other had a molecular weight above 100,000. The low-molecular-weight component was found to inhibit tumor cell destruction when incubated with the lymphocytes but had no effect when incubated with the tumor cells before the lymphocytes were added. The high-molecular-weight factor did not block when incubated with either the lymphocytes or the target cells. It was postulated that the smaller component contained tumor antigen, that the larger one contained antibody, and that the combination of the two contained antigen-antibody complexes (18). Subsequent work performed on human tumors gave similar findings (83).

Brawn reported in 1971 that destruction of plated mouse tumor cells by lymphocytes immune to their H-2 antigens could be abrogated if sera from mice carrying the same H-2 antigens were added (83). He postulated that soluble H-2 antigens were present in the sera and could act as specific blocking factors.

Brawn also showed (85) that antigenic extracts prepared from either mouse tumors or fetal mouse tissues could inhibit the cytotoxic effect of lymphocytes from multiparous mice on tumor target cells. He ascribed this inhibition to effector cell blockade by antigen. Currie and Basham (86), as well as Thomson et al. (87), subsequently reported similar findings—i.e., inhibition of lymphocyte-mediated target cell destruction by circulating tumor antigen.

Findings of Baldwin et al. have further implicated both tumor antigen and tumor antigen-antibody complexes as capable of abrogating specific cell-mediated antitumor reactivity in vitro (13,27,28). Baldwin et al. showed that tumor extracts, confirmed to contain antigen by a membrane immunofluorescence inhibition test, could block reactivity of lymphocytes which were incubated with the antigen containing extract and washed prior to the assay. Antibody alone, derived from serum of rats whose tumors had been excised, generally did not block when added to either the lymphocytes or the target cells. Mixtures of the appropriate antigen and its antibody, however, could block when added to either the lymphocytes or the target cells. Baldwin et al. concluded that both antigen and antigen-antibody complexes can block, with antigen acting only on lymphocytes, while complexes can act by combining with either lymphocytes or target cells (13,28).

This view has been further supported by more recent investigations. Gorczynski and Knight studied mice with Moloney sarcomas and showed that antigens, as well as antigen-antibody complexes, can block lymphocyte-mediated tumor cell killing (30). Both a specific T-cell-mediated destruction of tumor cells and a less specific cytotoxic effect of macrophages or K cells could be blocked by antigens and complexes.

Baldwin et al. have presented evidence for inhibition of lymphocyte-mediated reactivity to human tumor cells by exposure to extracts containing specific tumor antigens (88). Some evidence for inhibition of lymphocyte-mediated reactivity to cells from human colonic carcinomas by circulating antigens and antigen-antibody complexes has recently been reported by Nind et al. (89).

Jose et al. reported that lymphocyte-mediated destruction of autologous human neuroblastoma cells could be blocked by complexes between tumor antigens and specific IgG antibodies (90,91). They presented data which clearly indicated that antigen-antibody complexes were the essential blockers in sera from patients with neuroblastoma and were more efficient than tumor antigens alone. These findings were published fairly recently; final conclusions must await their independent confirmation.

Tamerius et al. studied the ability of sera from multiparous mice to abrogate destruction of syngeneic neoplastic cells by lymphocytes from multiparous mice (92). The blocking activity of such sera could be removed by passage through an immunoadsorbent which was prepared with a rabbit antiserum to mouse embryonic cells. It was also removed by passage of serum through an immunoadsorbent removing IgG2a or IgG2b immunoglobulins. From these findings the conclusion was drawn that the blocking factors had specificities corresponding to both embryonic antigens and IgG antibodies, and that they were most likely complexes between the two.

Recent work by Tamerius et al. on mice with chemically induced sarcomas has further supported this notion (93). Immunoadsorbents prepared from sera from mice hyperimmunized against a chemically induced mouse sarcoma could remove the blocking activity of sera from mice carrying the same sarcoma, whereas a control adsorbent prepared from normal control mouse serum could not. The blocking activity was recovered in the eluates from the immunoadsorbents and was shown to cofractionate with an IgG marker on a Sephadex G200 column. Greater than hundredfold purification of the blocking factors was obtained in this peak.

When sera from mice carrying a methylcholanthrene-induced sarcoma were recently studied further, using immunoadsorbents prepared from hyperimmune sera raised against the particular sarcoma, evidence was obtained that the blocking factor involved had a molecular weight of approximately 56,000 (94). These data suggest that the blocking factor operating in that particular system was either tumor antigen or some immunosuppressive substance that was neither antigen nor antibody, while the data do not fit the idea that the blocking factor in that system is an antigen-antibody complex. Work is presently ongoing to characterize the blocking factors further and to investigate the relative roles of antigens, antibodies, complexes, and other immunosuppressive substances in providing specific blocking of cell-mediated antitumor immunity.

Another approach which may also be useful for purifying blocking factors is to utilize the ability of "protein A," isolated from *Staphylococcus aureus,* to remove certain IgG antibodies from serum. Steele et al. have shown that sera from tumor-bearing rats, when treated with protein A, lose their specific blocking activity (95). A disadvantage of this approach is that it is more indirect than are techniques using immunoadsorbents prepared with specific antibodies (93).

Blocking Effects of Free Antigens Versus Complexes

It is not yet clear what proportion of the blocking effect of tumor bearer serum is due to free antigen, or to antigen present as immune complexes. Neither is it well established whether complexes or free antigens are more efficient as blockers.

The fact that the blocking effect of tumor bearer or multipara sera as tested at either the target cell or the lymphocyte level can be regularly removed by absorption with appropriate tumor cells (19,76,77,96) suggests that the blocking factors are more commonly complexes than free antigens. Findings of Baldwin et al. (97) indicate that soon after tumor transplantation, blocking factors are primarily free antigens, but they become complexes within the next few days and remain so for the life of animals carrying transplanted tumors; blocking complexes in antibody excess may be seen late.

Studies by Diener and Feldman on tolerization of B lymphocytes in vitro indicate that exposure of lymphocytes to antigen-antibody complexes more easily renders them nonreactive than exposure to free antigens (98). They have hypothesized that antibodies can cross-link the antigens to lymphocyte receptor sites (98). In tumor systems it has not been tested, however, whether antigen-antibody complexes are, indeed, more effective in blocking lymphocyte reactivity than are free antigens, except for the one study of Jose et al. (91), suggesting that complexes are more efficient blockers.

There is some evidence (mentioned above) that putatively embryonic tumor antigens more efficiently elicit blocking factor formation than do individually unique tumor-specific transplantation antigens (37,39). However, the difference between antigens stimulating a cytotoxic immune response in vivo or in vitro, and antigens inhibiting such a response, either alone or when complexed with antibodies, remains unclear. One may speculate that the molecular nature of the antigen, its dose, and its mode of presentation (in soluble form, as compared to antigens bound to a cell surface), as well as the immune competence of the host may all influence the kind of immune response obtained. Knowledge in this area seems fundamental to any attempt to modify the immune response in favor of tumor destruction.

Mode of Action of Blocking Factors

The mode of action of blocking factors is poorly understood. When T-cell-mediated tumor cell killing is inhibited (30,36,99,100), one may speculate that the blocking factors bind to receptors on T lymphocytes specific for target cell antigens and that this prevents the lymphocytes from damaging the tumor cells upon contact and/or from producing lymphokines. This inhibition has to be reversible to account for the finding that lymphocytes from tumor-bearing animals are often able to kill cells from the respective neoplasm in vitro, either immediately or after a short period of incubation in vitro (3). There is, however no proof that there is direct interaction between blocking factors and cytotoxic lymphocytes, or that blocking factors do not act in an indirect way, perhaps by a mechanism involving suppressor cells. Studies in this area are much needed.

The cytotoxic effect of K cells, acting in consort with lymphocyte-dependent antibodies, can be inhibited by complexes between specific antigens and their antibodies (99,101). The great sensitivity of the K lymphocyte effect also to nonspecific inhibition by various types of antigen-antibody complexes (101) is noteworthy, however. This may contribute to the apparently low efficiency of K cell killing of tumor cells in vivo, as contrasted to the greater efficiency of such killing in vitro.

Unblocking and Blocking Effects of Free Antibodies

Since tumor antigen, alone and as part of a complex with antibody, appears to be largely responsible for the blocking effect of tumor bearer serum, then antibodies to tumor antigen are likely to cancel this effect—i.e., to be "unblocking"—if present in sufficient concentrations. There is, indeed, experimental evidence for this: sera from animals and human patients whose tumors have regressed or have been excised can decrease the blocking activity of tumor bearers' sera (72,73). The unblocking effect has been shown to be specific, and the serum factors responsible for it to be antibodies to the respective tumor antigen (3). These antibodies can be used for preparing immunoadsorbents which will remove the blocking activity of tumor-bearing sera, and from which the blocking factors can be subsequently eluted (92,93; also see above).

That the unblocking effect and the removal of blocking factors by using antitumor antibodies for preparing immunoadsorbents is really due to an interaction between these antibodies and antigens forming part of the block factors has not been conclusively proven. It thus remains possible (albeit unlikely) that the unblocking effect is due to an interaction with some immunosuppressive substance which is not antigen.

Under certain circumstances, antibodies to tumor antigens, particularly antibodies present in hyperimmune sera, are not unblocking but can abrogate a cytotoxic antitumor immune response following interaction with the target cells (77,102). It is possible that these antibodies at certain dilutions facilitate the release of antigens from the tumor cells and form complexes with them (77). It is also possible, however, that they may mask target cell antigens and give an efferent form of enhancement (102). In vivo, similar antibodies may also give afferent enhancement, by binding to tumor cell antigens and preventing them from immunizing the host.

Antibodies which are unblocking in microcytotoxicity assays may, at the same time, inhibit a proliferative response of lymphocytes exposed to tumor antigens. Although such inhibition of proliferation has not been sufficiently studied in tumor systems, it is well documented that antibodies to alloantigens can inhibit proliferation in mixed leukocyte cultures (55).

Conclusions

Free tumor antigens, as well as antigen-antibody complexes, and possibly other immunosuppressive substances, can specifically block lymphocyte-mediated cytotoxic reactions to tumor antigens; they most commonly do so by interacting with the effector cells. This may represent a form of central enhancement. Antibodies to tumor antigens can be "unblocking" when tested in combination with immune lymphocytes. They may also inhibit proliferative lymphocyte responses in vitro, they may block target cell destruction in vitro by masking their antigens or by releasing antigens from the tumor cells, and they may participate in tumor enhancement in vivo.

MECHANISMS OF FORMATION OF THE ANTIBODY PART OF BLOCKING ANTIGEN-ANTIBODY COMPLEXES

Since the blocking factors in tumor bearer sera appear to be more often antigen-antibody complexes than free antigens, it is important to understand the mode of production of the antibody component. Relatively little is known about this. What is known comes primarily from studies performed by Nelson et al., using spleen cultures from tumor-bearing mice carrying chemically induced sarcomas (100, 103–105). Since these tumors have individually unique tumor-specific transplantation antigens, it was possible to demonstrate the specificity of blocking factors formed by performing criss-cross experiments, using the same spleen culture material with one type of tumor target cell as the experimental group, and the other as the control. The work by Nelson et al. is reviewed below.

Formation of Blocking Factors by Mouse Spleen Cultures

Cell cultures were prepared from the spleens of mice carrying sarcomas and were maintained in vitro under conditions ensuring their viability. Supernatants from such cultures were tested for factors which could specifically block cell-mediated destruction of the respective sarcomas. The immunization procedure used to produce effector cells for these assays was one which led primarily to the development of cytotoxic cells expressing Thy-1 antigens (100).

Blocking factors were regularly detected in culture supernatants from tumor bearer spleen cells in spite of the fact that these cells had been thoroughly washed and cultured in fresh medium at 2–3 day intervals (103, 105). Spleen cell supernatants from tumor-excised animals did generally not contain blocking factors (103).

Nelson et al. determined whether the blocking activity of the spleen culture supernatants resulted from active synthesis during culture or from passive release of preformed blocking factors in vitro (105). This was approached by adding tritium-labeled leucine to the culture medium and isolating IgG immunoglobulins from the supernatants 24–48 hours afterwards by using immunoadsorption procedures. The spleen cultures were found to produce labeled immunoglobulin molecules which could specifically bind to tumor cells from the same line as the ones carried by the spleen cell donors, and which could inhibit lymphocyte-mediated destruction of the respective tumor cells. These findings indicate that blocking factors were actively synthesized by the spleen cultures and contained at least in part immunoglobulin.

The next step was to study the effect of inhibitors of protein synthesis on blocking factor production by the spleen cultures. Both puromycin and cyclohex-imide inhibition of protein synthesis could completely shut off synthesis of the blocking factors (105). The results with cycloheximide were particularly interesting, since this drug can inhibit protein synthesis in a reversible way. Cultures receiving 5 μg or more cycloheximide per ml neither formed protein nor produced blocking factors. After cycloheximide was removed from the culture medium, both protein synthesis and blocking factor production resumed.

These findings further support the notion that production of blocking factors occurs in vitro. The sensitivity to antimetabolites of the in vitro production is particularly interesting. It suggests that exposure of an effector cell population to the appropriate antimetabolite might selectively increase its cytotoxic reactivity (in vitro), when the effector cell population consists of a combination of already reactive lymphocytes, which are resistant to the drug, and drug-sensitive cells producing blocking factors. Since the ability of immune lymphocytes to destroy their targets in vitro is resistant to inhibition of protein synthesis (106), such a situation may be actually achieved. There is some evidence to support this prediction: antitumor reactive cells have been found to be more capable of destroying their targets in the presence of cycloheximide or puromycin, which prevent the synthesis of blocking factors (107); one cannot conclude, however, that the increased reactivity seen in the latter case necessarily resulted from depressed blocking factor formation.

Nature of Cells Forming Blocking Factors in Mouse Spleen Cultures

Nelson et al. studied the nature of the cells involved in the synthesis of blocking factors by mouse spleen cultures (100). It was found that removal of macrophages and plasma cells by passage of spleen cells through Sephadex G-10 columns did not decrease this synthesis, nor did removal of cells which carried immunoglobulins at their surface. On the other hand, spleen cells incubated with antiserum to the Thy-1 antigen, in the presence of complement, no longer produced blocking factors. Production was fully restored if untreated lymphoid cells from the same tumor-bearing animals, enriched for Thy-1 bearing cells, were added back to the spleen cultures. Partial restoration was seen also when, instead, the cultures were reconstituted with T-enriched spleen cells from untreated syngeneic mice which had not been sensitized to the tumor.

These findings indicate that the synthesis by mouse spleen cultures of blocking factors capable of inhibiting a T-cell-mediated cytotoxic response is dependent on a T cell function. It remains uncertain whether the immunoglobulin part of the blocking factors is produced by T cells or by B (or plasma) cells as a T-cell-dependent event. The fact that removal of B cells, macrophages, and plasma cells from the same cultures entirely removed their ability to form lymphocyte-dependent antibodies (104), which are active at a much lower concentration than the blocking factors, suggests (but does not prove) that the immunoglobulin part of the blocking factors may, indeed, be synthesized by T lymphocytes.

It is interesting that a significant (but depressed) blocking factor synthesis was also seen when T cells from untreated animals were used (100) to reconstitute the T-cell-depleted cultures. A tentative interpretation of this finding is that previously unsensitized T cells quickly become able to make blocking factors in the presence of tumor antigen, or to collaborate with other cells making such factors. Spleen cells from mice whose tumors had been removed did not synthesize blocking factors in vitro (100,103). This indicates that a continued presence of tumor antigen (in the culture) may be crucial for blocking factor production.

Since T cells appear to play an important role in blocking factor synthesis, it is noteworthy that mice which are neonatally thymectomized develop fewer spontaneous mammary carcinomas than do sham-operated controls, and that Heppner found blocking serum factors specific for the mammary tumor antigens less frequently in the thymectomized mice than in the controls (108). This work has not been followed up, however, and a study of the mode of blocking factor production in vivo is much needed.

Suppressor Cells and Blocking Factor Production

In some cases lymphoid cells from tumor-bearing animals have been found to specifically abrogate the cytotoxic response of lymphocytes from tumor-immunized animals, when mixed together with these and tested with either the microcytotoxicity assay (109) or the macrophage migration inhibition technique (45,110). There is some evidence from studies using the latter assay that tumor bearer lymphoid cells release blocking factors into the culture medium (110).

It has recently been demonstrated that lymphoid cell populations from mice bearing sarcomas were initially cytotoxic but became nonreactive following 5 days of in vitro exposure to cells carrying the respective tumor antigens. Such cell populations had suppressive qualities, as detected by mixing the nonreactive cells with reactive cells and testing the mixtures in a microcytotoxicity assay (111). The suppression was at least partially specific.

In all these cases the tumor bearer lymphocytes can, operationally, be characterized as suppressor cells. Further studies are needed to clarify how these cells relate to suppressor cells found in other systems (112) and to the tumor bearer spleen cells shown to produce blocking factors in vitro (100,105).

One may speculate that some of the suppression seen with tumor bearer lymphoid cells is, indeed, mediated by antigen-antibody complexes and/or tumor antigen, released from cells present in the lymphocyte populations tested. It is, however, also possible that the suppression could be caused by other molecules or just by contact between appropriate cells. Some of the suppression may also be nonspecific. Indeed, tumor bearer lymphoid cells can, in some systems, suppress lymphocyte reactivity even to activators like PHA (103).

Finally, one should keep the possibility in mind that tumor growth facilitation, when seen in vitro, may be the outcome of tumor antigens or antigen-antibody complexes activating a suppressor cell mechanism, which enhances tumor growth by turning off effective antitumor immunity.

Conclusions

There is evidence that T lymphocytes are involved in the in vitro synthesis of blocking factors by spleen cultures from tumor-bearing mice. To what extent tumor bearer lymphoid cells can suppress an immune response by releasing blocking antigen-antibody complexes, or free antigens, remains unknown. The sensitivity of blocking-factor synthesis to certain antimetabolites may be exploited to increase effective antitumor reactivity.

IMMUNOLOGIC ENHANCEMENT OF ANTIGENIC TUMORS AND CONCOMITANT TUMOR IMMUNITY

Concomitant Tumor Immunity in Tumor-Bearing Individuals

Southam (114), Gershon et al. (115), and others have shown that tumor-bearing individuals often have a certain degree of transplantation resistance when challenged (outside the tumor site) with cells from the same neoplasm. This phenomenon has been called concomitant tumor immunity. As already discussed, lymphocyte-mediated reactivity against tumor antigens in vitro is also detectable in many individuals with tumor (3). Altogether these observations reflect a systemic immunity present in many tumor-bearing individuals to tumor antigens. They may explain why some patients do not develop generalized metastases even when circulating neoplastic cells are detectable in their blood stream.

Why Can Tumors Grow in an Individual Showing Concomitant Tumor Immunity?

The question arises why an antigenic tumor can grow in its original site and in the area to which it has metastasized but still be rejected when transplanted as a single cell suspension. A plausible answer is suggested by the finding that factors consisting in part of tumor antigens can prevent lymphocytes from attacking neoplastic cells.

In a tumor nodule a large amount of free antigen is likely to be present. Furthermore, antigen-antibody complexes with blocking activity can be eluted from tumors, both in experimental animals and in man (23,79,83). Whether these complexes are actually located on the neoplastic cells themselves, on lymphocytes infiltrating the tumors, or on some stromal cells is not clear; there is, however, evidence that cells derived from tumor biopsies often have immunoglobulin bound to their surface (116,117). The effect of blocking factors on antitumor activity is thus likely to be greater within a growing tumor and in its vicinity than elsewhere in the organism, where the concentration of these factors is smaller. In addition, blocking factors produced locally may be more important than any circulating complexes, which because of their size are likely to be restricted to the vascular compartments and may hence not reach tumor cells existing extravascularly.

Alexander et al. (118) have shown that lymphocytes from lymph nodes draining a tumor do not leave the nodes as long as a growing tumor is present and would, therefore, not be available in sufficient amounts in the area of a growing neoplasm. Free tumor antigens, as well as antigen-antibody complexes, localizing in the lymph nodes are likely candidates responsible for this effect. The finding that specific blocking factors can be eluted from lymph nodes and spleens of tumor-bearing animals (57) supports this notion.

The fact that there is a larger concentration of tumor antigens in the area of a growing neoplasm than elsewhere in the organism implies that blocking factors can be present in sufficient amounts to turn off local cell-mediated tumor destruction, even when tests for these factors in the serum are negative. It also means that even if unblocking antitumor antibodies are inoculated into tumor-bearing individuals in doses which are sufficient to abolish detectable serum blocking activity, blocking factors may still be active at the site of a growing neoplasm. If the tumor mass is large and/or the ability of the tumor cells to release antigens is high, it may be extremely difficult to abolish this local blocking effect. It may even increase if passively administered antibodies facilitate the release of tumor antigens from the neoplastic cells.

Formation of Blocking Factors upon Contact Between Tumor Cells and Antibodies

Hayami et al. showed that some sera from Japanese quail, whose Rous sarcomas had spontaneously regressed, had blocking activity when added to plated Rous sarcoma cells before exposure of these to immune lymphocytes (76,77). They hypothesized that these sera may combine with antigens present on the tumor cells, leading to the formation of blocking antigen-antibody complexes. Amos et al. (6) and Klein (7), studying hyperimmune sera which could enhance allogeneic tumor grafts in mice, had suggested an analogous phenomenon.

To test this possibility, Hayami et al. exposed cultivated Rous sarcoma cells for 24 hours to sera from regressor (or control) quail and tested the culture supernatants for their ability to inhibit specific lymphocyte-mediated destruction of Rous sarcoma cells. Immune lymphoid cells were incubated with these supernatants and were then washed and tested for reactivity to Rous sarcoma cells. It was found that Rous sarcoma cells exposed to regressor serum released blocking factors into the medium, which could inhibit lymphocyte-mediated killing of such target cells when added to the lymphocytes. No blocking activity was detected when the same regressor sera were tested in conjunction with the effector cells without previous incubation with tumor cells (77).

Observations of Thomson et al. (87) are also suggestive in this connection. These investigators showed that the blocking activity of sera from rats transplanted with tumor was reduced by sublethal irradiation of the animals prior to transplantation. They hypothesized that nonirradiated rats transplanted with tumor made antibodies which aided the release of tumor antigens into the circulation, and that antibody formation was reduced by irradiating the rats.

Antigen Release of Tumors as a Mechanism of Escape from Immunologic Control

One may speculate that the extent to which tumor cells can release (blocking) antigens into the surrounding tissue is largely responsible for their ability to escape from immunological control. There is evidence suggesting that embryonic tumor antigens might be more easily released from neoplastic cells than are their individually unique transplantation antigens, and this may explain why the embryonic antigens appear to be more effective as blockers of cell-mediated tumor immunity than the unique antigens (38). Experimental data on this point are, however, scanty.

Critical studies of the ability of various tumor lines to release antigens with blocking properties are needed, as are studies of the ability of antibodies, and immune lymphocytes, to aid the release of tumor antigens from cells. Modern techniques for labeling cell surface antigens (118) may be helpful for such studies.

Conclusions

The higher concentration of tumor antigens and of immune complexes in the area of a growing neoplasm may facilitate its escape from immunologic control. The lower concentration of these factors outside the area of a growing tumor may explain why circulating immune cells can succeed in rejecting transplanted neoplastic cells in many individuals with growing neoplasms.

POSSIBLE CLINICAL VALUE OF MONITORING BLOCKING SERUM FACTORS IN TUMOR-BEARING INDIVIDUALS

The fact that blocking serum factors can be detected in a large variety of animal and human tumor systems suggests that methods by which these factors can be quantitated may be useful for monitoring individuals with cancer undergoing therapy, and possibly also for diagnosing tumors.

Detection of Blocking Factors in Relation to Clinical Course of Tumors

Determination of blocking serum activity for monitoring individuals with cancer seems potentially feasible, since blocking factors are commonly detected in animals or human patients with small tumor loads (41), before a tumor recurrence can be demonstrated clinically (see below). Experiments by Steele et al. on chemically induced colonic carcinomas in rats illustrate this point (32). Rats given chemical carcinogens and subsequently developing primary colonic carcinomas often had tumor-specific blocking factors already before their tumors could be detected with a sensitive X-ray technique capable of demonstrating neoplastic nodules as small as 1–1.5 mm in diameter. Rats which had blocking serum factors developed colon carcinomas, while tumors were not detected in rats whose sera did not block.

Blocking factors have been detected in human patients in remission before they had clinically demonstrable relapses of their neoplasms (32,40). In one study, patients were tested with the microcytotoxicity assay within one to three months following surgery. Blocking serum activity was demonstrated in most of those patients who relapsed within a year, while it was only rarely seen in patients who did not relapse during the same time period (41). Analogous findings have recently been described by Halliday et al. in melanoma patients tested with the leukocyte adherence inhibition technique (49). Patients with growing tumors were found to have sera with blocking activity, thereby differing from patients who had no clinical evidence of tumor. Halliday et al. have also shown that blocking factors detectable with the leukocyte adherence inhibition test could be demonstrated prior to relapse in patients with hepatic carcinomas (130).

Need for Better Techniques to Assay Blocking Serum Factors

There is a great need in this area for techniques which are both more quantitative and more rapid, and which can be used in a routine setting to study blocking serum factors in animals and in human subjects. Perhaps the leukocyte adherence inhibition technique, or some modification of the macrophage migration inhibition assay, may become useful for this purpose, but further confirmation of published work with these techniques is needed before any judgments on their value can be made. Another, perhaps better, strategy might be to purify the tumor antigens so as to be able to develop radioimmunoassays (including assays for the antigen part of blocking complexes). One must realize, however, that we do not know at this time whether the use of improved immunologic techniques will make it possible to detect tumor recurrences any earlier than can be done with more conventional clinical methods.

Effector Cell Blockade by Antigen as Means to Study Tumor Specificity

Lymphocyte-mediated immune reactions to tumor antigens can be inhibited by exposure of the lymphocytes to preparations containing the specific tumor antigen, as reviewed in a preceding section. A possibly useful approach to studying human tumor immunity, therefore, may be to test which reactions can be inhibited by defined tumor antigens (or immune complexes). This approach might circumvent a major technical difficulty when studying cell-mediated tumor immunity in man—namely, nontumor-related reactions against various alloantigens and against contaminating antigens present on the cultivated tumor cells used for most of these studies. Reactions which can be blocked by incubating lymphocytes with specific tumor antigens are more likely to be tumor related than those which cannot. This might be then utilized when following the level of lymphocyte-mediated specific antitumor reactivity in human cancer patients.

Conclusions

Procedures for monitoring the levels of tumor antigens and antigen-antibody complexes in cancer patients may give prognostically useful information. However, tests for doing this which are both simple and reliable are still lacking. Tests for inhibition of lymphocyte-mediated immune responses by antigens may aid in establishing the specificity of such reactions.

POSSIBLE WAYS TO CIRCUMVENT THE BLOCKING MECHANISM IN VIVO

If, indeed, effector cell blockade by antigens and antigen-antibody complexes plays a major role in a tumor's escape from immunologic control, procedures which can circumvent such a blockade may counteract tumor growth in vivo.

Tumor Removal Decreases Blocking Serum Activity

Since the antigen part of the blocking factor seems crucial for its ability to inhibit lymphocyte-mediated tumor cell destruction, a logical approach is to try decreasing the amount of circulating tumor antigen (occurring in free form and/or as immune complexes). The simplest way to do this is to surgically remove the tumor or to destroy it by radiotherapy and/or chemotherapy. This is, of course, also the natural approach to a primary cure, irrespective of whether or not there is an immune response to the tumor.

For the same reason, removal (destruction) of as much tumor tissue as possible may decrease the impact of the blocking mechanism when a complete tumor removal is not feasible and might hence be expected to be therapeutically beneficial. It would follow that measures to reduce total tumor burden should be considered also in individuals whose tumors cannot be eradicated. However, we do not at this time advise such an approach in human patients, since it would be contrary to current clinical practice. Rather, we feel that one should test in animals whether removal of the bulk of incompletely eradicable tumors does decrease serum blocking activity and whether it does prolong survival. If, indeed, a therapeutic value of such an approach were substantiated, a similar trial in man might be considered.

Drugs capable of destroying neoplastic cells might also be used to diminish the impact of the blocking mechanism; if any drugs were available which could decrease the release of tumor antigens, they may lead to the same end. Stolfi et al. (33) could significantly reduce metastasis formation in mice bearing an immunogenic mammary carcinoma by giving combination chemotherapy following surgery. Mice bearing a nonimmunogenic tumor did not benefit from this therapy. Most likely, an immune response to a few neoplastic cells remaining after surgery and chemotherapy was needed for complete cure. The primary effect of the chemotherapy was then to decrease the number of such remaining tumor cells. As a result of this decrease, the amount of blocking tumor antigens (and complexes) also decreased.

Therapy with Unblocking Sera

Another approach to diminish blocking serum activity is to give antibodies in sufficient doses to neutralize all circulating tumor antigen, including the antigen part of immune complexes. Such an approach has been tried to some extent. Fewer mice died from primary Moloney sarcoma (121) and fewer rats died from transplanted polyoma tumors (122) when they were given unblocking (as compared to control) sera, capable of neutralizing the blocking effect of tumor bearer sera in the respective systems. Similar, but less impressive, effects were seen in rats with primary polyoma tumors (123), and the development of lung metastases was delayed following injection of unblocking sera to rats with subcutaneously transplanted polyoma tumors which normally metastasized to the lung (124). Perhaps the most interesting aspect of the latter studies was the finding of a correlation between decreased tumor growth in vivo and low blocking serum activity in vitro (23,24,123,124). This suggests that the serotherapy may have improved the antitumor immunity in the treated animals by decreasing the impact of the blocking mechanism. Alternative interpretations are, however, possible. The therapeutic effects may, e.g., have been the outcome of lymphocyte-dependent antibodies (75) present in the unblocking sera.

It is also apparent that most animals receiving unblocking sera ultimately died from their tumors and that the effects observed, although significant, were not remarkable. A possible explanation is that it may be impossible to neutralize all free antigens at the site of a growing neoplasm. Rather, as discussed above, sera which are unblocking in vitro may—particularly when given to animals with large antigen loads—create more, rather than less, blocking antigen-antibody complexes in the area of a growing tumor. Furthermore, inoculation of large doses of unblocking sera may produce afferent enhancement by decreasing the ability of the tumor antigens to immunize, so that more effector cells will be generated.

Treatment with unblocking sera during the latency period of primary tumor induction may demonstrate more remarkable effects. Preliminary experiments in which mice were given unblocking sera, followed by methylcholanthrene, are interesting in this context. The unblocking sera had been raised against common, putatively embryonic antigens present on most chemically induced mouse sarcomas; these antigens do not serve as good targets for an immune response in standard tests for tumor-specific transplantation immunity (13,38). Mice inoculated with unblocking sera during the first 22 weeks following injection of methylcholanthrene developed significantly fewer primary sarcomas than did control animals (57).

Some attempts to treat human cancer patients with unblocking sera have been made. So far, no convincing beneficial effects have been reported, but a large study to evaluate this mode of treatment is underway, studying patients with melanomas. This work has recently been reviewed (125) and will, therefore, not be covered here.

Depression of Antibody Formation as a Means to Decrease Blocking Serum Activity

As discussed in preceding sections, antibodies not only appear to be an integral part of most blocking factors found in the circulation, but they also seem to aid in the release of tumor antigens from neoplastic cells, thereby facilitating the formation of blocking factors. For these reasons, procedures capable of decreasing the production of those humoral antibodies which are most apt to combine with tumor antigens and form blocking complexes may decrease blocking-serum activity and may, thereby, be therapeutically beneficial.

As discussed above, the synthesis of blocking factors by spleen cells in vitro was found to be highly sensitive to inhibition of protein synthesis by puromycin or cycloheximide. Furthermore, mice receiving cytosine arabinoside (126), or combination chemotherapy (33), and rats getting cyclophosphamide (127), had a lower blocking serum activity than the controls. Some evidence has been presented in these studies that mice treated with chemotherapy did clinically better than the controls (33,126,128), while the treated rats did not benefit.

The decreased blocking activity of serum from mice or rats treated with antimetabolites seems most likely to be due to tumor destruction by the drugs. However, in the studies on spleen cultures discussed above, a direct effect on antibody production was apparently observed. For that reason, one should consider the possibility that some of the in vivo effects of chemotherapeutic drugs on blocking serum activity may be due to their ability to depress formation of certain antibodies. To what extent this is related to their therapeutic effects is unknown.

Generation of Cells Which Are Less Blockable

One of the most rational approaches to decrease the influence of the blocking mechanism is to try to generate effector cells which are relatively insensitive to blockade by antigens or complexes. There is some evidence suggesting that this can be achieved. Some of this evidence comes from studies on immunologic enhancement of renal allografts in rats. Rats bearing enhanced allogeneic kidneys were found to possess lymphocytes capable of destroying cells carrying the alloantigens present on the enhanced kidneys, when tested with a 30–40 hour microcytotoxicity assay (129). They also had serum factors which could block the lymphocyte effect, and similar factors could be eluted from the enhanced kidneys. This work was confirmed by subsequent studies, using a similar test (130). When, however, a short-term (4–6 hours) Cr^{51} test was used to assay the immune status of similar rats, neither cytotoxic lymphocytes nor blocking serum factors were found (130). A possible explanation of this discrepancy is that the microcytotoxicity assay measures a combination of two steps, namely an "activation" of immune lymphocytes upon contact with foreign antigens, and the subsequent killing of the target cells. The second step, which may be the only one measured by the Cr^{51} assay, may be less sensitive to blockade by antigens or complexes.

Recent data tend to support this notion (57). Immune lymphocytes which were brought in contact with tumor cells during a 24–48 hour period prior to testing in the microcytotoxicity assay were found to be less sensitive to blockade by tumor-bearer serum than similar lymphocytes tested initially. If the lymphocytes were exposed to tumor bearer serum during the period of contact with the target cells (prior to the test), their reactivity was very low.

Other evidence, indicating that some lymphocyte populations may not be sensitive to blockade by antigens and complexes, was reported by Gorczynski and Knight (30). They found that a subpopulation of T lymphocytes from mice whose Moloney sarcomas had regressed could not be blocked by tumor bearer serum, while most reactive T lymphocytes from similar mice could be easily blocked by antigens and complexes.

Physical Removal of Blocking Factors

One approach that has been suggested for decreasing blocking serum activity is to remove blocking factors from the blood stream by plasmaphoresis, or from the lymph following cannulation of the thoracic duct. Removal might be further accomplished by passage of the plasma (or lymph) through an immunoadsorbent, which removes antigens and complexes. A problem with such an approach, in addition to its obvious technical difficulties, is that those blocking factors which are firmly bound to lymphoid cells would not be removed. Another problem is that antigens would be continuously released from remaining tumor tissues and that antibodies to these antigens would be formed as well. Therefore, physical removal of blocking factors from the blood or lymph does not seem to represent a realistic approach at this time. Neither have the few attempts made in this area been very encouraging (131,132).

Splenectomy

Still another way of trying to decrease the quantity of circulating blocking serum factors in tumor-bearing individuals is to try removing the source of cells synthesizing the antibody part of these factors. There is evidence that the spleen plays a major role in blocking factor synthesis in the mouse and rat (23–25); whether it also does so in other species is unknown. It seems probable, however, that lymphoid cells other than those present in the spleen can synthesize the antibody part of blocking factors, too. It then does not appear likely that splenectomy, per se, is going to effectively decrease blocking serum activity over a sufficiently long period of time to be of therapeutic value.

Conclusions

There are several approaches by which the impact of the blocking mechanism in vivo may be decreased. These include removal of the source of tumor antigens, passive administration of "unblocking" antibodies, and attempts to generate effector cells which are resistant to the blocking effect.

GENERAL CONCLUSIONS

Sera from animals hyperimmune to tumor antigens can enhance (i.e., facilitate) the take of tumor cells transplanted into syngeneic animals. The evidence for an enhancement mechanism in the autochthonous host is more indirect and is primarily based on studies performed in vitro. Sera from tumor-bearing animals and human patients have been regularly found to block (inhibit) lymphocyte-mediated cytotoxic reactions against tumor antigens. A blocking effect of such sera has also been detected in studies performed in the macrophage migration inhibition test and the leukocyte adherence inhibition assay. We postulate that the blocking phenomenon detected in such experiments reflects a major mechanism of escape of antigenic tumors from immunologic control.

In a few instances tumor bearer sera have been shown to enhance tumor growth in vivo, while in other cases sera from tumor-bearing animals have not produced such enhancement. It is quite possible that in the latter cases the sera were given in too low a dose or too infrequently, since no tests were performed to prove that animals inoculated with tumor bearer sera had really developed detectable blocking serum activity as a result of this inoculation. Active enhancement of tumor growth following inoculation of antigen, rather than tumor bearer serum, has been more regularly detected.

The blocking serum factors are of at least three types: free tumor antigens; complexes between tumor antigens and their antibodies; and free antibodies. Free antibodies can block in vitro by "masking" target cell antigens and by aiding in the release of antigens from the tumor cells; in addition they may inhibit the proliferation of lymphocytes exposed to tumor antigens antisera. On the other hand, antisera to tumor antigens are often unblocking in vitro; i.e., they are capable of canceling the blocking effect of tumor bearer sera, probably by combining with the antigenic part of the blocking factors, but they might also enhance tumor growth.

There is evidence from spleen culture experiments in mice that T lymphocytes play a crucial role in the production of the antibody part of the blocking factors.

The fact that blocking serum factors are commonly found in animals and patients with growing tumors suggests that methods by which they can be measured quantitatively would provide useful information for monitoring various forms of tumor therapy.

Procedures by which blocking serum activity can be decreased in vivo may be useful for tumor therapy and, perhaps, also for tumor prevention.

REFERENCES

1. Kaliss, N., *Cancer Res.* **18,** 992 (1958).
2. Hellström, K. E., and Möller, G., *Progr. Allergy* **9,** 158 (1965).
3. Hellström, K. E., and Hellström, I., *Adv. Immunol.* **18,** 209 (1974).
4. Dresser, D. W., and Mitchison, N. A., *Adv. Immunol.* **8,** 129 (1968).
5. Elkins, W. L., Hellström, I., and Hellström, K. E., *Transplantation* **18,** 38 (1974).
6. Amos, D. B., Cohen, T., and Klein, W. J., Jr., *Transpl. Proc.* **2,** 68 (1970).
7. Klein, W. J., Jr., *J. Exp. Med.* **134,** 1238 (1971).
8. Bansal, S. C., Hellström, I., Hellström, K. E., and Sjögren, H. O., *J. Exp. Med.* **137,** 590 (1973).
9. Wright, P. W., Hargreaves, R. E., Bansal, S. C., Bernstein, I. D., and Hellström, K. E., *Proc. Nat. Acad. Sci.* **70,** 2539 (1973).
10. Wright, P. W., Hargreaves, R. E., Bernstein, I. D., and Hellström, I., *J. Immunol.* **112,** 1267 (1974).
11. Möller, G., *Nature* (London) **204,** 846 (1964).
12. Hellström, I., Hellström, K. E., Evans, C. A., Heppner, G. H., Pierce, G. E., and Yang, J. P. S., *Proc. Nat. Acad. Sci.* **12,** 362 (1969).
13. Baldwin, R. W., *Adv. Cancer Res.* **18,** 1 (1973).
14. Feldman, I., *Adv. Immunol.* **15,** 167 (1972).
15. Herberman, R. B., *Adv. Cancer Res.* **19,** 207 (1974).
16. Hellström, I., and Hellström, K. E., in *In Vitro Methods in Cell-Mediated Immunity* (B. R. Bloom and P. R. Glade, eds.), Academic Press, New York, 1971, p. 409.
17. Jagarlamoody, S. M., Aust, J. E., Tew, R. H., and McKhann, C. F., *Proc. Nat. Acad. Sci.* **68,** 1346 (1971).
18. Sjögren, H. O., Hellström, I., Bansal, S. C., and Hellström, K. E., *Proc. Nat. Acad. Sci.* **68,** 1372 (1971).
19. Hellström, I., and Hellström, K. E., *Int. J. Cancer* **4,** 587 (1969).
20. Heppner, G. H., *Int. J. Cancer* **4,** 608 (1969).
21. Hellström, I., Evans, C. A., and Hellström, K. E., *Int. J. Cancer* **4,** 601 (1969).
22. Sjögren, H. O., and Borum, K., *Cancer Res.* **31,** 890 (1971).
23. Sjögren, H. O., and Bansal, S. C., in *Progress in Immunology* (B. Amos, ed.), Academic Press, New York, 1971, p. 921.
24. Bansal, S. C., and Sjögren, H. O., *Fed. Proc. Amer. Soc. Exp. Biol.* **32,** 165 (1973).
25. Hellström, I., Hellström, K. E., and Sjögren, H. O., *Cell. Immunol.* **1,** 18 (1970).
26. Baldwin, R. W., Glaves, D., and Pimm, M. V., in *Progress in Immunology* (B. Amos, ed.), Academic Press, New York, 1971, p. 907.
27. Baldwin, R. W., Price, M. R., and Robins, R. A., *Nat. New Biol.* **238,** 185 (1972).
28. Baldwin, R. W., Embleton, M. J., and Robins, R. A., *Int. J. Cancer* **11,** 1 (1973).
29. Baldwin, R. W., Price, M. R., and Robins, R. A., *Int. J. Cancer* **11,** 527 (1973).
30. Gorczynski, R., and Knight, R. A., *Brit. J. Cancer* **31,** 387 (1975).
31. Steele, G., Jr., and Sjögren, H. O., *Cancer Res.* **34,** 1801 (1974).
32. Steele, G., Jr., Sjögren, H. O., Rosengren, J. E., Lindström, C., Larsson, A., and Leandoer, L., *J. Nat. Cancer Inst.* **54,** 959 (1975).
33. Stolfi, R. L., Fugmann, R. A., Stolfi, L. M., and Martin, D. S., *Int. J. Cancer* **13,** 389 (1974).
34. Dierlam, P., Anderson, N. G., and Coggin, J. H., Jr., *Proceedings of the First Conference and Workshop on Embryonic and Fetal Antigens in Cancer*, Oak Ridge National Laboratory, Oak Ridge, Tenn., 1971, p. 203.
35. Baldwin, R. W., and Embleton, M. J., *Int. J. Cancer* **13,** 433 (1974).
36. Hellström, I., and Hellström, K. E., *Int. J. Cancer* **15,** 1 (1975).
37. Hellström, I., and Hellström, K. E., *Int. J. Cancer* **15,** 30 (1975).

38. Hellström, K. E., and Hellström, I., in *Critical Factors in Cancer Immunology* (J. Schultz and R. C. Leif, eds.), Miami Winter Symposia, Vol. 10 (1975), p. 211.

39. Hellström, I., Sjögren, H. O., Warner, G., and Hellström, K. E., *Int. J. Cancer* **7**, 226 (1971).

40. Hellström, I. Warner, G. A., Hellström, K. E., and Sjögren, H. O., *Int. J. Cancer* **11**, 280 (1973).

41. Hellström, I., and Hellström, K. E., *Cancer* **34**, 1461 (1974).

42. Baldwin, R. W., Embleton, M. J., Jones, S. P., Jr., and Langman, M. J. S., *Int. J. Cancer* **12**, 73 (1973).

43. Avis, F., Mosonov, I., and Haughton, G., *J. Nat. Cancer Inst.* **52**, 1041 (1974).

44. Halliday, W. J., *J. Immunol.* **106**, 855 (1971).

45. Halliday, W. J., *Cell. Immunol.* **3**, 113 (1972).

46. Poupon, M.-F., Lespinats, G., and Kolb, J.-P., *J. Nat. Cancer Inst.* **52**, 1127 (1974).

47. Halliday, W. J., Maluish, A., and Miller, S., *Cell. Immunol.* **10**, 467 (1974).

48. Maluish, A., and Halliday, W. J., *J. Nat. Cancer Inst.* **52**, 1415 (1974).

49. Halliday, W. J., Maluish, A. E., Little, J. H., and Davis, N. C., *Int. J. Cancer* **16**, 645 (1975).

50. Vanky, F., Stjernswärd, J., Klein, G., and Nilsonne, V., *J. Nat. Cancer Inst.* **47**, 95 (1971).

51. Wright, P. W., and Bernstein, I. D., to be published.

52. Knight, R. A., Mitchison, N. A., and Shellam, G. R., *Int. J. Cancer* **15**, 417 (1975).

53. Deckers, P. J., Davis, R. C., Parker, G. A., and Mannik, J. A., *Cancer Res.* **33**, 33 (1973).

54. Gutterman, J. U., Rossen, R. D., Butler, W. T., McCredie, K. B., Bodey, G. P., Sr., Freireich, E. J., and Hersh, E. M., *N. Engl. J. Med.* **288**, 169 (1973).

55. Bernstein, I. D., Hamilton, B. L., Wright, P. W., Burstein, R., and Hellström, K. E., *J. Immunol.* **114**, 320 (1975).

56. Hattler, B. G., Jr., and Soehnlen, B., *Science* **184**, 1374 (1974).

57. Hellström, K. E., and Hellström, I., *J. Ann. N.Y. Acad. Sci.*, **276**, 176 (1976).

58. De Landazuri, M. O., and Herberman, R. B., *J. Exp. Med.* **136**, 969 (1972).

59. Laux, D., and Lausch, R. N., *J. Immunol.* **112**, 1900 (1974).

60. Blasecki, J. W., and Tevethia, S. S., *Int. J. Cancer* **16**, 275 (1975).

61. Barski, G., and Youn, J. K., *J. Nat. Cancer Inst.* **43**, 111 (1969).

62. Barski, G., Youn, J. K., LeFrancois, D., and Belehradek, J., Jr., *Israel J. Med. Sci.* **10**, 913 (1974).

63. Belehradek, J., Jr., Barski, G., and Thonier, M., *Int. J. Cancer* **9**, 461 (1972).

64. Paranjpe, M. S., and Boone, C. W., *Int. J. Cancer* **13**, 179 (1974).

65. Howell, S. B., Dean, J. H., and Law, L. W., *Int. J. Cancer* **15**, 152 (1975).

66. Mikulska, Z. B., Smith, C., and Alexander, P., *J. Nat. Cancer Inst.* **46**, 981 (1971).

67. Paranjpe, M. S., and Boone, C. W., *Cancer Res.* **35**, 1209 (1975).

68. Vaage, J., *Cancer Res.* **33**, 493 (1973).

69. Youn, J. K., LeFrancois, D., Hue, G., Santillana, M., and Barski, G., *Int. J. Cancer* **16**, 629 (1975).

70. Apffel, C. A., and Peters, J. H., *Progr. Exp. Tumor Res.* **12**, 1 (1969).

71. Simmons, R. L., Rios, A., Ray, P. V., and Lundgren, G., *J. Nat. Cancer Inst.* **47**, 1087 (1971).

72. Hellström, I., and Hellström, K. E., *Int. J. Cancer* **5**, 195 (1970).

73. Hellström, I., Hellström, K. E., Sjögren, H. O., and Warner, G. A., *Int. J. Cancer* **8**, 185 (1971).

74. Stjernswärd, J., *J. Nat. Cancer Inst.* **40**, 13 (1968).

75. Pollack, S., Heppner, G., Brawn, R. J., and Nelson, K., *Int. J. Cancer* **9**, 316 (1972).

76. Hayami, M., Hellström, I., and Hellström, K. E., *Int. J. Cancer* **12**, 667 (1973).

77. Hayami, M., Hellström, I., Hellström, K. E., and Lannin, D. R., *Int. J. Cancer* **13**, 43 (1974).

78. Pierce, G. E., *Int. J. Cancer* **8**, 22, (1971).

79. Bansal, S. C., Hargreaves, R., and Sjögren, H. O., *Int. J. Cancer* **9**, 97 (1972).

80. Vaage, J., *Cancer Res.* **32**, 193 (1972).

81. Proctor, J. W., Rudenstam, C. M., and Alexander, P., *Nature* **242**, 29 (1973).

82. Hellström, I., and Hellström, K. E., *Tranpl. Proc.* **3**, 721 (1971).

83. Sjögren, H. O., Hellström, I., Bansal, S. C., Warner, G. A., and Hellström, K. E., *Int. J. Cancer* **9**, 274 (1972).

84. Brawn, R. J., *Proc. Nat. Acad. Sci.* **68**, 1634 (1971).

85. Brawn, R. J., in *Proceedings of the First Conference and Workshop on Embryonic and Fetal Antigens in Cancer*, Oak Ridge National Laboratory, Oak Ridge, Tenn., 1971, p. 143.

86. Currie, G. A., and Basham, C., *Brit. J. Cancer* **26**, 427 (1972).

87. Thomson, D. M., Steele, K., and Alexander, P., *Brit. J. Cancer* **27**, 27 (1973).

88. Baldwin, R. W., Embleton, M. J., and Price, M. R., *Int. J. Cancer* **12**, 84 (1973).

89. Nind, A. P. P., Matthews, N., Pihl, E. A. V., Rolland, J. M., and Nairn, R. C., *Brit. J. Cancer* **31**, 620 (1975).

90. Jose, D. G., and Skvaril, F., *Int. J. Cancer* **13**, 173 (1974).

91. Jose, D. G., and Seshadri, R., *Int. J. Cancer* **13**, 824 (1974).

92. Tamerius, J., Hellström, I., and Hellström, K. E., *Int. J. Cancer* **16**, 456 (1975).

93. Tamerius, J., Nepom, J., Hellström, I., and Hellström, K. E., *J. Immunol.* **116**: 724 (1976).

94. Nepom, J. T., Hellström, I., and Hellström, K. E., *J. Immunol.*, in press.

95. Steele, G., Jr., Ankerst, J., and Sjögren, H. O., *Int. J. Cancer* **14**, 83 (1974).

96. Steele, G., Jr., and Sjögren, H. O., *Int. J. Cancer* **14**, 435 (1974).

97. Baldwin, R. W., and Price, M. R., *Ann. N.Y. Acad. Sci.* **276**, 3 (1976).

98. Diener, E., and Feldmann, M., *Transplant, Rev.* **8**, 76 (1971).

99. Gorczynski, R. M., Kilburn, D. C., Knight, R. A., Norbury, C., Parker, D. C., and Smith, J. B., *Nature* **254**, 141 (1975).

100. Nelson, K., Pollack, S. B., and Hellström, K. E., *Int. J. Cancer* **16**, 539 (1975).

101. Perlmann, P., Perlmann, H., and Wigzell, H., *Transplant. Rev.* **13**, 91 (1972).

102. Robins, R. A., and Baldwin, R. W., *Int. J. Cancer* **14**, 589 (1974).

103. Nelson, K., Pollack, S. B., and Hellström, K. E., *Int. J. Cancer* **15**, 806 (1975).

104. Nelson, K., Pollack, S. B., and Hellström, K. E., *Int. J. Cancer* **16**, 292 (1975).

105. Nelson, K., Pollack, S. B., and Hellström, K. E., *Int. J. Cancer* **16**: 539 (1975).

106. Henney, C., *Transplant. Rev.* **17**, 37 (1973).

107. Hellström, I., Hellström, K. E., Nepom, J. T., *Int. J. Cancer* **116**: 724 (1976).

108. Heppner, G. J., in *Immunity and Tolerance in Oncogenesis* (L. Severi, ed.), Division of Cancer Research, Perugia University, Perugia, Italy, 1970, p. 503.

109. Hayami, M., Hellström, I., Hellström, K. E., and Yamanouchi, K., *Int. J. Cancer* **10**, 507 (1972).

110. Blasecki, J. W., and Tevethia, S. S., *J. Immunol.* **114**, 244 (1975).

111. Kall, M. A., Hellström, I., and Hellström, K. E., *Proc. Natl. Acad. Sci.* **72**: 5086 (1975).

112. Gershon, R. K., in *Contemporary Topics in Immunology* (M. D. Cooper and N. L. Warner, eds.), Vol. 3, Plenum Publishing Co., New York, 1974, p. 1.

113. Gorczynski, R. M., *J. Immunol.* **112**, 1826 (1974).

114. Southam, C. M., *Progr. Exp. Tumor Res.* **9**, 1 (1967).

115. Gershon, R. K., Carter, R. L., and Kondo, K., *Nature* (London) **224**, 277 (1969).

116. Ran, M., and Witz, I. P., *Int. J. Cancer* **6**, 361 (1970).

117. Irie, K., Irie, R. F., and Morton, D. L., *Cancer Res.* **35**, 1244 (1975).

118. Alexander, P., Bensted, J., DeLorme, E. J., Hall, J. G., and Hodgetts, J. B., *Proc. Roy. Soc.* **B 174**, 237 (1969).

119. Juliano, R. L., and Behar-Bannelier, M., *Biochem. Biophys. Acta* **375**, 249 (1975).

120. Halliday, W. J., Halliday, J. W., Campbell, C. B., Maluish, A., and Powell, L. W., *Brit. Med. J.* **2**, 349 (1974).

121. Hellström, I., Hellström, K. E., Pierce, G. E., and Fefer, A., *Transpl. Proc.* **1**, 90 (1969).

122. Bansal, S. C., and Sjögren, H. O., *Nat. New Biol.* (London) **233**, 76 (1971).

123. Bansal, S. C., and Sjögren, H. O., *Int. J. Cancer* **9**, 490 (1972).

124. Bansal, S. C., and Sjögren, H. O., *Int. J. Cancer* **12,** 179 (1973).

125. Wright, P. W., Hellström, K. E., Hellström, I., and Bernstein, I. D., *Med. Clin. of North America* **60,** 607 (1976).

126. Heppner, G. H., and Calabresi, P., *J. Nat. Cancer Inst.* **48,** 1161 (1972).

127. Steele, G., Jr., Sjögren, H. O., and Ankerst, J., *Int. J. Cancer* **14,** 743 (1974).

128. Steele, G., Jr., and Pierce, G. E., *Int. J. Cancer* **13,** 572 (1974).

129. Stuart, F. P., Fitch, F. W., Rowley, D. A., Biesecker, J. L., Hellström, K. E., and Hellström, I., *Transplantation* **12,** 331 (1971).

130. Biesecker, J. L., Fitch, F. W., Rowley, D. A., Scollard, D., and Stuart, F. P., *Transplantation* **16,** 421 (1973).

131. Noonan, F. P., Gardner, M. A. H., Clunie, G. J. A., Isbister, W. H., and Halliday, W. J., *Int. J. Cancer* **13,** 640 (1974).

132. Isbister, W. H., Noonan, F. P., and Halliday, W. J., *Cancer* **35,** 1465 (1975).

Chapter Seven

Existence of Tumor Immunity in Man

RONALD B. HERBERMAN

Laboratory of Immunodiagnosis, National Cancer Institute, Bethesda, Maryland

The concept of the existence of tumor immunity, even in experimental animal systems, only began to develop solid support about 20 years ago. A series of studies were performed, mainly with chemically induced sarcomas of inbred mice, which clearly demonstrated that tumor-bearing individuals develop specific immunity to tumor antigens (1–4). Since these important in vivo studies, a large body of in vitro evidence supporting the concept of humoral and cell-mediated immunity against tumors in experimental animals has developed (e.g., see recent reviews in 5,6 and Chapters 3 and 4). The accumulation of strong evidence for the existence of tumor immunity in man has occurred at a slower pace. This has certainly not been due to a relative lack of interest in this question, but rather to the difficulties in performing the appropriate, well-controlled studies with human tumor materials and cancer patients.

For many years some clinical features of cancer have suggested that host defense mechanisms play a role in human neoplasia. The rare occurrence of well-documented cases of spontaneous regressions of cancer (7,8) and the more frequent instances of prolonged survival of tumor-bearing patients, not accountable for by any therapeutic intervention, have been cited as presumptive evidence for the existence of tumor immunity in man (9). Another clinical observation, pointing more directly to immune reactions against tumors, has been the infiltration of some primary tumors with cells mediating immune responses, i.e., lymphocytes, macrophages, and plasma cells. This has been most extensively studied in breast cancer, where such infiltration has correlated to some extent with a good prognosis (10,11, also Chapter 1).

Over the last ten years there has been a considerable increase in evidence for humoral and cell-mediated immunity against a variety of human tumors. The rate of progress has been dramatic. In 1967 a review of tumor immunology stated that "although numerous attempts have been made, there is no certain evidence for the antigenicity of any given tumor in man" (12). Just five years later the same authors were much more optimistic, pointing to "direct evidence that human patients respond immunologically to their own tumors" (13). At present it is widely accepted that human tumor immunity exists (14–17).

One of the principal objectives of this review is to examine in detail the evidence supporting this concept, and its implications. First, it is important to ask what is meant by "tumor immunity in man." In one sense, and the one most important to the patient with cancer, this means host resistance, mediated by the immune system, against the autochthonous tumor. This form of immunity must be directed against tumor-specific or tumor-associated transplantation antigens (TATA's, see 6 for discussion of definition). In experimental tumor systems it has been relatively simple to perform in vivo protection experiments and gather evidence for TATA's. In man, however, it has been very difficult, for ethical and logistical reasons, to perform comparable in vivo experiments and therefore direct evidence for immunity to TATA's is quite limited. The data on this critical issue will be reviewed below.

Most of the evidence for the existence of tumor immunity is less focused and concerns immunity against any tumor-associated antigens. It is often assumed that the tumor antigens detected by various immunologic assays, particularly those antigens expressed on the cell surface, are TATA's. In most cases, however, little or no evidence for this relationship is given. In fact it is quite difficult to demonstrate, particularly in man, that a given cell surface antigen detected by an in vitro technique is the same as the TATA (18). Despite our limited knowledge about the in vivo relevance of many of the assays, the data do support the general concept of tumor immunity, and most of this review will discuss this type of evidence. The characteristics of the immune reactions, particularly the specificity, and the limitations of the available data will be considered in detail.

IN VIVO EVIDENCE FOR TUMOR IMMUNITY IN MAN

A series of early in vivo experiments provide the most direct evidence for host resistance against growth of autochthonous tumor. These studies, performed in the 1960s, concerned the behavior of autologous viable tumor cells when inoculated subcutaneously (19–21). In all these studies it was noted that small doses of tumor cells did not grow, and that large numbers (greater than 10^8 cells) were usually needed to produce a nodule. This observation suggested that the patients were resistant to autologous tumor cell growth, but it provided no evidence for an immunologic reaction against human TATA's. Southam and his associates also performed neutralization studies (19,21), very similar to the Winn assays which have been performed in experimental animals and which have provided evidence for immune reactions against TATA's (4,22–24). In 20 of 44 patients the autologous leukocytes inhibited nodule formation by the tumor cells. Leukocytes from healthy donors were used as the control, and these had little or no effect. Unfortunately, although these results suggested cell-mediated immunity against TATA's on the autologous tumor, no definite conclusions could be made because of the inadequacy of the controls (21).

In addition to the above approaches, which potentially could yield important information about human immunity to TATA's, studies involving active immunotherapy could also provide this needed evidence. If immunotherapy with tumor cells or tumor extracts could be shown to prolong survival or disease-free intervals, and if the study were properly controlled, strong support for the role of human TATA's would be obtained. At present little such information exists. Immunotherapy trials involving only active immunotherapy with tumor materials either have been poorly controlled or uncontrolled or have given unimpressive results (25–30). Most of these studies were performed in patients with advanced disease, at a time when immunotherapy would not be expected to succeed (e.g., 31). The successful trials with allogeneic tumor cells have also included systemic administration of BCG (32,33), and it is therefore not possible to determine the mechanism for the apparent therapeutic effects.

In the past few years a number of studies of delayed hypersensitivity to extracts of human tumors have been performed. Such studies have been somewhat crude and difficult to quantitate. Skin tests lack the precision and sophisticated technology of modern in vitro immunologic procedures. However, it is important to consider that these in vivo skin tests may be closer reflections of the state of immunity in cancer patients than are many of the in vitro assays. In fact, in vitro assays of cellular immunity to tuberculin and similar, well-studied soluble antigens have generally been validated by looking for the extent of correlation with delayed hypersensitivity skin reactions (34–38), and not vice versa.

Delayed hypersensitivity skin reactions to extracts of a variety of human tumors have been observed. The early studies involved the use of crude autologous extracts of carcinomas (39–41). Positive reactions were seen in about 25% of the patients. Reactivity either did not correlate well with clinical state (39,40) or positive reactions actually were associated with decreased survival (41). The specificity of the reactions seen in these studies was not well characterized. Some extracts of normal control tissues also gave positive reactions, and bacterial contamination in some of the preparations might have contributed to the reactions.

In several subsequent studies of patients with acute leukemia or Burkitt's lymphoma (42–44) an emphasis was placed on defining the nature and the specificity of the observed reactions. The reactions had all the features of typical delayed hypersensitivity reactions. Only patients who were not anergic—i.e., reacted to one or more recall antigens—had positive reactions with the tumor extracts. Biopsies of positive reactions showed perivascular mononuclear infiltration in the upper dermis, indistinguishable from reactions to tuberculin or other recall antigens (42,44). The specificity of the reactions to crude membrane extracts of leukemic cells was not completely defined, but the antigens appeared to be tumor associated. When tests were performed with extracts at 0.1 mg of protein or less, many positive reactions to autologous and allogeneic tumor extracts occurred. There were virtually no reactions to extracts of normal leukocytes. In the allogeneic tests (44) leukemic patients reacted to extracts of blast cells from patients with the same type of leukemia but did not react to extracts of allogeneic remission cells, or blast cells from the other form of acute leukemia. In addition, only one of 60 normal individuals tested with extracts of allogeneic normal leukocytes gave a positive reaction. Therefore it seemed quite unlikely that the observed reactions were to normal histocompatibility antigens or to normal leukocyte antigens. It is still possible that the antigens involved were differentiation antigens, present on immature normal blast cells as well as on leukemic blasts. In any event, the reactivity of patients to these extracts had a significant correlation with disease status. Patients in remission had much higher reactivity than did patients in relapse (42–44). In addition, Burkitt's lymphoma patients with positive reactions remained in remission significantly longer than those with negative reactions (45).

Skin testing of patients with intestinal cancer has also demonstrated reactivity to antigens which appear to be tumor associated (46,47). Soluble materials, obtained by low-frequency sonication of membrane extracts of intestinal cancer cells, or of fetal intestinal or liver cells, gave positive reactions in autologous or allogeneic patients with intestinal cancer. Comparable preparations from normal intestinal tissues gave negative reactions in these patients. Although the skin-reactive antigen could be found in fetal cells as well as in cancer cells, it was shown to be distinct from the carcinoembryonic antigen of Gold (47).

Skin tests on patients with malignant melanoma have given a more complex pattern of reactivity. In a preliminary report on patients in Uganda (48), the observed reactions were thought to be tumor associated, since extracts of autologous tumors were positive and those from autologous lymphocytes were negative. However, in a more extensive study, using an additional control extract from normal skin, several positive reactions were obtained (49). It appeared from this study, and from a study with American melanoma patients (50), that some of the reactivity was directed against tissue-associated antigens, probably present on normal skin and absent on lymphocytes. These findings emphasize the importance, in all studies of tumor immunity, of having control tissues as close in type to the tumor as possible, in order to distinguish between tumor-associated and tissue-associated antigens. When the crude membrane extracts of melanoma were sonicated and soluble materials fractionated by Sephadex chromatography and polyacrylamide gel electrophoresis (50), evidence for two separate skin-reactive antigens was obtained. The higher molecular weight antigen appeared to be tumor associated. It gave positive reactions in 17 of 22 patients with early stage melanoma and in 7 of 19 patients with advanced disease; it gave no positive reactions in 22 tests of patients with other types of cancer. The other antigen, of lower molecular weight, was isolated from normal skin as well as from melanoma cells and gave positive reactions in both melanoma patients and breast cancer patients. It is of interest to note that this non-tumor-associated antigen also yields a significantly different incidence of reactions in early stage (9 of 21 positive) versus advanced stage (13 of 18 positive) melanoma patients. Based on the finding of a separated soluble melanoma antigen which appeared to be tumor associated (i.e., the higher molecular weight antigen), a group of patients suspected of having ocular melanoma were tested, along with control patients with other types of cancer, and the skin-test responses were found to clearly distinguish between patients with ocular melanoma and those with other diseases (51). Eighteen out of 19 patients with pathologically confirmed melanoma were positive, as were eight other patients with clinical diagnoses of choroidal melanoma. All seven control patients gave negative reactions, as did five patients who were initially thought to have ocular melanomas but who, on extensive work-up, were considered to have other, nonmelanoma, ocular lesions.

Tests for delayed hypersensitivity reactions in breast cancer patients have also provided evidence for separate antigens, one apparently breast-tumor-associated and the other associated with both malignant and normal breast tissues (52,53). The first antigen was detected in breast cancer extracts and not in control breast extracts. It elicited reactivity in patients with either localized or metastatic breast cancer and was negative with patients with other types of carcinomas. The tissue-associated antigen produced skin reactions mainly in breast cancer patients with localized disease, but it also reacted in some patients with other types of gynecologic cancer (53).

Black and Leis (11) used a different approach to study delayed hypersensitivity reactions in breast cancer patients. Their skin-window technique, employing cryostat sections of autologous breast tissues, yielded reactions to apparently breast-tumor-associated antigens and the reactivity correlated with the clinical state. Patients with in situ carcinoma were most reactive, and those with extensive tumor involvement had decreased reactivity.

All of the skin-test assays for tumor immunity have been limited by a few major problems. The most serious one is that the procedures involve inoculation with materials usually derived from neoplastic tissues. The attendant possible hazards have required the limitation of testing only cancer patients with the neoplastic extracts. It has generally not been possible to perform tests in normal individuals and in patients with nonmalignant diseases, and therefore the specificity of the reactions has not been fully determined. It is possible that a tumor extract which produces positive reactions in patients with cancer of various types may still contain tumor-associated antigens, but ones which are not restricted to a particular histologic type. Another major limitation has been the lack of sufficient material from one tumor to perform extensive testing with large numbers of patients, or to perform frequent serial tests on the same patients. This problem is particularly important, since only some extracts elicit good reactivity, whereas others are virtually inactive (44). It would be very helpful to identify large, reactive extracts which could be used as standard preparations for detailed specificity testing and for isolation and characterization of the skin reactive antigens. Preparation of extracts from tissue culture cell lines which contain skin reactive antigens would seem to offer a solution. Some lymphoid tissue culture cell lines appear to contain tumor-associated antigens, which elicit delayed skin reactions in patients with leukemia, lymphoma, and nasopharyngeal carcinoma (54,55). However, the specificity of the skin reactive antigens in the extracts of lymphoid cell lines appeared broader than that seen with extracts of fresh tumor cells, and we have seen considerable variation in the incidence of reactivity to different extracts prepared from the same cell line. Once these problems are resolved, skin testing of tumor patients may be a very practical and reliable method for monitoring of cell-mediated immunity to tumor-associated antigens.

ANTIBODIES TO HUMAN TUMOR-ASSOCIATED ANTIGENS

For many years investigators have searched in the sera of cancer patients for humoral antibodies which would react with tumor-associated antigens. Many of the earlier studies have been previously reviewed (21,56,57). We will not discuss these here, particularly because most of the reports failed to convincingly demonstrate antibodies to tumor-associated antigens. In the last few years there have been many reports of antibodies in the sera of patients with Burkitt's lymphoma, malignant melanoma, and sarcomas which appear to react with tumor-associated antigens. These studies will be briefly summarized below.

A variety of antibodies have been described that react with Burkitt's lymphoma cells or with tissue culture cell lines derived from the tumors. Most of these antibodies have been associated with Epstein-Barr virus (EBV). This virus has been very closely linked with Burkitt's lymphoma (reviewed recently in 58). Although not limited to Burkitt's lymphoma patients, antibodies to membrane antigen, viral capsid antigen, early antigen, and nuclear antigen have been found with higher incidence and titers in these patients than in controls. Some investigators have used these data to support the etiologic role of EBV in Burkitt's lymphoma (e.g., 58). However, it is quite difficult to establish a causal relationship by even strong correlative serologic data. Studies have also been performed to relate the anti-EBV antibody titers to disease status in Burkitt's lymphoma. Several patients in long-term remission showed a fall in antibodies to membrane antigen some time before recurrence of tumor (59,60). It was suggested that loss of these antibodies permitted regrowth of tumor. These authors based this on the assumption that the serologically defined cell surface antigen functions as a TATA. This was not, however, proven, and the correlation between relapse and change in antibody titers was not complete. Antibodies to early antigen have also been suggested to have prognostic implications (61), with high titers associated with poor prognosis. Again, however, the correlation has not been complete. In recent studies in Ghana, the skin reactivity to extracts of a cell line derived from Burkitt's lymphoma has correlated better with disease status than have any of the anti-EBV antibodies (F. Nkrumah and R. Depue, personal communication).

Antibodies in the sera of patients with malignant melanoma have been detected by assays of complement-dependent cytotoxicity and by immunofluorescence. Cytotoxic antibodies against melanoma cells were first detected by Lewis and his colleagues (62,63) in the sera of 35% of melanoma patients. The antigens involved appeared to be individual specific, present only on the cell surface of the tumor cells of the serum donor. In a later study, Nairn et al. (64) also noted individual specificity. Such individually distinct antigens are very unusual in human tumor immunology. Most antigens have been found to be shared by many tumors. Using immunofluorescence, antibodies to membrane antigens and also to cytoplasmic antigens have been described (63–69). Most of these studies showed reactions to common cytoplasmic antigens shared by most melanoma cells. Antibodies were found in the sera of a majority of melanoma patients and also in the sera of about 20% of normal controls. The cytoplasmic antigens appeared to be tumor associated, since they were not found in a variety of established cell lines derived from other types of cancer or in normal skin. However, in a recent study of coded sera, a number of positive reactions were seen with an osteogenic sarcoma cell line (M. Lewis and R. Herberman, unpublished observations). With the antibodies to membrane antigens, some controversy exists. Lewis and his associates (63,69) found these antigens, like those detected by cytotoxicity assays, to be individual-specific and distinct from the cytoplasmic antigens. However, others found common membrane antigens and no individual specificities (65,67). It is clear that further studies, and exchange of reagents between laboratories, are needed to characterize the specificity of these antibodies.

There have been some differences among the studies regarding the correlation of antibodies with clinical course of disease. Some workers found a loss of detectable antibodies in advanced disease (70), whereas others did not see a correlation with disease status (64,65).

A series of studies by Morton and associates (71–74), and by others (75–77), has also demonstrated antibodies in the sera of patients with sarcoma. Initially, antibodies were detected by indirect immunofluorescence assays with fixed tumor cells (71) in the sera of most patients with sarcomas, their family members, and their close associates. Very few sera from normal individuals were positive. Cultured cells containing the antigen were shown to contain type-C virus particles (75,78), and the antigen could be induced in cultures of normal human cells by cell-free supernates of positive sarcoma cultures (79). On the basis of these findings a viral etiology for human sarcomas was suggested. Subsequent studies by Giraldo, Hirshaut, and associates (76,77,80) have indicated several problems with this interpretation. They have distinguished between two separate cytoplasmic antigens, one punctate (S_1, 80) and the other diffusely distributed (S_2, 77). S_1 was found in cultured sarcoma cells and in fibroblasts exposed to filtrates of positive lines, but not in fresh biopsies of sarcomas. The antibody was found with equal frequency in the sera of normal individuals, sarcoma patients, and patients with other types of cancer. The S_2 antigen system appeared to be analogous to the system originally described by Morton and Malmgren (71). Patients with sarcoma and their family members had a high frequency of positive reactions, and only 10% of normal donors reacted. However, many patients with other types of cancer, particularly those with carcinomas of the breast, lung, and ovary, also had antibodies to the S_2 antigen. The antigen was shown not to be tumor associated but was found in cultures of embryos and of normal adult skin as well as in cultures of some sarcomas (77).

Antibodies in the sera of sarcoma patients have also been detected by complement fixation (73) and cytotoxicity assays (74). However, the relationship of these antibodies and those previously described by immunofluorescence assays is not clear. More detailed studies of the distribution of the antibodies and of the antigenic specificities will be needed to determine whether any of these antibody reactions represent immunity to tumor-associated antigens.

Despite the questions of specificity which have been raised in the sarcoma studies, measurement of antibodies in the sera of patients with sarcoma appears to have some value in monitoring the course of disease. Patients who had definitive surgery and remained tumor free had high levels of antibody, as measured by the complement-fixation assay (81). In contrast, recurrence of disease or metastatic spread was associated with declining antibody titers.

IN VITRO EVIDENCE FOR CELL-MEDIATED IMMUNITY TO HUMAN TUMORS

Studies of cell-mediated immunity to human tumors have been performed most extensively with assays of cytotoxicity. Several studies (e.g., 82–88) initially indicated that patients with cancer had significantly more cytotoxic reactivity than normal individuals against tissue culture cells derived from tumors of the same histologic type (designated histologic type specific reactivity) and not against cultures derived from normal cells or from tumors of other histologic types. Few or no normal controls were shown to have significant cytotoxic reactivity. Recently the specificity of the observed reactions and the relative lack of normal reactivity in these assays have been increasingly called into question (89). Although many of the problems have been attributed to a variety of technical features of the assays, it now seems likely that the reactivity of lymphocytes from cancer patients may not be entirely directed against histologic type specific tumor-associated antigens, and also that normal human cytotoxic reactivity is a real and not particularly rare phenomenon.

A central factor determining the pattern of results appears to be the study design of the experiments themselves. Most of the reports of microcytotoxicity assays with human tumor systems have been summaries of varying numbers of small individual experiments. Each of the experiments typically consisted of effector cells from a few cancer patients, one normal donor, and 2–3 target cells. The types of target cells usually were: ones derived from the same type of cancer as the patients'; normal cells, usually skin or tissue fibroblasts, from the same or different patients; and perhaps cells derived from a different type of cancer. The normal fibroblasts have been the most frequent negative control; very few cancer patients had cytotoxic reactivity against them. However, such cells may be quite resistant to cytotoxicity, and they are not adequate specificity controls. Experiments designed along these lines, although performed many times, would probably not detect normal reactivity, and they may not be likely to clearly document the specificity of the assays.

It is very desirable to set up experiments involving a large "checkerboard" design, with lymphocytes from several patients with cancer of different histologic types, from patients with benign diseases of the same organs, and from several normal individuals, tested against an equally large array of target cells derived from various types of cancer and normal cells. All of the target cells used in an assay, including those used as specificity controls, need to be susceptible to cytotoxicity by lymphocytes from some patients or from normal controls. The use of target cells which are resistant to cytotoxicity would obviously bias the control results in the desired direction of histologic type specificity. In order to directly study the frequency and range of normal cytotoxic reactivity, it is particularly necessary to design experiments to look for such reactivity. Several normal donors, not selected on the basis of previous reactivity or lack of reactivity in the assay, need to be tested concurrently, and significant differences between their activities examined. Studies performed along these lines have demonstrated a considerable degree of normal reactivity and lack of histologic type specific reactivity by cancer patients (90,91). Also, the change in the pattern of results in some laboratories (92–94), from apparently good specificity and no normal reactivity to considerable cross-reactivity and normal reactivity, without any changes in test methodologies, can probably be ascribed to changes in study design of the kind we have just described.

In addition to the cytotoxicity assays with cultured target cells described above, it has been possible to perform tests with fresh or cryopreserved leukemia and lymphoma target cells, using a ^{51}Cr-release assay. Lymphocytes from some patients with acute lymphocytic leukemia and with acute myelogenous leukemia were found to have significant cytotoxic reactivity against autologous blast cells (95,96). The observed reactivity appeared to be directed against leukemia-associated antigens, since no positive reactions were obtained against autologous remission leukocytes. However, there was no correlation between reactivity and clinical state, with as many positive reactions in relapse as in remission. In order to study allogeneic cell-mediated reactivity in leukemia using freshly harvested cells, and to have available comparable normal cells as controls for those from the leukemia patients, some experiments were performed with identical twins, one member of each pair having leukemia (97). Leukemia-associated antigens were detected on the cells of several leukemic patients. Allogeneic reactions were seen against remission cells of the leukemic patients, as well as against blast cells; no positive reactions were seen with the target cells from the normal twins. Leukemia patients, their family members, and even unrelated normal adults were found to have allogeneic reactivity against cells from leukemic patients (96–98). The finding of normal reactivity against leukemic target cells and against tissue cultures derived from human tumors may be analogous to the observation of natural cell-mediated reactivity in mice and rats against tumor-associated and virus-associated antigens (99–101).

Lymphocytes from some patients with cancer have been shown to have proliferative responses to autologous tumor cells. Stjernswärd and his colleagues have done extensive testing with this assay, using fresh or frozen tumor cells, treated with mitomycin C. They found positive reactions with some patients with Burkitt's lymphoma (102), sarcomas (103), brain tumors (104), and a variety of carcinomas (104–107). In studies of renal carcinomas the specificity of stimulation by tumor cells was indicated by the lack of stimulation by normal kidney cells (105). In most of the other studies, however, control tests with appropriate normal cells were not performed. In these studies there was no apparent correlation between positive stimulation and the clinical state of the patients. In studies with a variety of solid-tumor patients, Mavligit et al. (108) observed higher degrees of stimulation among patients with localized disease, as compared to those with systemic disease.

In acute leukemia, peripheral blood lymphocytes were stimulated by autologous, viable blast cells which had been stored in liquid nitrogen (95,109–112). The specificity of the antigens detected on the leukemic cells is not completely clear. Several workers have incubated remission bone marrow cells with autologous peripheral blood lymphocytes, and usually negative results were obtained (95,98,113). However, in some instances remission bone marrow cells did produce stimulation (95,113), and this appeared to correlate with the presence of residual disease (113). Whereas stimulation of lymphocytes by leukemic blast cells did not correlate with clinical condition at the time of testing (95), there was a correlation with good prognosis (112,114). One dissenting note in stimulation studies in acute leukemia was offered by Schweitzer et al. (115). They observed some stimulation by autologous blast cells but did not feel that the assay could be reliably used to detect cell-mediated immunity.

Lymphocyte stimulation has been produced by extracts of human tumors as well as by intact tumor cells. Savel (116) and Fischer et al. (117) obtained stimulation of autologous lymphocytes by crude saline extracts of tumors. In the latter study, stimulation was also seen with allogeneic lymphocytes of cancer patients. However, this could have been due to normal histocompatibility antigens, since these extracts also stimulated the lymphocytes of some normal controls. Jehn et al. (118) reported the stimulation of autologous and allogeneic lymphocytes by crude extracts of melanomas. The degree of stimulation in this study was remarkable: in some patients, stimulation was as high as, or higher than, that produced by phytohemagglutinin. Soluble extracts of tumor cells, prepared by treatment with 3M potassium chloride, have recently been reported to stimulate autologous lymphocytes of leukemia patients (119) and of solid-tumor patients (108,120). Patients also reacted to KCl extracts of allogeneic tumors (108,119,120), and it has been postulated that the soluble antigens could stimulate lymphocytes only of immune individuals, in contrast to the ability of antigens on intact cells to elicit primary proliferative responses in vitro (108,119). However, some KCl extracts of tumors and of normal leukocytes could stimulate normal lymphocytes (121), and it seems likely that the presence of histocompatibility antigens in such extracts can confuse the interpretation of any observed reactions.

Reactivity to tumor-associated antigens has also been detected by the leukocyte migration inhibition assay, in patients with breast cancer (122–129), malignant melanoma (124,125,130,131), intestinal cancer (123,128,132,133), kidney cancer (134,135), lung cancer (123,136), medullary thyroid cancer (137), leukemia, and lymphoma (124,134,138). In most of these studies the reactions have been against common antigens on tumors of the same histologic type. However, the cross-reactivity has not been complete. Some extracts have elicited more reactions than others (130), and it has generally been necessary to test patients with several different extracts. In studies of patients with breast cancer, Black et al. (129) found very little reactivity to allogeneic invasive tumors but did find more reactivity to in situ cancers. A few studies have observed reactivity almost completely limited to autologous tumors (124,133). The specificity of the migration inhibition reactions has been examined in some detail. In most reports, patients only rarely reacted to extracts of other types of cancer or to extracts of benign or normal tissues (122,126,127,131,135). Only a small proportion of normal controls reacted to the tumor preparations. However, the nature of the detected antigens is still not well defined. All of these studies have been performed with either whole cells or with crude particulate or soluble extracts.

It is possible that normal tissue-associated antigens play a role in these reactions. The tumors may have a higher concentration of such antigens than the normal control tissues. Patients with benign breast diseases reacted to breast tumor extracts with a higher frequency than did normal controls (126). One study found that normal blacks reacted frequently to an extract of a cell line derived from melanoma, and normal controls reacted as frequently to lung cancer extracts as did patients with lung cancer (128). Cochran (personal communication) found frequent reactions of melanoma patients to some extracts of benign nevi. Such reactivity to tissue-associated antigens could be explained by circulation of these materials under certain conditions, e.g., necrosis of tumor, followed by sensitization. Sensitization to normal kidney antigens has been noted in migration inhibition studies of patients with glomerulonephritis or kidney transplants (139,140). Fetal antigens may also play a role in the reactions of cancer patients. Kjaer (135) observed frequent reactivity of kidney cancer patients to extracts of fetal kidney. However, carcinoembryonic antigen of Gold does not seem to be involved in these assays of cell-mediated immunity (141). Black and associates have noted reactivity of breast cancer patients to mouse milk containing mammary tumor virus and have suggested that the common breast tumor antigens may be virus associated (142,143). Although the nature of this cross-reaction is not yet clear, other laboratories have confirmed the reactivity to mouse mammary tumor virus preparations (e.g., McCoy, Parks, Maurer, and Herberman, unpublished observations).

Several groups have examined the correlation of reactivity in migration inhibition assays with clinical parameters, but the results have been divergent. Cochran et al. (125,127) found decreased reactivity in patients with advanced disease and in most patients in the immediate postoperative period. McCoy et al. (126,131) also observed the effect of surgery but did not find a good correlation of reactivity with stage of disease. Black et al. (129,143) observed that reactivity to breast tumors and to mouse milk was associated with early disease and good prognosis. Kjaer (135) found reactivity in renal cancer patients with localized disease but not in those with metastatic disease. In contrast, workers in the same laboratory found no correlation of reactivity of breast cancer patients with extent of disease (122). Bull et al. (132) detected reactivity only around the time of intitial surgery; patients with no evidence of disease for 6 months or more were uniformly unreactive.

Migration inhibition assays have been shown to correlate well with delayed cutaneous hypersensitivity to tuberculin and other soluble protein antigens (e.g., 126,144). However, the relationship between migration inhibition by human tumor extracts and skin tests is not clear. In one study which looked at simultaneous reactivity in both tests, the correlation was not complete (130). It is quite possible that assays for migration inhibition measure different antigens than skin tests and may be influenced by a variety of technical factors. These tests are still quite difficult to perform and are not yet standardized or completely reproducible.

Because of the technical difficulties with the migration inhibition assays, the leukocyte adherence inhibition assay has been developed (145,146). The results obtained thus far have been encouraging. Patients with malignant melanoma and hepatocellular carcinoma have given positive results with tumors of the same histologic type. Virtually no normal reactivity has been seen. The presence of blocking serum factors has been correlated with the presence of tumor. Another assay with some similarities to the leukocyte migration inhibition assay is that of macrophage electrophoretic mobility (147,148). The pattern of results in this test has been quite different from that seen with the cellular immunity assays described above. Most cancer patients, and virtually no normal controls, have reacted to an antigen, cancer basic protein, which appears to be common to a wide variety of tumors. However, more patients with various benign diseases need to be tested before the significance of these reactions can be evaluated. Cercek et al. (149) have also observed stimulation of lymphocytes of cancer patients by cancer basic protein.

CONCLUDING REMARKS

A large body of evidence has now accumulated which clearly indicates that many patients with cancer have immune reactions with antigens on tumor cells. The central issue which remains after all these studies is the nature of the detected antigens. It has been particularly difficult in these clinical studies to clearly define the specificity of the tumor antigens. We lack several of the tools which have been so helpful in comparable studies of tumor immunity in experimental animals. The ready availability of large numbers of syngeneic rodents has only been matched by the infrequent availability of normal identical twins of cancer patients. The ethical and logistical difficulties involved in testing for the effects of tumor antigens on in vivo protection against tumor growth hinders the determination of which human tumor antigens can function as TATA's. The best evidence now available concerning this important problem is indirect: the correlation of some tests for tumor immunity with clinical course of disease. Immunotherapy trials with tumor cells or with extracts of tumor cells, which are now being initiated, may help to determine whether human TATA's exist and how frequently they are expressed. Parallel studies of patients with various assays of immunity should indicate which tests correlate with in vivo induction of resistance to tumor growth.

It has been possible to ask whether immune reactions are directed against tumor-associated antigens or against other types of antigens on human tumor cells. However, most studies performed thus far have not been conclusive. A large number of controls and a large number of tests need to be done to determine whether some tumor antigens are organ-associated, differentiation, virus-associated, or fetal antigens. Since common human tumor-associated antigens have often been restricted to a particular histologic type of tumor, the occurrence of reactivity to organ-associated antigens needs to be examined very carefully. The growth of tumors and necrosis may lead to sensitization against such normal-tissue antigens. Similar reactivity may also occur with benign inflammatory diseases of the same organ, and such control patients should be included in studies of human tumor immunity.

It may be very helpful to look to the experimental animal tumor systems for possible analogies with, and insight into, the complex human tumor systems, which are so difficult to analyze. This may be particularly useful with the microcytotoxicity assays, where many reactions are being seen against antigens on histologically dissimilar tumors. In the animal tumor systems, common tumor-associated antigens have usually been related to expression of fetal antigens or of antigens associated with a virus. These common tumor-associated antigens have usually not been restricted to a particular histologic type of tumor, but rather the same antigen might be found in leukemias, sarcomas, and even carcinomas. It should therefore not be too surprising to find cytotoxic or other forms of immune reactivity against antigens which are expressed on diverse types of human tumor cells. However, detailed studies will be needed to determine whether these antigens are found in fetal tissues or are associated with some virus.

The issue of cytotoxicity or other immune reactivity by some normal individuals against tumor cells or tumor antigens may also be analogous to natural humoral immunity and cell-mediated cytotoxicity which has been detected in murine tumor systems (see 150). Many normal mice and rats have been found to have specific immune reactivity against a variety of leukemias, lymphomas, and mammary carcinomas. In the systems described thus far, most of the natural reactivity appears to be directed against virus-associated antigens. It is intriguing to postulate that some of the normal human reactivity is directed against antigens associated with ubiquitous viruses. Alternatively, some of the natural immune reactivity to human tumors may reflect an important immune surveillance mechanism against tumors.

REFERENCES

1. Gross, L., *Cancer Res.* **3,** 326 (1943).
2. Foley, E. J., *Cancer Res.* **13,** 835 (1953).
3. Prehn, R. T., and Main, J. M., *J. Natl. Cancer Inst.* **18,** 769 (1957).
4. Klein, G., Sjögren, H. O., Klein, E., and Hellström, K. E., *Cancer Res.* **20,** 1561 (1960).
5. Ting, C. C., and Herberman, R. B., *Int. Rev. Exper. Pathol.* (G. W. Richter and M. A. Epstein, eds.), Vol. 15, Academic Press, New York, 1976, pp. 93–152.
6. Herberman, R. B., *Adv. Cancer Res.* **19,** 207 (1974).
7. Everson, T. C., and Cole, W. H., *Spontaneous Regression of Cancer,* W. B. Saunders Co., Philadelphia and London, 1966.
8. Sumner, W. C., and Foraker, A. G., *Cancer* **13,** 79 (1960).
9. Southam, C. M., *Cancer Res.* **20,** 271 (1960).
10. Black, M. M., and Speer, F. D., *Surg. Gynec. Obstet,* **109,** 105 (1959).
11. Black, M. M., and Leis, H. P., Jr., *Cancer* **28,** 263 (1971).
12. Old, L. J., and Boyse, E. A., *Med. Clin. N. Amer.* **50,** 901 (1966).
13. Oettgen, H. F., Old, L. J., and Boyse, E. A., *Med. Clin. N. Amer.* **55,** 761 (1971).
14. Hamilton-Fairley, G., *Brit. Med. J.* **4,** 483 (1970).
15. Smith, R. T., *N. Eng. J. Med.* **287,** 439 (1972).
16. Hellström, K. E., and Hellström, I. *Adv. Immunol.* **18,** 209 (1973).
17. Green, I., and Shevach, E. M., in *Mechanisms of Cell-Mediated immunity* (R. T. McCloskey and S. Cohen, eds.) John Wiley & Sons, New York, 1974.
18. Herberman, R. B., in *Pathobiology Annual* (H. L. Ioachim, ed.), Vol. 3, Appleton-Century-Crofts, New York, 1973, p. 291.
19. Brunschwig, A., Southam, C. M., and Levin, A. G., *Ann. Surg.* **162,** 416 (1965).
20. Grace, J. T., Perese, D., Metzgar, R. S., Sasabe, T., and Holdredge, B. J., *Neurosurg.* **28,** 159 (1961).
21. Southam, C. M., *Progr. Exp. Tumor Res.* **9,** 1 (1967).
22. Old, L. J., Boyse, E. A., Clarke, D. A., and Carswell, E. A., *Ann. N.Y. Acad. Sci.* **101,** 80 (1962).
23. Sjögren, H. O., Hellström, I., and Klein, G., *Cancer Res.* **21,** 329 (1961).
24. Fefer, A., McCoy, J. L., and Glynn, J. P., *Cancer Res.* **27,** 2207 (1967).
25. Graham, J. B., and Graham, R. M. *Surg. Gynec. Obstet.* **114,** 1 (1962).
26. Aswaq, M., Richards, V., and McFadden, S. *Arch. Surg.* **89,** 485 (1964).
27. Gorodilova, V. V., Silina, I. G., and Saraeva, Z. M., *Vopr. Onkol.* **2,** 22 (1965).
28. Nadler, S. H., and Moore, G. E., *Ann. Surg.* **164,** 482 (1966).
29. Nadler, S. H., and Moore, G. E., *Arch. Surg.* **100,** 244 (1970).
30. Czajkowski, N. P., Rosenblatt, M., Wolf, P. L., and Vasquez, J. *Lancet* **2,** 905 (1967).
31. Mathé, G., Pouillart, P., and Lapeyraque, F., *Brit. J. Cancer* **23,** 814 (1969).
32. Mathé, G., Amiel, J. L., Schwarzenberg, L., Schneider, M., Cattan, A., Schlumberger, J. R., Hayat, M., and de Vassal, F., *Lancet* **1,** 697 (1969).
33. Powles, R. L., Crowther, D., Bateman, C. J. T., Beard, M. E. J., McElwain, T. J., Russell, J., Lister, T. A., Whitehouse, J. M. A., Wrigley, P. F. M., Pike, M., Alexander, P., and Hamilton-Fairley, G., *Br. J. Cancer* **28,** 365 (1973).
34. Bloom, B. R., *Adv. Immunol.* **13,** 101 (1971).
35. David, J. R., *Fed. Proc.* **30,** 1730 (1971).
36. Thor, D., Jureziz, R. E., Veach, S. R., Miller, E., and Dray, S., *Nature* **219,** 755 (1968).

37. Rocklin, R. E., Meyers, O. L., and David, J. R., *J. Immunol.* **104,** 95 (1970).

38. Rosenberg, S. A., *Natl. Cancer Inst. Monogr.* **37,** 143 (1973).

39. Hughes, L. E., and Lytton, B., *Brit. Med. J.* **1,** 209 (1964).

40. Stewart, T. H. M., *Cancer* **23,** 1368 (1969).

41. Stewart, T. H. M., and Orizaga, M., *Cancer* **28,** 1472 (1971).

42. Oren, M. E., and Herberman, R. B., *Clin. Exp. Immunol.* **9,** 45 (1971).

43. Fass, L., Herberman, R. B., and Ziegler, J., *N. Eng. J. Med.* **282,** 776 (1970).

44. Char, D. H., Lepourhiet, A., Leventhal, B. G., and Herberman, R. B., *Int. J. Cancer* **12,** 409 (1973).

45. Bluming, A. Z., Ziegler, J. L., Fass, L., and Herberman, R. B., *Clin. Exp. Immunol.* **9,** 713 (1971).

46. Hollinshead, A., Glew, D., Bunnag, B., Gold, P., and Herberman, R., *Lancet* **1,** 119 (1970).

47. Hollinshead, A., McWright, C. G., Alford, T. C., Glew, D. H., Gold, P., and Herberman, R. B., *Science* **177,** 887 (1972).

48. Fass, L., Herberman, R. B., Ziegler, J. L., and Kiryabwire, J. W. M., *Lancet* **1,** 116 (1970).

49. Bluming, A. Z., Vogel, C. L., Ziegler, J. L., and Kiryabwire, J. W. M., *J. Natl. Cancer Inst.* **48,** 17 (1972).

50. Hollinshead, A. C., Herberman, R. B., Jaffurs, W. J., Alpert, L. K., Minton, J. P., and Harris, J. E., *Cancer* **34,** 1235 (1974).

51. Char, D. H., Hollinshead, A., Cogan, D. G., Ballentine, E. J., Hogan, M. J., and Herberman, R. B., *N. Eng. J. Med.* **291,** 274 (1974).

52. Alford, C., Hollinshead, A. C., and Herberman, R. B., *Ann. Surg.* **178,** 20 (1973).

53. Hollinshead, A. C., Jaffurs, W. T., Alpert, L. K., Harris, J. E., and Herberman, R. B., *Cancer Res.* **34,** 2961 (1974).

54. Herberman, R. B., McCoy, J. L., and Levine, P. H., *Cancer Res.* **34,** 1222 (1974).

55. Herberman, R. B., Char, D., Oldham, R., Levine, P., Leventhal, B. G., McCoy, J. L., Ho, H. C., and Chau, J. C. W., in *Comparative Leukemia Research* (Y. Ito and R. M. Dutcher, eds.), University of Tokyo Press, 1974, p. 585.

56. Lewis, M. G., *Med. Clin. N. Amer.* **56,** 481 (1972).

57. Herberman, R. B., Lepourhiet, A., Hollinshead, A., Char, D., McCoy, J. L., and Leventhal, B. G., in *Twenty-sixth Annual M. D. Anderson Symposium on Fundamental Cancer Research. Immunological Aspects of Neoplasia.* Williams & Wilkins Co., Baltimore, Md., 1975, pp. 423–438.

58. Henle, W., and Henle, G., *Cancer* **34,** 1368 (1974).

59. Klein, G., Clifford, P., Henle, G., Henle, W., Geering, G., and Old, L. J., *Int. J. Cancer* **4,** 416 (1969).

60. Gunvén, P., Klein, G., Henle, W., Henle, G., Rocchi, G., Hewetson, J. F., Guerra, A., Clifford, P., Singh, S., Demissie, A., and Svedmyr, E., *Int. J. Cancer* **12,** 115 (1973).

61. Henle, W., Henle, G., Gunvén P., Klein, G., Clifford, P., and Singh, S., *J. Natl. Cancer Inst.* **50,** 1163 (1973).

62. Lewis, M. G., *Lancet* **2,** 921 (1967).

63. Lewis, M. G., Ikonopisov, R. L., Nairn, R. C., Phillips, T. M., Hamilton-Fairley, G., Bodenham, D. C., and Alexander, P., *Brit. Med. J.* **3,** 547 (1969).

64. Nairn, R. C., Nind, A. P. P., Guli, E. P. G., Davies, D. J., Little, J. H., Davis, N. C., and Whitehead, R. H., *Med. J. Austr.* **1,** 397 (1972).

65. Morton, D. L., Malmgren, R. A., Holmes, E. C., and Ketcham, A. S., *Surgery* **64,** 233 (1968).

66. Muna, N. M., Marcus, S., and Smart, C., *Cancer* **23,** 88 (1969).

67. Romsdahl, M. M., and Cox, I. S., *Arch. Surg.* **100,** 491 (1970).

68. Oettgen, H. R., Aoki, T., Old, L. J., Boyse, E. A., de Harven, E., and Mills, G. J., *Natl. Cancer Inst.* **41,** 827 (1968).

69. Lewis, M. G., and Phillips, T. M., *J. Natl. Cancer Inst.* **49,** 915 (1972).

70. Lewis, M. G., Phillips, T. M., Cook, K. B., and Blake, J., *Nat. New Biol.* **232,** 52 (1971).

71. Morton, D. L., and Malmgren, R. A., *Science* **162,** 1279 (1968).

72. Morton, D. L., Eilber, F. R., Joseph, W. L., Wood, W. C., Trahan, E., and Ketcham, A. S., *Ann. Surgery* **172**, 740 (1970).

73. Eilber, F. R., and Morton, D. L., *J. Natl. Cancer Inst.* **44**, 651 (1970).

74. Wood, W. C., and Morton, D. L., *N. Eng. J. Med.* **284**, 569 (1971).

75. Priori, E. S., Wilber, J. R., and Dmochowski, L. *J. Natl. Cancer Inst.* **46**, 1299 (1971).

76. Giraldo, G., Beth, E., Hirshaut, Y., Aoki, T., Old, L. J., Boyse, E. A., and Chopra, H. C., *J. Exp. Med.* **133**, 454 (1971).

77. Mukherji, B., and Hirshaut, Y., *Science* **181**, 440 (1973).

78. Morton, D. L., Hall, W. T., and Malmgren, R. A., *Science* **165**, 813 (1968).

79. Morton, D. L., Malmgren, R. A., Hall, W. T., and Schidlovsky, G., *Surgery* **66**, 152 (1969).

80. Hirshaut, Y., Tsien, D., Marcone, R. C., and Essner, E. S., *Proc. Amer. Assoc. Cancer Res.* **13**, 114 (1972).

81. Morton, D. L., Holmes, E. C., Eilber, F. R., and Wood, W. C., *Ann. Intern. Med.* **74**, 587 (1971).

82. Hellström, I., Hellström, K. E., Pierce, G. E., and Bill, A. H., *Proc. Natl. Acad. Sci.* **60**, 1231 (1968).

83. Hellström, I., Hellström, K. E., Sjögren, H. O., and Warner, G. A., *Int. J. Cancer* **7**, 1 (1971).

84. Fossati, G., Colnaghi, M. I., Della Porta, G., Cascinelli, W., and Veronesi, U., *Int. J. Cancer* **8**, 344 (1971).

85. O'Toole, C., Perlmann, P., Unsgaard, B., Moberger, G., and Edysmyr, F., *Int. J. Cancer* **10**, 77 (1972).

86. Levy, N. L., Mahaley, M. S., and Day, E. D., *Cancer Res.* **32**, 477 (1972).

87. Heppner, G. H., Stolbach, L., Byrne, M., Cummings, F. J., McDonough, E., and Calabresi, P., *Int. J. Cancer* **11**, 245 (1973).

88. Sinkovics, J. G., Dreyer, D. A., Shirato, E., Cabiness, J. R., and Schullenberger, C. C., *Texas Rep. Biol. Med.* **29**, 227 (1971).

89. Herberman, R. B., and Oldham, R. K., *J. Natl. Cancer Inst.* **55**, 749 (1975).

90. Takasugi, M., Mickey, M. R., and Terasaki, P. I., *J. Natl. Cancer Inst.* **53**, 1527 (1974).

91. Oldham, R. K., Herberman, R. B., Djeu, J. Y., and Cannon, G. B., **55**, 1305 (1975). 1975.

92. Heppner, G., Henry, E., Stolbach, L., Cummings, F., McDonough, E., and Calabresi, P., *Cancer Res.* **35**, 1931 (1975).

93. Canevari, S., Fossati, G, and Della Porta, G., *J. Natl. Cancer Inst.* **56**, 705 (1976).

94. Thota, H., Sinkovics, J. G., Carrier, S. K., and Kay, H. D., *Proc. IX Inter. Pigment Cell Confer.* (in press, 1975).

95. Leventhal, B. G., Halterman, R. H., Rosenberg, E. B., and Herberman, R. B., *Cancer Res.* **32**, 1820 (1972).

96. Herberman, R. B., *Fed. Proc.* **32**, 160 (1973).

97. Rosenberg, E. B., Herberman, R. B., Levine, P. H., Halterman, R. H., McCoy, J. L., and Wunderlich, J. R., *Int. J. Cancer* **9**, 648 (1972).

98. Anderson, P. N., Klein, D. L., Bias, W. B., Mullins, G. M., Burke, P. J., and Santos, G. W., *Israel J. Med. Sci.* **10**, 1033 (1974).

99. Herberman, R. B., Ting, C. C., Kirchner, H., Holden, H., Glaser, M., Bonnard, G. D., and Lavrin, D., *Prog. Immunol.* II **3**, 285 (1974).

100. Kiessling, R., Klein, E., and Wigzell, H., *Eur. J. Immunol.* **5**, 112 (1975).

101. Blair, P. B., Lane, M. A., and Yagi, M. J., *J. Immunol.* **112**, 693 (1974).

102. Stjernswärd, J., Clifford, P., Singh, S., and Svedmyr, E., *East Afr. Med. J.* **45**, 484 (1968).

103. Vánky, F., Stjernswärd, J., and Nilsonne, U., *J. Natl. Cancer Inst.* **46**, 1145 (1971).

104. Stjernswärd, J., and Vánky, F., *Natl. Cancer Inst. Monogr.* **35**, 237 (1972).

105. Stjernswärd, J., Almgard, L. E., Franzen, S., von Schreeb, T., and Wadstrom, L. B., *Clin. Exp. Immunol.* **6**, 963 (1970).

106. Stjernswärd, J., Johansson, B., Svedmyr, E., and Sundblad, R., *Clin. Exp. Immunol.* **6**, 429 (1970).

107. Stjernswärd, J., and Clifford, P., in *Immunity and Tolerance in Oncogenesis* (L. Severi, ed.), Div. Cancer Res., Perugia, 1970, p. 749.

108. Mavligit, G. M., Ambus, U., Gutterman, J. U., and Hersh, E. M., *Nat. New Biol.* **243,** 188 (1973).

109. Fridman, W. H., and Kourilsky, F. M., *Nature* **224,** 277 (1969).

110. Viza, D. C., Bernard-Degani, O., Bernard, C., and Harris, R. C., *Lancet* **2,** 493 (1969).

111. Powles, R. L., Balchin, L. A., Hamilton-Fairley, G., and Alexander, P., *Brit. Med. J.* **1,** 486 (1971).

112. Gutterman, J. U., Rossen, R. D., Butler, W. T., McCredie, K. B., Bodey, G. P., Freireich, E. J., and Hersh, E. M., *N. Eng. J. Med.* **288,** 169 (1973).

113. Gutterman, J. U., Mavligit, G., Burgess, M. A., McCredie, K. B., Hunter, C., Freireich, E. J., and Hersh, E. M., *J. Natl. Cancer Inst.* **53,** 389 (1974).

114. Leventhal, B. G., Lepourhiet, A., Halterman, R. H., Henderson, E. S., and Herberman, R. B., *Natl. Cancer Inst. Monogr.* **39,** 177 (1973).

115. Schweitzer, M., Melief, C. J. M., and Eijsvogel, V. P., *Int. J. Cancer* **11,** 11 (1973).

116. Savel, H., *Cancer* **24,** 56 (1969).

117. Fischer, P., Golub, E., Holzner, H., and Kunze-Mühl, E., *Z. Krebsforsch.* **72,** 155 (1969).

118. Jehn, U. M., Nathanson, L., Schwartz, R. B. S., and Skinner, M., *N. Eng. J. Med.* **283,** 329 (1970).

119. Gutterman, J. U., Hersh, E. M., Freireich, E. J., Rossen, R. D., Butler, W. T., McCredie, K. B., Bodey, G. P. Sr., Rodriguez, V., and Mavligit, G. M., *Natl. Cancer Inst. Monogr.* **37,** 153 (1973).

120. Vánky, F., Klein, E., Sternswärd, J., and Nilsonne, U., *Int. J. Cancer* **14,** 277 (1974).

121. Dean, J. H., Silva, J. S., McCoy, J. L., Leonard, C. M., Middleton, M., Cannon, G., and Herberman, R. B., *J. Natl. Cancer Inst.* **54,** 1295, (1975).

122. Andersen, V., Bjerrum, O., Bendixen, G., Schiodt, T. and Dissing, I., *Int. J. Cancer* **5,** 357 (1970).

123. Wolberg, W. H., and Goelzer, M. L., *Nature* **229,** 632 (1971).

124. Segall, A., Weiler, O., Genin, J., Lacour, J., and Lacour, F., *Int. J. Cancer* **9,** 417 (1972).

125. Cochran, A. J., Spilg, W. G. S., Mackie, R. M., and Thomas, C. E., *Brit. Med. J.* **4,** 67 (1972).

126. McCoy, J. L., Jerome, L. F., Dean, J. H., Cannon, G. B., Alford, T. C., Doering, T., and Herberman, R. B., *J. Natl. Cancer Inst.* **53,** 11 (1974).

127. Cochran, A. J., Grant, R. M., Spilg, W. G., Mackie, R. M., ross, C. E., Hoyle, D. E., and Russell, J. M., *Int. J. Cancer* **14,** 19 (1974).

128. Ax, W., and Tautz, C., *Behring Inst. Mitt.* **54,** 72 (1974).

129. Black, M. M., Leis, H. P., Jr., Shore, B., and Zachrau, R. E., *Cancer* **33,** 952 (1974).

130. Herberman, R. B., Hollinshead, A., Char, D., Oldham, R., McCoy, J., and Cohen, M., *Behring Inst. Mitt.* **56,** 131 (1975).

131. McCoy, J. L., Jerome, L. F., Dean, J. H., Perlin, E., Oldham, R. K., Char, D. H., Cohen, M. H., Felix, E., and Herberman, R. B., *J. Natl. Cancer Inst.* **55,** 19 (1975).

132. Bull, D. M., Leibach, J. R., Williams, M. A., and Helms, R. A., *Science* **181,** 957 (1973).

133. Elias, E. G., and Elias, L. L., *Cancer* **36,** 1393 (1975).

134. Hilberg, R. W., Balcerzak, S. P., and Lo Buglio, A. F., *Cell. Immunol.* **7,** 152 (1973).

135. Kjaer, M., *Europ. J. Cancer* **10,** 523 (1974).

136. Boddie, A. W., Jr., Holmes, E. C., Roth, J. A., and Morton, D. L., *Int. J. Cancer* **15,** 823 (1975).

137. George, J. M., Williams, M. a., almorey, R., and Sizemore, G., submitted for publication, 1975.

138. Braun, M., Sen, L., Bachmann, A. E., and Pavlovsky, A., *Blood* **39,** 368 (1972).

139. Bendixen, G., *Acta Med. Scand.* **184,** 99 (1968).

140. Weeke, E., Weeke, B., and Bendixen, G., *Acta Med. Scand.* **188,** 307 (1970).

141. Straus, E., Vernace, S., Janowitz, H., and Paronetto, F., *Proc. Soc. Exp. Biol. Med.* **148,** 494 (1975).

142. Black, M. M., Zachrau, R. E., Shore, B., Moore, D. H., and Leis, H. P., Jr., *Cancer* **35,** 121 (1975).

143. Black, M. M., Moore, D. H., Shore, B., Zachrau, R. E., and Leis, H. P., Jr., *Cancer Res.* **34,** 1054 (1974).

144. Bloom, B. R., *Adv. Immunol.* **13,** 101 (1971).

145. Maluish, A., and Halliday, W. J., *J. Natl. Cancer Inst.* **52,** 1415 (1974).

146. Halliday, W. J., Halliday, J. W., Campbell, C. B., Maluish, A. E., and Powell, L. W., *Brit. Med. J.* **2,** 349 (1974).

147. Caspary, E. A., and Field, E. J., *Brit. Med. J.* **2,** 613 (1971).

148. Pritchard, J. A. V., Moore, J. L., Sutherland, W. H., and Joslin, C. A. F., *Brit, J. Cancer* **27,** 1 (1973).

149. Cercek, L., Cercek, B., and Franklin, C. I. V., *Brit. J. Cancer* **29,** 345 (1974).

150. Herberman, R. B., Nunn, M. E., and Lavrin, D. H., *Int. J. Cancer* **16,** 216 (1975).

Chapter Eight

Immunotherapy of Experimental Animals

RONALD M. FERGUSON, JON R. SCHMIDTKE,
AND RICHARD L. SIMMONS

Department of Surgery, University of Minnesota, Minneapolis

Most animal and human tumors possess tumor-specific transplantation antigens on their cell surfaces that are capable of inducing immunity in their hosts (1). The first clear evidence that syngeneic tumors could be specifically reacted against by the immune system were studies in which mice were first immunized by inoculation of syngeneic tumor cells. The tumors were then totally excised or otherwise destroyed and the host survived (2). However, subsequent transplants of the same tumor into the same host were rejected (2,3). Lymphoid cells from such immune animals were shown to prevent growth of tumors when mixed together either in vivo or in vitro (4,5). However, a syngeneic tumor antigenically unrelated to the immunizing tumor could kill a host resistant to the first tumor, demonstrating the immunospecificity of the animal's immune response (6).

It is not necessary to excise or destroy a neoplasm to induce an immune response to the tumor in syngeneic hosts. If a second inoculum of tumor is given to a host already bearing this tumor, the second challenge will grow less well (7). A state of immunity has been established concomitant with the growth of the primary inoculum. Animals bearing small transplantable tumors can be shown to have both antibodies to their tumor cells and lymphoid cells capable of killing tumor cells in vitro (8). If the primary tumor is allowed to grow, however, concomitant immunity appears to wane, and lymphoid cells from hosts bearing larger tumors in some cases may no longer kill tumor cells in vitro (9). Not only is the intrinsic cytotoxic ability of these cells lost, but serum of the tumor-bearing host appears to be capable of specifically blocking the cytotoxic capabilities of

This work was supported by NIH Grant #CA 11605.

preimmunized cells (10). In addition, there appear to be severe limitations to the degree of tumor immunity. Not only is concomitant immunity lost as tumor size increases, but even strong preexisting immunity can be overcome by large challenging doses of tumors. The specific immune response of a host against a syngeneic tumor is depressed by large tumors, and there is an apparent nonspecific depression of many of the components of the immune system as well.

In brief, "once established, a tumor and the host act synergistically in favoring the growth of the tumor" (3). Cancer immunotherapy seeks to reverse this trend by augmenting those elements of the immune response that are inhibitory to tumor growth or by suppressing those components that appear to counteract the effect of tumor cell destruction. In evaluating any demonstration of cancer immunotherapy among the many models available, it is important to distinguish the difference between immunoprophylaxis and true immunotherapy. Immunoprophylaxis seeks to prevent the establishment of an infectious group of cells or oncogenic organisms. Immunotherapy attempts to enable the host to destroy an established growing tumor. A primary difference here is that the established tumor has already developed in a system of "immunologic accommodation" which must be broken during immunotherapy, a far more complex and difficult task than immunoprophylaxis.

It is theoretically possible to augment the effective immune response to tumor antigens in several ways:

1. *Specific active immunization* using tumor antigens whose immunogenicity is increased.

2. *Nonspecific active stimulation* of the immune apparatus with various adjuvant substances.

3. *Adoptive transfer* of immunologically competent, specifically sensitized cells.

4. *Passive administration* of antibodies to tumor antigens or antitumor antibodies conjugated to toxic substances.

5. *Passive administration of informational substances* which can transmit specific immunity to a nonimmune population of immunocompetent cells, i.e., "immune RNA" or "transfer factor."

Various combinations of these methods with each other or with other therapeutic modalities are possible.

SPECIFIC ACTIVE IMMUNOTHERAPY

Tumor antigens are generally poor immunogens capable of eliciting only a low degree of incomplete or ineffective immunity. In fact, some tumor antigens are so weak that they produce a state of relative immunologic unresponsiveness analogous to immunologic tolerance. Virus-induced tumors, in particular, may arise as a result of neonatally or congenitally acquired unresponsiveness to the virus itself, or to latent tumor viruses. It is possible to increase the immunogenicity of tumor antigens, thus supplementing an ineffective degree of immunity or even breaking the unresponsive state.

Antigens can be rendered more immunogenic by altering the dose, physical state, or route of administration, but most attempts to alter immunogenicity have been made by altering the chemical nature of the antigenic groupings themselves, or the "carrier" substances also borne by the tumor cell. Unfortunately, immunotherapeutic protocols have almost never been utilized. In most cases only the effect of an immunizing inoculum on subsequent tumor challenge has been investigated. In fact many studies have confined themselves to the chemical modification of the cell surface antigens as determined by in vitro assays (11,12). The use of modified antigens to immunize animals bearing established tumors has only recently come under intensive investigation. The entire field of modified tumor cell immunogenicity has been reviewed by Prager and Baechtel (13).

Modification of Tumor Cells in situ

A number of investigators have attempted to modify the immunogenicity of in situ tumors by subjecting the tumor cell mass in the case of solid tumors to various physical stimuli. For example, the effect of irradiation on the tumor mass and the immune response to the tumor has been tested, as have the effects of ligation of the tumor's blood supply with subsequent release (14), exposure of the tumor to cryosurgical control (exposure to severe destructive amounts of cold), and exposure of the tumor to heat in its various forms, including ultrasonic treatment and local heat (15). It is not clear from the results of these experiments whether the effect of the local tumor treatment acts by virtue of its nonspecific augmentation of the immune response or whether actually altering the tumor cell antigens in some way renders them more immunogenic. The protocols demand that comparisons be carried out with animals whose tumors have been surgically excised as well as those surgically excised plus the local treatment. The most extensive such studies utilized cryosurgery (16). Animals treated with methylcholanthrene-induced fibrosarcomas showed no local recurrence after cryosurgery and demonstrated increased lymphocyte-mediated cytotoxicity and serum-mediated cytotoxicity against the tumor. The effect was specific for the animal bearing the tumor and could not be elicited by merely freezing normal tissue. This does not demonstrate that the effect is specific for the tumor, merely that the animal who was bearing the tumor becomes more immune to the tumor when the tumor is destroyed by cryosurgery rather than eliminated by excision (17). The studies utilizing cryosurgery for carcinoma of the prostate have revealed increased IgG levels and antitumor antibodies in the sera of patients treated by this method, and for certain selected solid tumors such techniques may provide promise (18–20). In studying the mechanism by which heightened tumor immunity can be induced by cryosurgery, Faraci et al. (16) have demonstrated that similar degrees of immunity, as detected by cell-mediated cytotoxicity tests in vitro, can be induced by cryosurgery of the primary tumor or by treating the tumor-amputated mice with frozen exogenous tumor antigen. The mechanism now appears that the frozen tumor in some way has an augmented immunogenicity (16).

Physical Modification of Tumor Cells

As noted above, if a growing syngeneic tumor is excised or destroyed, the animal is frequently rendered specifically immune to the TSTA on the tumor. Therefore, it is not surprising that inoculating animals with tumor cells which cannot grow also renders them immune. Thus, tumors irradiated in vitro with X-rays, gamma rays, or even ultraviolet rays before injection into susceptible recipients can immunize animals to subsequent normal tumor cells. Naturally, these mice frequently will demonstrate immune capacity to the tumor cells in vitro (21–32), and lymphoid cells from these animals can adoptively transfer immunity (30). There is evidence, however, even in immunoprophylactic systems, that a loss of immunogenicity results from certain irradiation doses (33).

However, several immunotherapeutic studies have demonstrated (30) that irradiated cells injected into animals bearing small tumors will slow tumor growth and permit occasional tumor regression. We have evidence (unpublished) that cells irradiated with 10,000 R in vitro and injected subcutaneously into mice bearing small palpable transplanted syngeneic MCA sarcomas will show some tumor regression. Irradiation of the tumor cells with 2,000 R or 20,000 R had no effect.

Even though irradiated vaccines injected soon after tumor challenge are of some use, irradiated cells have never been shown to have any immunotherapeutic effect in animals bearing advanced tumors. It is uncertain whether irradiation actually increases the immunogenicity of the tumor cells or whether its effect is due solely to its ability to render the tumor nontransplantable, thereby increasing the dose of cells and tumor antigens which can be given (34). The favorable results claimed in some human experiments are difficult to interpret, since BCG is usually given as part of the immunotherapy. Nevertheless, the combined use of BCG and irradiated cells has become a popular approach to experimental immunotherapy in man. Most often allogeneic tumor cells have been used in these attempts, since there is some evidence that allogeneic tumors share some TSTA with each other.

Other tumor cell alterations have also been studied. Vaccination has been attempted utilizing cells disrupted by freezing and thawing, lyophilization, high pressure, and mechanical homogenization. Subcellular fractions and various cellular extracts have also been used, but none of these methods has produced results which appear clearly superior to the use of intact cells (13).

Coupling Immunogens to Tumor Cells

If a nonimmunogenic hapten is attached to a strongly immunogenic protein, antibodies can be elicited which bear antihaptenic specificities. In accordance with this principle, Czajkowski and associates (35) coupled rabbit gamma globulin (RGG) to tumor cells using bis-diazotized benzidine (BDB) to create a tumor vaccine with increased immunogenicity. When the tumor cells were used to treat mice with spontaneous mammary adenocarcinomas, the tumor growth was markedly retarded but no tumor regression was seen. In patients with advanced malignancy, the results using similar methods have been less impressive (36). Other attempts have coupled bovine serum albumin, ovalbumin, and methylated bovine gamma globulin to treat cells. In some cases the antibody response was augmented; in others there was a mild tumor-inhibitory effect.

Mitchison has suggested that a strong immunogen bound to the tumor cell surface may frequently act as a "helper" substance in increasing the immunogenicity of weaker (i.e., TSTA) antigens on the cell surface (37). Whether the actual mechanism by which immunogenicity to tumor antigens is increased by the chemical modifications discussed below involves the chemical creation of immunogens remains to be determined.

Chemical Modification of Tumor Cells

The chemical modification of the tumor cell surface by reagents specific for molecular components on the cell surface has been extensively described by Prager and Baechtel (13). The advantage of this method is that both antigenically strong and weak haptens on the cell surface can be selected for modification. One can vaccinate against a number of tumor lines using tumor cells treated with sulphydryl-blocking agents (iodoacetate, iodoacetamide, N-ethylmaleimide, and p-hydrozymercuribenzoate). The latter agent, which is a good hapten, when coupled to a carrier was ineffective in increasing the immunogenicity of tumor cells, whereas the former three agents were effective. Consequently, merely blocking the sulphydryl groups on the cell surface is not effective in increasing their immunogenicity, but the specific agent used as a blocker is important. Unfortunately, although iodoacetate and iodoacetamide-modified tumors can be used for immunoprophylaxis, only one experiment describes a therapeutic effect after tumor growth has been established (38). Even less effective vaccines appear to result from treatment of tumor cells with periodate to alter the hydroxyl groups, or with dinitrophenol or formaldehyde to react with surface amino groups (13).

Similar studies using other surface active agents have also revealed increased immunogenicity of cells (32,38–43). Prager and his colleagues have continued to analyze this problem (44) and have pointed out that the spontaneous immune response to certain tumors may modify the effectiveness of modified tumor tissue. Mice who manifest concomitant immunity to growing tumors become immune in response to altered tumor cells more easily. When a natural host response cannot be uncovered, immunity with altered cells is difficult but not impossible to elicit (44). In some systems, changes in tumor or host over several generations may alter host-tumor immunologic interactions, and one cannot assume that tumors with the same name maintain the same immunologic relationship to the host in different laboratories, or in the same laboratory over time.

Viral Oncolysis of Tumor Cells

Some tumors are susceptible to lysis by specific viruses. Kaprowski et al. (45) demonstrated that mice treated with certain viruses which destroyed their tumors were subsequently resistant to implants of the same tumor. Lindenmann and Klein (46) later showed that mice injected with influenza virus oncolysate of Ehrlich's ascites tumors were protected against subsequent challenge with a lethal dose of tumor cells.

Though Ehrlich's ascites tumor is an allogeneic tumor, the extensive studies utilizing either intact syngeneic tumor cells infected with influenza virus or homogenates of virally infected tumor cells have confirmed the immuno-prophylactic effect of these and other virally infected cells (32, 46–51). Until recently, few attempts at immunotherapy with virally infected cells have been carried out.

Surface Alterations by Enzymes

A number of enzymes—trypsin, pepsin, bromolin, collagenase, and chymotrypsin—have been used to modify the immunogenicity of tumor cells (13). Only *Vibrio cholerae* neuraminidase (VCN) has proven to be of value in the immunotherapy of established cancer. Currie and Bagshawe (52) first suggested that the sialic acid content on the surface of tumor cells might act in some way as a barrier to the detection of antigens by the host organism, thus explaining the immunologic paradox implicit in the growth and development of potentially antigenic tumors. Apffel and Peters (53) have even suggested that this masking of antigens is one of the normal biological roles of glycoproteins in nature and that sialoglycoproteins might act as a distinct system of immunoregulation. On the basis of these theoretical considerations, Sanford and Codington (54) showed that treatment of TA-3 cells with neuraminidase reduced their transplantability in the allogeneic C3H mouse. Currie and Bagshawe (55) demonstrated a similar effect with allogeneic Landschutz ascites tumors and L1210 leukemias as well as syngeneic methylcholanthrene-induced sarcomas. Subsequent experiments by Simmons and associates (56,57) demonstrated that VCN is capable of increasing the immunogenicity of a variety of strong and weak transplantation antigens in vivo and in vitro. In the case of strong histocompatibility antigens, no increase in the ability of VCN-treated cells to adsorb anti-H-2 antibody was noted; i.e., there was no unmasking of new antigenic histocompatibility sites to accompany the increase in apparent immunogenicity of the cells.

On the basis of these observations Simmons et al. (58) demonstrated that small, but firmly established, methylcholanthrene-induced fibrosarcomas could be made to regress by inoculation of tumor-bearing mice with tumor cells treated with VCN in vitro. The effect could not be induced with cells treated with heat-inactivated VCN (IVCN) or cells incubated with VCN in either an excess of sialic acid (product inhibition) or N-neuramino lactose (substrate inhibition). The regression was immunospecific and could be induced only with VCN-treated cells identical in type to the growing tumor. The successful treatment of other syngeneic and allogeneic tumors have also been demonstrated using a vaccine of VCN-treated tumor cells. In murine leukemia systems tumor regression induced by VCN-treated leukemia cells has been obtained (59,60). In fact Bekesi and Holland (61) have shown that spontaneous AKR lymphoma will respond to a combination of chemotherapy and immunotherapy with VCN-treated AKR lymphoma cells.

As an extension of these observations, Simmons et al. (62) observed that transplantable tumors could be made to regress by intratumor inoculations of VCN. The injections, however, must be repeated over a long period in order to induce total regression. Inhibition of tumor growth could not be induced by injection with IVCN or when the animal was injected with VCN in locations distant from the tumor. The inhibition of tumor growth induced by direct injection of VCN was shown to be immunospecific, since regression could be induced in uninjected tumors immunologically identical with the injected tumor in the same recipient. Tumors which were not identical in type to the injected tumor would not regress. It is even possible to induce regression of an injected tumor when the animal is dying of an immunologically distinct tumor.

The regression of established spontaneous mammary tumors was induced by the combined intratumor injections of BCG and VCN (63). Surprisingly, animals that demonstrated the best immunoregressive response to intratumor injections of VCN and BCG developed new tumors of identical histological types of uninjected mammary glands. If the treatment of the primary tumor had induced immunity to the mammary tumor virus (MTV)-associated antigen always found on mammary tumors of this type, the secondary tumors should not have developed. Subsequent experiments clearly demonstrated that VCN can increase the immunogenicity of the "private" TSTA on the mammary carcinoma but cannot increase the immunogenicity of the strong MTV-associated antigen. It is not clear, however, whether VCN destroys the MTV antigen.

Immunotherapeutic models utilizing VCN have been combined with other antitumor modalities. For example, the combination of chemotherapy and immunotherapy with VCN-treated cells has been found to be antagonistic in some systems—a finding which might be expected, since most chemotherapeutic agents are immunosuppressants. However, the proper use of chemotherapy to reduce tumor mass and of immunotherapy to "mop up" surviving tumor cells has been shown to be possible (61) using the spontaneous AKR lymphoma.

It has been shown that VCN-treated tumor cells can also prevent local recurrences of tumor after excision. There is no synergistic effect, however, unless near-total excisions of the tumor mass are performed, thereby proving once more that the effects of immunotherapy are limited by the mass of the tumor.

The mechanism by which VCN increases the immunogenicity of weak cellular antigens is unknown, but several possibilities suggest themselves:

1.   Since VCN removes sialic acid from the cell surface, the sialic acid may sterically interfere with the perception of TSTA or with the contact between antigen-bearing and antigen-handling cells.

2.   VCN also reduces the negative charge on the cell surface; a negatively charged antigen-handling or antigen-responsive cell might be more easily attracted to a less highly charged tumor cell.

3.   Reducing the negative charge also reduces the rigidity of the cell surface, since the mutually repellent negative charges on the surface are removed. The increased deformability of the antigenic cell itself might allow an increased area of contact between it and the antigen-responsive cell.

4.   VCN-treated cells are more extensively opsonized and phagocytosed, which in turn may aid antigen processing and the development of immunity.

5.   VCN-treated cells are much more susceptible to complement lysis.

6.   There is little evidence that VCN truly "unmasks" obscured tumor antigens, but VCN apparently unmasks neoantigens on the cell surface, to which even the autochthonous host may have preformed antibodies. Thus, the weak TSTA on the cell surface may behave like a hapten on a cellular carrier to which the host is already immune. Immunity to carrier proteins is known to alter the immunologic responses to haptens on the carrier.

7.   VCN-treated cells may act as mitogens in tissue culture. Mitogens on the cell surface might supplement an inadequate number of specific antigens in triggering specific clones of immunoreactive cells in the host.

8.   Immunolysis of mastocytoma target cells by immunized spleen cells was not augmented by VCN treatment of target cells. These data suggested that VCN treatment of tumor cells does not enhance the contact of, or destruction by, killer cells.

Other considerations in the actions of VCN to increase tumor immunogenicity have been discussed recently by Weiss (64).

Concanavalin A

Concanavalin A (Con A) is a jackbean globulin that can bind to cell surface carbohydrates. Con A may act as a specific T cell mitogen even after being bound to lymphocytes. Con A-treated tumor cells have been used to vaccinate against subsequent inoculations of tumor and to produce heightened levels of antitumor antibody. Simmons and associates (65) have shown that Con A-treated tumor cells injected into mice bearing either methylcholanthrene-induced fibrosarcomas or transplantable mammary adenocarcinomas will induce the immunospecific regression of some tumors. The effectiveness (roughly equivalent to that obtained with VCN-treated cells) depends, in part, on the concentration of Con A—very high or very low concentrations have no effect on the immunogenicity of the treated cell.

NONSPECIFIC ACTIVE IMMUNOTHERAPY

Nonspecific stimulation of cell-mediated immunity or humoral antibody production by adjuvants is usually accompanied by increased host resistance to infectious agents and/or the appearance of copious amounts of antibody to antigens compared to responses evoked without concomitant administration of adjuvants. Nonspecific stimulation of the immunologic apparatus may be a reasonable modality to augment the host's ability to react to a tumor antigen(s), eventually leading to host-mediated rejection of a tumor or destruction of residual tumor remaining after surgery, chemotherapy, or X-ray. Bacterial and nonbacterial agents have been utilized as adjuvants to increase host resistance to tumors.

While Coley first described the use of crude bacterial toxins to treat advanced malignancy (66), the most promising and clinically tested bacterial adjuvant to date is the bacillus Calmette-Guerin (BCG) strain of *Mycobacterium bovis* or its products. BCG was first used to interfere with the growth of allogeneic but not syngeneic tumors in mice (67–69). Later studies showed that local injection of BCG prevented the establishment (immunoprophylaxis) of intradermal syngeneic murine tumors (70) and suppressed the growth (immunotherapy) of syngeneic 3-methylcholanthrene-induced rat fibrosarcomas (71) and murine fibrosarcomas (72). BCG has also been used immunoprophylactically to prevent the growth of spontaneous tumors or those induced by viral or chemical carcinogens (reviewed in refs. 70 and 71). The most extensively studied animal model for immunotherapy in a syngeneic system has been developed in the guinea pig (73). In general, the ability of BCG to mediate or augment host-induced antitumor effects depends on the substrain of BCG, the number of viable organisms, the dose, route of administration, and timing with respect to tumor inoculation. The antitumor effect of BCG is considered to be local, not systemic, not due to cytotoxic effects on tumor cells, and to require stimulation of the host immune mechanism, resulting in some degree of host participation in antitumor immunity. Usually BCG has proven ineffective when given systemically more than a few days after tumor inoculum, although the growth of well established neoplasms may be temporarily inhibited. Later studies have focused on the methanol extraction residue (MER) of BCG, which has been shown to augment resistance of mice to syngeneic tumor grafts and inhibit development of spontaneous mammary carcinomas in mice (74). In rats, MER has been shown to be effective in inducing immunity to chemically induced sarcomas and a hepatoma when cells were inoculated with an admixture of MER (75).

While the exact mechanism(s) of BCG-mediated immunostimulation and its role in tumor immunotherapy are unknown, the association of BCG-induced macrophage activation and tumor resistance is well established. BCG has been shown to act in combination with a growing tumor to augment macrophage production in murine bone marrow cells (76). Murine peritoneal exudate macrophages from mice infected with BCG nonspecifically inhibited the growth of and killed tumor targets at ratios as low as 1 : 1 (77). Data derived from studies using other mycobacteria showed a correlation between adjuvant activity and the capacity to activate macrophages with tumoricidal activity (78). BCG also has been shown to augment T cell function in mice by counteracting the normally induced inhibition of T cells mediated by products of the humoral response (79).

More recent experimental evidence has suggested that another bacterium, *Corynebacterium parvum,* can exert immunopotentiative effects, activate macrophages, and display significant antitumor activity (80). In mice *C. parvum* functioned immunoprophylactically by inhibiting the establishment of fibrosarcomas and immunotherapeutically with this tumor when given three days after tumor injection (81). In rats *C. parvum* injected directly into growing subcutaneous mammary adenocarcinomas was followed by tumor regression and the histological presence of an infiltrate consisting mostly of macrophages (82). An extensive study by Fisher et al. (83), using a murine immunotherapy model of a combination of *C. parvum* and cyclophosphamide (CY), concluded that the time interval between the administration of immunostimulating agents and chemotherapeutic agents was not as critical as previously suggested. While most evidence relating to the immunotherapeutic use of BCG indicated that viable organisms should be used, other studies indicated that killed *C. parvum* vaccine could be used immunoprophylactically and immunotherapeutically in murine and rat systems (84). Other bacterial species and products which have been examined in tumor systems include *Bordetella pertussis* (85), bacterial endotoxins (86), *Listeria monocytogenes* (87,88), certain viral agents, and zymosan (89).

Nonbacterial products also have been examined for their ability to nonspecifically enhance the immune response and to mediate antitumor effects. Chemically defined nucleic acid complexes, polyadenylic and polyuridylic acid (poly A:U) (90), and polyinosinic and polycytidylic acid poly (I:C) (91) have been shown to augment host responses to a variety of antigens. Poly A:U was effective in mediating host immunologic control of a murine leukemia (92). In mice poly I:C administered prior to carcinogenic chemicals inhibited the formation of tumors compared to untreated controls (93). When mice were hyperimmunized

with poly I:C complexed to methylated bovine serum albumin, they were protected against challenge with Friend leukemia virus (94), suggesting that immunization with polynucleotide complexes may provide a means of augmenting host
responses to oncornaviruses. Another nonbacterial agent, levamisole, was shown
to reduce the number of metastases by HSV-1-transformed cells in a model
hamster system even when the drug was inoculated after development of tumor at
the site of tumor cell inoculation (95). However, Fidler and Spitler (96) concluded
that levamisole did not protect mice against a syngeneic melanoma and adenocarcinoma. Other nonbacterial substances with adjuvant properties which have use in
immunotherapy include small organic molecules such as vitamin A (97), fatty
acids, and lipids, pyran copolymer (98), and inorganic molecules such as alum,
bentonite, and beryllium sulfate (66).

Immunopotentiators or adjuvants are effective only when given at a critical
time with respect to antigenic or tumor cell stimulus. Usually, this time is before
tumor challenge, or less often after tumor transplantation but before the tumor is
firmly established. In a few tumor systems adjuvants can also stimulate tumor
growth. The mechanisms of adjuvant action stimulating host responses are very
complex, but most of these substances stimulate the reticuloendothelial system
and activate macrophages in vitro (99). Thymus-derived cells may also be affected
by adjuvant-stimulated macrophages. However, before any of the above agents
can be utilized effectively to augment either cellular or humoral antitumor activity, more evidence related to the mechanism of adjuvant action must be made
available.

Far more effective than the systemic administration of these substances is the
local administration of some adjuvants into the region of growing tumor. Once
more, BCG is the most thoroughly studied agent; the most extensively studied
system involves the treatment of intradermal transplants of certain carcinogen-
induced hepatomas in guinea pigs (100). Such tumors metastasize promptly to the
regional nodes, and even animals treated by local excision succumb from progressive growth of metastatic disease. When small tumors are injected with live BCG
organisms, however, both the local tumor and the regional metastases totally
regress without recurrence; such animals are immunologically resistant to challenge by the same tumor. The animals need not be preimmunized against BCG.
Dead organisms are not as effective as living organisms; however, lipid-free cell
walls of the organism in oil droplets have shown limited effectiveness.

There are severe limitations even to this truly immunotherapeutic model. BCG
must be injected into the primary tumor site. The larger the tumor, the less
effective is the treatment. Not every carcinogen-induced hepatoma is susceptible
to this treatment. And, if the primary tumor is situated deeper than the intradermal tissues, it will not regress.

The principle of adjuvant injection into cutaneous metastases has been vigorously applied to humans with skin metastases. BCG organisms are most frequently
used, but vaccinia virus and other adjuvants have also been tried. The responses to
treatment are not uniform and appear to depend on an intact immune system in
the host. If the patient is already immunosuppressed, no beneficial response will
be obtained. The most frequent favorable response is local necrosis of the injected
tumor; however, a few patients will manifest regression of both injected and
uninjected metastases. Visceral metastases have almost never responded to this

treatment, although there is experimental evidence that intravenous injection of the BCG might be more effective in reaching visceral metastases.

Klein (101) has observed that cutaneous and mucosal cancers in man will regress if the skin overlying the lesions is painted with certain contact allergens such as PPD, DNCB (dinitro chlorobenzene), and TEIB (triethylene imion-benzo quinone) when the patient has been presensitized to the allergen. The concentrations used were insufficient to elicit delayed hypersensitivity reactions in normal skin, but the neoplastic tissue did manifest a reaction and regress.

Mechanisms involved in the therapeutic effects of local adjuvants may delineate from the demonstration that macrophages can be stimulated by adjuvants like endotoxin into cytotoxic activities against tumor cells (102). Sometimes tumor cells can be preferentially killed, leaving normal cells intact. The adjuvant may act by increasing the attraction of inflammatory cells to the tumor, then activating these cells, thus leading to local tumor death. At the same time, systemic immunity can be induced, since the activated killer cells themselves still participate in the immune response. It is important to recognize that the two functions, local tumor necrosis and the induction of systemic immunity, may be independent functions of the same or even of differing cell populations in the inflammatory mixture. It is also important to recognize that the intratumor inoculation of nonspecific adjuvant agents results in a method of active specific immunotherapy which differs in essence from the systemic administration of adjuvant substances.

ADOPTIVE IMMUNOTHERAPY

The fact that tumor rejection is mediated largely by lymphoid cells and that animals bearing tumors lose both specific antitumor as well as general immune competence during tumor growth has prompted attempts to adoptively transfer immunocompetent lymphoid cells as a method of immunoprophylaxis or immunotherapy against cancer. Such an approach offers a unique opportunity to obtain killing of residual tumor cells preferentially with a high degree of antitumor specificity due to tumor-associated antigens. Several approaches to adoptive immunotherapy have been taken. One deals with the transfer of syngeneic cells from one animal immune to a tumor to a syngeneic animal bearing the tumor (immunotherapy) or one shortly to be challenged with the tumor (immunoprophylaxis). Another approach (less promising but not to be dismissed without trial) involves the use of allogeneic immunocompetent cells. It is apparent that each of these adoptive immunotherapeutic approaches can be combined with other anticancer modalities and that each alone has its own defined limitations and restrictions in terms of practical immunotherapeutic potential for man.

Immune syngeneic lymphocytes either incubated with tumor cells (103–107) or administered to animals shortly before or shortly after challenge with a small number of tumor cells (108–115) have consistently been shown to inhibit tumor growth. Such immunoprophylaxis models have firmly established that tumor immunity, like allograft immunity, can be much more easily transferred by cells than by serum. However, as discussed above, there is a great difference between immunoprophylaxis and immunotherapy. The ability of adoptively transferred specifically immune cells to protect against subsequent inocula of certain tumors is well established. The ability of such adoptively transferred cells to kill established tumors is less clear and is currently the subject of a number of investigations.

The earliest of these studies were developed from a model of whole body X-irradiation plus lymphoid cell reconstitution of mice with disseminated lymphoma. Attempts to treat animal lymphomas with lethal X-irradiation plus normal nonimmune syngeneic bone marrow or spleen yielded inconsistent and variable results, probably dependent on the radiosensitivity and antigenic quality of the lymphoma model system being tested (116). The aggregate of results suggested, however, that "the maximum irradiation dose that can be survived with a marrow graft is not enough to destroy all leukemic cells" (117). Subsequent studies using a combined approach model as above, but utilizing tumor-immune syngeneic lymphocytes, have shown more promising results. Fass and Fefer (103) combined chemotherapy with cytoxan followed by transfer of syngeneic tumor-immune spleen cells to the treatment of Friend virus-induced lymphoma in mice. Striking results were obtained, in that untreated mice or mice treated only with spleen from immune or nonimmune donors always died of the tumor within 15 days. Similarly, mice treated with chemotherapy alone or chemotherapy plus nonimmune cells died within 20–30 days. However, if mice were first treated with chemotherapy followed by tumor-immune spleen cells, 85% of the mice survived more than 100 days. Subsequently, in several other tumor models (110,118,119) lymphoid cells were quite effective in inhibiting or eradicating disseminated antigenic tumors if the adoptive immunotherapy was preceded by sublethal but noncurative chemotherapy to reduce the tumor load. An essential requirement for success in such a system was that the adoptively transferred lymphoid cells be viable and immune to the specific tumor being studied.

The vast majority of studies dealing with adoptive transfer of syngeneic immune lymphocytes have been carried out in inbred strains of animals. The donor animal was sensitized to a particular syngeneic tumor and his lymphocytes were transferred to a second syngeneic tumor-bearing animal. Such syngeneic in vivo sensitizations are impossible in man. A second difficulty with the above models is that the tumor load able to be eliminated by adoptive immunotherapy using syngeneic immune cells is small. Alone, syngeneic immune cell transfer is ineffective, but when combined with procedures that will decrease the tumor load (i.e., chemotherapy or radiation therapy) it seems to be much more efficacious. In a study designed to determine whether tumor metastasis could be prevented by immunologic manipulation Treves (120) implanted Lewis lung carcinomas on the foot pad of syngeneic mice. If the local tumors were removed at 7 days after inoculation, most mice died of lung metastases within 4 to 6 weeks. If, however, one day following tumor excision the mice were treated with syngeneic lymphocytes that had been sensitized against tumor cells in vitro, a drastic reduction in the number of metastases and an increase in survival was observed. Thus, once a solid tumor mass has been removed, it is apparent that metastatic foci, not yet discernible by histologic means, can be destroyed by specifically sensitized syngeneic lymphocytes. In addition, the need for in vivo sensitization and syngeneic donors is obviated by this model.

Although the results reviewed above appear promising, the problems of obtaining large numbers of specifically sensitized tumor-immune lymphocytes to be used in human tumor immunotherapy still remains.

The use of tumor-immune allogeneic cells for adoptive immunotherapy has also been employed in experimental animals. Fass and Fefer (121) successfully combined such adoptive immunotherapy with chemotherapy in the treatment of established systemically disseminated viral leukemia. Mice that were untreated or treated only with spleen cells from immune or nonimmune donors always died with the tumor. Similarly, mice treated with chemotherapy or chemotherapy plus nonimmune allogeneic cells always died. By contrast, mice treated with chemotherapy plus allogeneic immune cells frequently survived their tumors. The essential elements of this immunotherapy model appeared to be (1) reduction of the tumor load by chemotherapeutic agents (as similar to the syngeneic model), (2) reduction of the capacity of the host to reject the allogeneic donor spleen cells by chemotherapeutic agents, and (3) avoidance of the graft-versus-host reaction of the donor spleen cells against the immunosuppressed host by proper choice of F_1 hybrid donor spleen cells incapable of mounting a GVH reaction against the parental strain. Subsequent models in other murine tumor systems (MSV leukemia, SL12 leukemia, methylcholanthrene sarcoma) have confirmed these results. Unfortunately, success in this model is contingent upon the absence of GVH reaction induced by the allogeneic tumor-sensitive cells. This condition is currently difficult to achieve in man, though some successful attempts at treatment of leukemia utilizing matched (at HLA-A, B, and D subloci) nonimmune marrow have been achieved. The sensitizing of marrow in vitro to the tumor antigens of the marrow recipient without aggravating subsequent GVH reactions may be difficult, however.

If allogeneic cells are to be used in immunotherapy, one must utilize the GVH reaction as an immunotherapeutic tool. In recent years, graft-versus-host reactions have been shown to produce a variety of effects on immunologic processes. It has been reported that GVH (1) enhances primary and secondary antibody response to hapten protein conjugates in guinea pigs and mice (122,123), (2) suppresses the primary and secondary antibody response to sheep red blood cells, E. coli, LPS, Salmonella H antigen, and T_2 bacteriophage in mice (124–126), (3) prolongs the survival of first- and second-set skin allografts in mice (124,127), and (4) prolongs the survival of guinea pigs inoculated with syngeneic leukemia (128,129). This last observation led to the use of GVH reactions as immunotherapeutic tools in immunotherapy. Singh (130) demonstrated that during the induction and expression of the GVH reaction in mice two separate cytotoxic reactions were detectable. One component represented specific sensitization of donor cells to antigens of the recipient, leading to the lysis of the recipient cells. The other component was nonspecific cytodestruction of unrelated tumor cells by the host spleen cells. Okubo (131) has pointed out, however, that the ultimate immunologic effect of the GVH reaction is related to several factors: (1) the strain combinations and animals used, (2) the number of cells transferred in the induction of the GVH, and (3) the interval between the induction of GVH and immunologic or antigenic challenge. There seems to be a crucial importance to the time interval between the transfer of lymphoid cells and, in the model of immunotherapy, the inoculation of leukemia cells. If GVH is induced too long after challenge of the leukemia cells or immediately before challenge of the acute leukemia cells, the protective effect induced by the GVH reaction is abolished and, indeed, in some cases tumor growth is enhanced (131).

Thus, there seem to be two crucial problems inherent in the use of GVH reactions in adoptive immunotherapy. These are (1) ultimate control of the GVH reaction once it has been induced, and (2) appropriate timing of induction of the GVH so as to achieve maximal therapeutic benefit. Several attempts have been made at control of the GVH reaction. Bach (132) has suggested that potential donor lymphoid cells be sensitized in vitro to normal allogeneic patient cells. The responding clones of donor cells that would ultimately be the GVH-reactive cells would then be inactivated by 5BUDR or radioactive isotopes, thereby eliminating that clone capable of initiating the GVH. This theoretically would not affect the antitumor clones. The remaining cells could be infused into patients having already been treated with massive doses of irradiation or chemotherapeutic drugs. A second approach at control of GVH proposed by Mandel (133) involves the physical separation of GVH-reactive cells from a heterogenous immune population. Using a murine system, spleen cell populations were fractionated by centrifugation on a high-density bovine serum albumin gradient. The GVH cells localized in the denser layers, while cells responsible for immune memory and immunoglobulin production were found in other layers. If further investigations support these observations, this method of immune cell fractionation could be useful in the clinical application of adoptive immunotherapy utilizing tumor-immune allogeneic cells. A third proposed method of GVH control is given by Bortin (134) and utilizes a three-step therapy approach to spontaneous leukemia in AKR mice. The leukemic load was first reduced with chemotherapy followed by induction of graft-versus (leukemia)-host reaction using immunocompetent allogeneic cells; the third step was that of controlling or "rescuing" the animals from GVH by destruction of allogeneic GVH cells with chemotherapy and reconstruction of hematopoiesis with cells H-2 identical with the host. Using this complicated combination chemoimmunotherapy approach, significant therapeutic benefits were achieved in this murine leukemia model.

There have been several attempts to apply adoptive immunotherapy to human tumors. Nonspecific adoptive immunotherapy was first attempted by Woodworth and Nolan (135), who treated eight patients with advanced cancer with intravenous infusions of all the cells from a normal allogeneic human spleen. All patients were pretreated with cytotoxic chemotherapy in an attempt to inhibit the ability to reject the adoptively transferred cells. This attempt was met with limited success. Some improvement was reported in all eight cases but the benefits were brief and of no permanence. Schwartzenberg (136) reported treating 21 chemotherapy-resistant acute leukemias with 10^{12} leukocytes collected from patients with chronic myelocytic leukemia. Of the 21 patients treated, six experienced complete and three partial remissions, but again of only short duration. Specific adoptive immunotherapy—i.e., transfusion of "immune" lymphocytes specifically reactive against the tumor being treated—has shown somewhat more promising results. Andrews (137) reported cross-immunizing pairs of cancer patients with tumor tissue and subsequently exchanging their sensitized lymphocytes. Thoracic duct lymphocytes were then collected and infused. Although a massive number of cells was able to be collected, no therapeutic benefit was observed among four patients so treated. Nodler and More (138), utilizing a similar cross-sensitization technique between patients with malignant melanoma, collected peripheral blood lymphocytes, presumably sensitized to the allogeneic melanoma, and infused them into the donor tumor-bearing patients. Thirteen of the 53 patients were noted to have objective regressions of cutaneous lesions, two of which were complete.

Assuming that autologous lymphocytes from tumor-bearing patients were sensitive to their own tumors, Cheema (139) collected lymphocytes from peripheral blood of tumor-bearing patients and incubated them in vitro with phytohemagglutinin, thus "activating" potentially tumor-specific cytotoxic cells. Following reinfusion therapy of 29 patients with a variety of tumors, two were noted to regress completely; of the remaining 27, 25 had partial regressions. Using a similar protocol of in vitro activation of autologous lymphocytes, Frenster (140) has reported objective regressions of solid metastatic lesions in three out of five patients so treated.

Although the experimental studies and human trials have resulted in limited success, the ultimate therapeutic potential of adoptive immunotherapy has not yet been tested. The ideal circumstances of such a model would be large numbers of syngeneic cells containing an enriched population of cells cytotoxic to antigens present on the tumor. The use of these cells in a setting of limited tumor load would test the ultimate therapeutic capability of this form of therapy.

PASSIVE IMMUNOTHERAPY

The passive administration of cytotoxic antitumor serum might be expected to inhibit tumor growth. Cytotoxic antibodies have been found following the cure of various experimental tumors; they are frequently found in patients currently free of disease, and even in the relatives of cancer patients (141). Similarly, xenogenic antitumor sera might be developed and rendered specific for tumor antigens by absorption. Many tumors, however, are not readily susceptible to the cytotoxic effects of antisera in vitro, and it is possible that blocking factors (antibody?) rather than toxic agents could be administered; then, instead of producing tumor regression, the growth of the tumor would be enhanced. Such an enhancing effect has been repeatedly demonstrated in allogeneic tumor systems and can be deliberately induced with sera with demonstrated in vitro blocking activity or with tumor eluates. This fear of enhancing tumor growth, coupled with the inability to distinguish clearly between cytotoxic and blocking antibodies in vitro, has markedly inhibited the development of this experimental pathway.

Immune serum is rarely an effective prophylaxis against challenge with a large number of tumor cells or against clinically detectable tumors; the most prominent exception is the unusual Moloney sarcoma system in which young mice with palpable sarcomas can be effectively treated with serum from adult animals which have rejected their tumors. Another model utilized enormous volumes of "unblocking" serum to induce the regression of established polyoma tumor in rats (142).

In human patients many attempts have been made to use passively administered serum to inhibit or induce regression. Sera from personnel deliberately sensitized to allogeneic tumors have not met with much clinical success (143). Smith (144), in reviewing this problem, points out that infusion or perfusion with immune sera of areas involved by tumors has not been tried.

Nevertheless, there are sporadic convincing reports that serum therapy may, on occasion, provide an immunotherapeutic response. Gorer and Amos (145) immunized CBA mice with C57BL leukemia. CBA immune serum thereafter not only protected C57BL mice against subsequent challenge with the tumor, but also retarded growth of tumor injected two days prior to the serum injection. Immune serum incubated with tumor cells or administered a few days before or after a small number of tumor cells retards the growth of most lymphoid tumors and an occasional nonlymphoid tumor. Similarly, xenogeneic sera rendered specific for antibody to tumor antigens by various means can be effective against certain leukemias, but heterologous antinormal lymphocyte sera have not proved useful against leukemias and lymphomas.

These quite impressive benefits have not been shown in other experimental tumor model systems, however. The rationale for passive antitumor antibody therapy has assumed that tumor protection or therapy was the result of tumor-antibody interaction with complement, thus causing tumor cell lysis. This is certainly one possible mechanism. An alternative explanation may explain some of the disparate experimental results with passive immunotherapy.

Antibody complexed to target cells can induce killing of the target cell by certain nonimmune lymphoid cells. Several studies have shown that antibody having this activity [lymphocyte-dependent antibody (LDA)] is of the IgG class and that the effector cells are thymus-independent, nonimmune lymphoid cells bearing fc receptors (146). This cytotoxic mechanism has been described in xeno-, allo-, and autoimmune situations and more recently has been implicated in tumor rejection (147). Hershey (148) has recently reported that the in vivo protective effect of rabbit antirat tumor cell serum in a syngeneic rat lymphoma system correlated very well with the LDA activity of the serum but showed no correlation with complement-mediated tumor cell lysis activity. Further investigations on the role of antibody-dependent cell-mediated lysis in a syngeneic tumor system are required to more accurately define the role of this cytotoxic mechanism in tumor rejection.

Although passive immunotherapy alone with antitumor antisera has shown little clinical benefit to date, recent encouraging results have been obtained by using cytotoxic substances conjugated to antitumor antibodies, thereby concentrating these substances around tumor cells. In the first decade of this century Ehrlich dreamed of using diptheria toxin bound to antitumor antibodies as a "magic bullet" against malignant tumors. Ghose (149) revived this concept and reported that by utilizing a chlorambucil-bound antitumor antibody successful treatment of the EL4 lymphoma in mice could be achieved. This has recently been extended to early but encouraging results with human cutaneous malignant melanoma (150). Similar studies showing positive results as well have utilized antibody conjugated with such toxic substances such as methotrexate (151), radioactive iodine (149), boron (152), and the enzyme glucose oxidase (153). This has been shown to be efficacious in the therapy of small murine leukemia lymphomas as well as the Novikoff hepatoma (154).

Although early studies utilizing the passive transfer of antitumor antibody to obtain specific prophylactic or therapeutic benefits met with little success, the use of such passive therapy might be reconsidered in light of the recent findings.

In addition, the role of "blocking" and "unblocking" sera might be reevaluated with reference to LDA activity as a mechanism. Indeed, recent evidence suggests the need for cellular elements in the facilitation of antibody-mediated suppression of a murine lymphoma (155).

PASSIVE TRANSFER OF INFORMATIONAL SUBSTANCES

In an attempt to bypass the problems involved in the adoptive transfer of lympho-cytes or in the passive transfer of immune serum, subcellular components from sensitized cell populations may be used to confer a state of immunity. Alexander et al. (156) suggested that the effectiveness of lymphocytes passively transferred is due not to their direct cytotoxic properties but rather to the transfer of a subcellu-lar component or messenger capable of recruiting host cells to antitumor activity. RNA extracted from sheep immunized with rat benzypyrene-induced sarcomas was effective in slowing the growth and causing temporary regression in rats following footpad injection (156,157). RNA was extracted from the spleens of rats immunized with sarcomas and incubated with normal nonimmune syngeneic spleen cells. The syngeneic recipients of RNA-treated spleen cells were resistant to the growth of sarcoma isografts. These results have been repeatedly confirmed. Immune RNA from syngeneic, allogeneic, and even xenogeneic hosts can be used (158). The RNA can be incubated with syngeneic lymphoid cells, which are then transferred to the recipient, thereby obviating the problems of HVG or GVH reactions. Alternatively, immune RNA can be injected directly into the tumor-bearing host. There is good evidence that the passively transferred immunity is a property of immune RNA. Nonimmune RNA is ineffective; RNase destroys the activity, and various proteolytic agents do not interfere with the specific transfer of immunity (159).

In vitro studies have also demonstrated that nonimmune murine spleen cells can be made specifically cytotoxic to a chemically induced tumor by in vitro incubation of RNA extracted from lymphoid organs of specifically immunized guinea pigs (160). In these studies, RNA extracted from guinea pigs immunized with a different tumor or normal murine tissue failed to induce immune cytolysis. Most early studies using passive transfer of immune RNA dealt with immune prophylaxis models (161). In other earlier studies, RNA-treated lymphoid cells were injected after tumor regression was observed (156). Recently, however, com-plete tumor-specific regression of established guinea pig hepatoma tumors has been accomplished by a combination of therapy utilizing (1) xenogeneic immune RNA extracted from immune animals, (2) unsensitized syngeneic peritoneal exudate cells, and (3) immunization with tumor-specific antigen preparation. Individually, each of these therapeutic modalities had no, or very little effect on established tumors, but when all three were given together, tumors of 3–4mm diameter regressed completely following local subtumor injection (162). In addi-tion, specific tumor regression of tumors at a distant site also have been shown to regress under such combined therapy (163). An attractive feature of this model is its applicability to the human situation and obviation of graft-versus-host reac-tions in the use of other forms of allogeneic adoptive immunotherapy. Further studies utilizing immune RNA and its application to human tumors are currently under investigation.

Several other subcellular products that may have potential in immunotherapy are the various biochemicals associated with states of delayed hypersensitivity, collectively called lymphokines. They have been incompletely characterized, and they may ultimately prove to be identical or related to one another. The most widely studied substance is transfer factor (TF)—a dialyzable substance derived from lymphocytes capable of conferring antigen-specific, cell-mediated (but not antibody-mediated) immunity on the recipients. The goal in using TF is to provide the patient with a means of instructing a clone of his own lymphocytes to recognize and reject the tumor. Four potential sources of antitumor TF have been suggested: (1) TF from normal donors, (2) TF from patients in "remission" from tumors which share antigen with the recipient's tumor, (3) TF from persons deliberately immunized to allogeneic tumor antigens, and (4) TF prepared from and reinjected into the same tumor-bearing host. Since the immunity conferred by TF is only transient, repeated injections may be necessary. The fact that TF has no propensity for conferring humoral immunity (i.e., blocking activity) is considered a theoretical advantage. Unfortunately, TF appears to be detectable only in human systems, and animal models have not yet been developed (164).

DISCUSSION

A model is a representation or a substitute for the real thing. Herein lies the dilemma of experimental immunotherapy models. There exists no animal model of tumor immunotherapy that truly reflects the situation in man. Human tumors almost always present a mass of established malignant cells which have arisen and adapted to the immunological environment of the host. Spread of such tumors involves either direct extension or spreading of metastatic foci by the blood stream or lymphatics to distant sites or regional lymph nodes. Human cancers take months or years to kill the host. By contrast most tumor models are not spontaneously occurring tumors but involve the transfer of quite small numbers of tumor cells into usually abnormal, although conveniently measured, sites. The lethality of such tumors does not correspond to that in humans; they kill the host in a few days or at most a few months. Metastatic disease may or may not appear. In addition, such tumor transfer models are forced upon a normal immunologic environment of a host and therefore perhaps represent an altered immunologic adaptation as contrasted to a spontaneously occurring tumor. In addition, successful models of immunotherapy can only operate when the tumor load is small and has been in residence for only a few days to weeks.

Further difficulty arises in the type of tumors studied in experimental model systems. These are generally well-established and multiply transferred generation tumors that are perhaps not truly autochthonous. Indeed, total isogenicity of such tumors is probably never achieved, and some contribution of histoincompatibility in most syngeneic tumor transfer systems probably does exist.

The uncertainties of the relevance of experimental models to human cancer are compounded by incomplete understanding of how a normal host immune response, both cellular and humoral, is altered in adaptation to an autochthonous growing tumor and how at various stages of tumor growth the degree of antigenic load or tumor size affects such immunologic adaptation.

Thus, it is difficult to conceive that even the most successful models of immunotherapy in experimental animals can be directly adapted to trials of human immunotherapy. At present the restrictions defined by the successful immunotherapy models limit the tumor load able to be destroyed by immunologic maneuvers. In addition, regression of tumors via immunotherapy can be achieved only shortly after induction of tumor growth. Such limitations would predict only limited success of the defined immunotherapeutic models available to human tumors. A certain human urgency regarding the cancer problem, however, presents a compelling argument against any delay in applications of what is presently known concerning immunologic intervention. It is apparent that animal models at this juncture are the only rational means by which effective immunological manipulations can be assessed. To utilize any empirical technique in human immunotherapy that has not been demonstrated to be effective in animal models seems to be a dangerous proposition. Even techniques shown to be effective in animal models may prove to enhance human tumors. Until conditions for tumor enhancement or rejection can be predicted, such dangers will persist. There is considerable evidence to support the idea that tumor immunogens are weak, that the immunologic response they evoke may be misdirected, and that tumor immunotherapy as a primary means of treatment is highly unlikely. There is hope, however, that immunologic manipulations can induce a degree of truly effective immunity in a tumor-bearing host which will permit destruction of a few tumor cells remaining after surgery, radiotherapy, or chemotherapy.

REFERENCES

1. Hellström, K. E., and Hellström, I.; *Adv. Cancer Res.* **12,** 167 (1969).
2. Old, L. A., and Boyse, E. A., *Ann. Rev. Med.* **15,** 167 (1964).
3. Smith, R. T., *N. Eng. J. Med.* **278,** 1207 (1968).
4. Klein, G., Sjögren, H. O., Klein, E., and Hellström, K. E., *Cancer Res.* **20,** 1561 (1960).
5. Winn, H. J., *Nat. Cancer Inst. Monogr.* **2,** 113 (1959).
6. Allison, A. C., *Ann. Inst. Pasteur, Paris* **122,** 619 (1972).
7. Simmons, R. L., unpublished observation.
8. Hellström, I., and Hellström, K. E., *Int. J. Cancer* **4,** 587 (1969).
9. Leclerc, J. C., Gomard, E., and Levy, J. P., *Int. J. Cancer* **4,** 587 (1969).
10. Hellström, K. E., and Hellström, I., *Adv. Immunol.* **18,** 208 (1973).
11. Ohno, S., Natsu-ume, S., and Migita, S., *J.N.C.I.* **55,** 569 (1975).
12. Hyman, R., Ralph, P., and Sarkar, S. *J.N.C.I.* **48,** 1973 (1972).
13. Prager, M. D., and Baechtel, F. S., *Methods in Cancer Res.* **9,** 339 (1973).
14. Suit, H. D., and Kastelan, A., *Cancer* **26,** 232 (1970).
15. Dickinson, J. A., *Cancer Chemo. Repts.* **58,** 294 (1974).
16. Faraci, R. P., Bagley, D. H., Marrone, J. C., Ketcham, A. S., and Beazley, R. M., *Amer. Surg.* **41,** 309 (1975).
17. Faraci, R. P., Bagley, D. H., Marrone, J. C., and Beazley, R. M., *Surgery* **77,** 433 (1975).
18. Drylie, D. M., Jordan, W. P., and Robbins, J. B., *Invest. Urol.* **5,** 619 (1968).
19. Aibin, R. J., Pfeiffer, L., Gonder, M. J., and Soanes, W. A., *Exp. Med. Surg.* **27,** 406 (1969).
20. Neel, H. B., Ketcham, A. S., and Hammond, W. G., *Laryngoscope* **83,** 376 (1973).
21. Johnson T. S., Hudson, J. L., Feldman, M. E., and Irvin, G. L., *J.N.C.I.* **55,** 561 (1975).
22. Belehradek, J., Jr., Barski, G., and Thonier, M., *Int. J. Cancer* **9,** 461 (1972).
23. Glynn, J. P., Humphreys, S. R., Trivers, G., Bianco, A. R., and Goldin, A., *Cancer Res.* **23,** 1008 (1963).
24. Mathe, G., Pouillart, P., and Lapeyraque, F., *Brit. J. Cancer* **23,** 814 (1969).
25. Natale, N., Reiner, J., and Southam, C. M., *Cancer* **28,** 1118 (1971).
26. Kasakura, S., *Transplantation* **11,** 117 (1970).
27. Rockwell, S. C., Kallman, R. F., and Fajardo, L. F., *J.N.C.I.* **49, 735 (1972).**

28. Porteous, D. D., and Munro, T. R., *Int. J. Cancer* **10,** 112 (1972).

29. Gebhardt, B., *Cell. Immunol.* **8,** 290 (1973).

30. Ellman, L., and Green, I., *Cancer* **28,**647 (1971).

31. Lumsden, T., *Amer. J. Cancer* **15,** 563 (1931).

32. Boone, C. W., and Blackman, K., *Cancer Res.* **32,** 1018 (1972).

33. Alexander, P., *Prog. Exp. Tumor Res.* **10,** 22 (1968).

34. Currie, G. A., *Brit. J. Cancer* **26,** 141 (1972).

35. Czajkowski, N. P., Rosenblatt, M., Wolf, D. L., and Vazquez, J., *Lancet* **ii,** 905 (1967).

36. Cunningham, T. J., Olson, K. B., Laffin, R., Horton, J., and Sullivan, J., *Cancer* **24,** 932 (1969).

37. Mitchison, N. A., *Transplant. Proc.* **2,** 92 (1970).

38. Apffel, C. A., Arnason, B. G., and Peters, J. H., *Nature* **209,** 694 (1966).

39. Martin, W. J., Wunderlich, J. R., Fletcher, F., and Inman, J. K., *P.N.A.S.* **68,** 469 (1971).

40. Prager, M. D., Der, I. Swann, A., and Cotropia, J., *Cancer Res.* **31,** 1488 (1971).

41. Mousseron-Canet, M., Magous, R., Lecou, C., and Levallois, C., *Cancer* **36,**1309 (1975).

42. Drake, W. P., Ungaro, P. C., and Mardiney, M.R., Jr., *Cancer Res.* **32,** 1042 (1972).

43. Frost, P., and Sanderson, C. J., *Cancer Res.* **35,** 2646 (1975).

44. Prager, M. D., Baechtel, F. S., Ribble, R. J., Ludden, C. M., and Mehta, J. M., *Cancer Res.* **34,** 3203 (1974).

45. Kaprowski, H., Lover, R., and Kaprowska, I., *Texas Rep. Biol. Med.* **15,** 559 (1957).

46. Lindenmann, J., and Klein, P. A., *Rec. Results Cancer Res.* **9,** 1 (1967).

47. Axler, D. A., and Girardi, A. J., *Proc. Amer. Assoc. Cancer Res.* **11,** 4 (1970).

48. Boone, C., Blackman, K., and Brandchaft, P., *Nature* **231,** 265 (1971).

49. Hakkinen, I., and Halonen, P., *J.N.C.I.* **46,** 1161 (1971).

50. Kobayashi, H., Senodo, F., Kaji, J., Shirai, T., Saito, H., Takeichi, N., Hosokawa, M., and Kodama, T., *J.N.C.I.* **44,** 11 (1970).

51. Lindenmann, J., and Klein, P. A., *J. Exp. Med.* **126,** 93 (1967).

52. Currie, G. A., and Bagshawe, K. D., *Brit. J. Cancer* **22,** 843 (1968).

53. Apffel, C. A., and Peters, J. H., *J. Theoret. Biol.* **26,** 47 (1970).

54. Sanford, B. H., and Codington, J. F., *Tissue Antigens* **1,** 153 (1971).

55. Currie, G. A., and Bagshawe, K. D., *Brit. J. Cancer* **23,** 141 (1969).

56. Simmons, R. L., Lipschultz, M. L., Rios, A., and Ray, P. K., *Nature* **231,**111 (1971).

57. Simmons, R. L., Rios, A., Ray, P. K., *Nature* **231,** 179 (1971).

58. Simmons, R. L., Rios, A., Lundgren, G., Ray, P. K., McKhann, C. F., and Haywood, G. R., *Surgery* **70,** 38 (1971).

59. Bekesi, J. G., Arneault, G., and Walter, L., *J.N.C.I.* **49,** 107 (1972).

60. Kollmorgen, G. M., Erwin, D. N., and Killion, J. J., *Proc. Amer. Assoc. Cancer Res.* **14,** 69 (1973).

61. Bekesi, J. G., and Holland, J. F., *Rec. Results in Cancer Res.* **47,** 357 (1974).

62. Simmons, R. L., Rios, A., and Kersey, J. H., *J. Surg. Res.* **12,** 57 (1972).

63. Simmons, R. L., and Rios, A., *Surgery* **71,** 556 (1972).

64. Weiss, L., *J.N.C.I.* **50,** 3 (1973).

65. Simmons, R. L., and Rios, A., *Transplant. Proc.* **VII,** 247 (1975).

66. Yashphe, D. J., in *Immunological Parameters of Host-Tumor Relationships* (D. W. Weiss, ed.), Academic Press, New York, 1971, p. 90.

67. Hersh, E. M., Gutterman, J. U., Mavligit, G. M., Reed, R. C., and Richman, S. P., *J. Amer. Med. Assoc.* **235,** 646 (1976).

68. *Conference on the Use of BCG in Therapy of Cancer,* National Cancer Institute Monograph, No. 39 (T. Borsos and H. J. Rapp, eds.), 1973.

69. Old, L. J., Clark, D. A., and Benacerraf, B., *Nature* **184,** 291 (1959).

70. Bart, R. C., Zbar, B., Borsos, T., and Rapp, H. J., *N. Eng. J. Med.* **290,** 1413 (1974).

71. Baldwin, R. W., and Pimm, M. W., *Conference on the Use of BCG in Therapy of Cancer,* National Cancer Institute Monograph, No. 39, 1973, p. 11.

72. Tokunaga, T., Yamamoto, S., Nakamura, R. M., and Kataoka, T., *J.N.C.I.* **53,** 459 (1973).

73. Zbar, B., Ribi, E., and Rapp, J. H., *Conference on the Use of BCG in Therapy of Cancer,* National Cancer Institute Monograph, No. 39, 1973, p.3.

74. Kuperman, O., Yashphe, D. J., Sharf, S., Ben-Efraim, S., and Weiss, D. W., *Cell Immunol.* **3,** 277 (1972).

75. Hopper, D. G., Pimm, M. V., and Baldwin, R. W., *Brit. J. Cancer* **31,** 176 (1975).

76. Fisher, B., Taylor, S., Levine, M., Saffer, E., and Fisher, E. R., *Cancer Res.* **34,** 1668 (1974).

77. Germain, R. N., Williams, R. M., and Benacerraf, B., *J.N.C.I.* **54,** 709 (1975).

78. Juy, D., and Chedid, L., *Proc. Natl. Acad. Sci., USA* **72,** 4105 (1975).

79. Mackaness, G. B., LaGrange, P. H., and Ishibashi, T., *J. Exp. Med.* **139,** 1540 (1974).

80. Halpern, B., *Rec. Results in Cancer Res.* **47,** 262 (1974).

81. Milas, L., Gutterman, J. U., Basic, I., Hunter, N., Mavligit, G. M., Hersh, E. M., and Withers, H. R., *Int. J. Cancer* **14,** 493 (1974).

82. Likhite, U. V., *Int. J. Cancer* **14,** 684 (1974).

83. Fisher, B., Wolmark, N., Rubin, H., and Saffer, E., *J.N.C.I.* **55,** 1147 (1975).

84. Likhite, V. V., and Halpern, B. N., *Int. J. Cancer* **12,** 699 (1973).

85. Pernell, D. M., Kreider, J. W., and Bartlett, G. L., *J.N.C.I.* **55,** 123 (1975).

86. Nigam, V.N., *Cancer Res.* **35,** 628 (1975).

87. Bast, R. C., Zbar, B., Mackanness, G. B., and Rapp, H. J., *J.N.C.I.* **54,** 749 (1975).

88. Bast, R. C., Zbar, B., Miller, T. E., Mackaness, G. B., and Rapp, H. J., *J.N.C.I.* **54,** 757 (1975).

89. Simartin, O. D., Fugmann, R. A., and Hayworth, P., *J.N.C.I.* **29,** 817 (1962).

90. Schmidtke, J. R., and Johnson, A. G., *J. Immunol.* **106,** 1191 (1971).

91. Levy, H. B., Law, L. W., and Rabson, A. S., *Proc. Nat. Acad. Sci.* **62,** 357 (1969).

92. Pendergrast, W. J., Drake, W. P., and Mardiney, *J.N.C.I.* **55,** 1223 (1975).

93. Gelboin, H. V., and Levy, H. B., *Science* **167,** 205 (1970).

94. Fourcade, A., Friend, C., Lacour, F., and Holland, J. G., *Cancer Res.* **14,** 1749 (1974).

95. Sadowshi, J. M., and Rapp, F., *Proc. Soc. Exp. Biol. Med.* **149,** 219 (1975).

96. Fidler, I. J., and Spitler, L. E., *J.N.C.I.* **55,** 1107 (1975).

97. Felix, E. L., Loyd., B., and Cohen, M. H., *Science* **189,** 887 (1975).

98. Harmel, R. P., and Zbar, B., *J.N.C.I.* **54,** 989 (1975).

99. Unanue. E. R., *Adv. Immunol.* **15,** 95 (1972).

100. Zbar, B., and Tanaka, T., *Science* **12,** 271 (1971).

101. Klein, E., *N.J.S.J. Med.* **68,** 900 (1968).

102. Alexander, P., Delorme, E. J., Hamilton, L. D. C., and Hall, J. C., *Nucleic Acids in Immunology* (O. J. Plescia and W. Brown, eds.), Springer-Verlag, New York, 1968, p. 527.

103. Fass, L., and Fefer, A. *Cancer Res.* **32,** 997 (1972).

104. Fefer, A., McCoy, J. L., and Glynn, J. P., *Cancer Res.* **27,** 2207 (1967).

105. Klein, G., *Ann. Rev. Microbiol.* **20,** 223 (1966).

106. Old, L. J., and Boyse, E. A., *Ann. Rev. Med.* **15,** 167 (1964)

107. Rosenau, W., and Morton, D. L., *J.N.C.I.* **36,** 825 (1966).

108. Vadlamudi, S., Padarathsingh, M., Bonmassar, E., and Goldin, A. *Int. J. Cancer* **7,** 160 (1971).

109. Deckers, P. J., Edgerton, B. W., Thomas, B. S., and Pilch, Y. H., *Cancer Res.* **31,** 734 (1971).

110. Mihich, E., *Cancer Res.* **29,** 848 (1969).

111. Ellman, L., and Green, G., *Cancer* **28,** 647 (1971).

112. Old, L. J., Boyse, E. A., Clarke, D. A., and Carswell, E. A., *Ann. N.Y. Acad. Sci.* **101,** 80 (1962).

113. Cater, D. B., and Waldmann, H., *Brit. J. Cancer* **21,** 124 (1967).

114. Ellman, L., Katz, D. H., Green, I., Paul, W. E., and Benacerraf, B., *Cancer Res.* **32,** 141 (1972).

115. Katz, D. H., Ellman, L., Paul, W. E., and Benacerraf, B., *Cancer Res.* **32,** 133 (1972).

116. Fefer, A., *Israel J. Med. Sci.* **9,** 350 (1973).

117. Barnes, D. W. H., Loutit, J. F., and Neal, F. E., *Brit. Med. J.* **2,** 626 (1956).

118. Fefer, A., *Int. J. Cancer* **8,** 364 (1971).

119. Vadlamudi, S., Padarathsingh, R., Bonmassar, E., and Goldin, A., *Int. J. Cancer* **7,** 160 (1971).

120. Treves, A., Cohen, I., and Feldman, M., *J.N.C.I.* **54,** 777 (1975).

121. Fass, L., and Fefer, A., *Cancer Res.* **32,** 2427 (1972).

122. Katz, D. H., Paul, W. E., Goidl, E. A., and Benacerraf, B., *J. Exp. Med.* **133,** 169 (1971).

123. Osborne, D. P., and Katz, D. H., *J. Exp. Med.* **136,** 439 (1972).

124. Howard, J. G., and Woodruff, M. A. S., *Proc. Roy. Soc.* **B/154,** 532 (1961).

125. Moller, G. *Immunology* **20,** 597 (1971).

126. Blaese, M., Martinez, C., and Good, R. A., *J. Exp. Med.* **119,** 211 (1964).

127. Lapp, W. S., and Moller, G., *Immunology* **17,** 339 (1969).

128. Katz, D. H., Ellman, L., Paul, W. E., Green, I., and Benacerraf, B., *Cancer Res.* **32,** 133 (1972).

129. Ellman, L., Katz, D. H., Green, I., Paul, W. E., and Benacerraf, B., *Cancer Res.* **32,** 141 (1972).

130. Singh, J. N., Sabbadini, E., and Sehon, A. M. *J. Exp. Med.* **136,** 39 (1972).

131. Okubo, S., Ottengen, H. F., Ciliozza, S. S., and Ovary, Z., *Proc. Nat. Acad. Sci.* **71,** 4264 (1974).

132. Boeh, M. L., Bach, F. H., and Zoschke, D. C., *Israel J. Med.* **9,** 344 (1973).

133. Mandel, M., and Usofsky, R., *J. Surg. Res.* **16,** 546 (1974).

134. Bortin, M., Rose, W., Truitt, R., Pimm, A., Saltzstein, E., and Rodey, G., *J.N.C.I.* **55,** 1227 (1975).

135. Woodruff, M. F. A., and Nolan, B., *Lancet* **ii,** 426 (1963).

136. Schwarzenberg, L., Mathe, G., Schneider, M., Amiel, J. L., Cattan, A., and Schlumberger, J. R., *Lancet* **ii,** 365 (1966).

137. Andrews, G. A., Congdon, C. C., Edwards, C. L., Gengozian, N., Nelson, B., and Vodopick, H., *Cancer Res.* **27,** 2535 (1967).

138. Nadler, S. H., and Moore, G. E., *Arch. Surg.* **99,** 376 (1969).

139. Cheema, H. R., and Hersh, E. M., *Cancer* **29,** 982 (1972).

140. Frenstar, J. H., and Rogoway, W. M., personal communication.

141. Klein, E., *Europ. J. Cancer* **6,** 15 (1970).

142. Bansal, S. C., Hargreaves, R., and Sjogren, H. O., *Int. J. Cancer* **9,** 97 (1972).

143. Currie, G. A., *Brit. J. Cancer* **26,** 141 (1972).

144. Smith, R. T., *N. Eng. J. Med.* **287,** 439 (1972).

145. Gorer, P. A., and Amos, D. B., *Cancer Res.* **16,** 338 (1956).

146. Perlmann, P., Perlmann, H., and Wigzell, H., *Transplant. Dev.* **13,** 91 (1972).

147. Lamon, E. W., Skurzak, A. M., Klein, E., and Wigzell, H., *J. Exp. Med.* **137,** 1072 (1973).

148. Hersey, P., *Nature* **244,** 22 (1973).

149. Ghose, T., Cerini, M., Carter, M., and Nairn, R., *Brit. Med. J.* **1,** 90 (1967).

150. Oon, C. J., Apsey, M., Buckleton, K. B., Cooke, I., Hanham, I., Hazarika, P., Hobbs, J., and McLeod, B., *Behring Inst. Mitt.* **56,** 352 (1974).

151. Mathe, G., and TranBaLoc, B. J., *Acad. Sci. Paris* **246,** 1626 (1958).

152. Hawthorne, M., Wiersema, R., and Takasuji, M., *J. Med. Chem.* **15,** 449 (1972).

153. Philpott, G., Bower, R. J., and Parker, C. W., *Surgery* 74, 51 (1973).

154. Smith, G. V., Grogan, J., Stribling, J., and Lockard, J., *Am. J. Surg.* **129,** 146 (1975).

155. Shin, H., Hayden, M., and Gotely, C. *Proc. Nat. Acad. Sci.* **71,** 163 (1974).

156. Alexander, P., Delorme, E. J., Hamilton, L. D. G., and Hall, J. G., *Nucleic Acids in Immunology* (O. J. Plescia and W. Brown, eds.), Springer-Verlag, New York, 1968, p. 527.

157. Alexander, P., Delorme, E. J., Hamilton, L. D. G., and Hall, J., G. *Nature* **213,** 569 (1967).

158. Pilch, Y. H., Ramming, K. P., and Deckers, P. J., *Methods in Cancer Res.* **9** (1973).

159. Pilch, Y., Veltman, L., and Kern, D., *Surgery* **76,** 23 (1974).

160. Ramming, K. P., and Pilch, Y., *Science* **168,** 492 (1970).

161. Kennedy, C., Cater, D., and Hartveit, F., *Acta Pathol. Microbiol. Scand.* **77,** 196 (1969).

162. Paque, R. E., Meltzer, M., Zbar, B., Rapp, H., and Dray, S., *Cancer Res.* **33,** 3165 (1973).

163. Schlayer, S. I., Paque, R. E., and Dray, S., *Cancer Res.* **35,** 1907 (1975).

164. Lawrence, H. W., *Adv. Immunol* **11,** 195 (1970).

Chapter Nine

Immunologic Treatment of Neoplasms in Man

BRIGID G. LEVENTHAL AND GERALDINE S. KONIOR

Pediatric Oncology Branch, National Cancer Institute, National Institutes of Health, Bethesda, Maryland

There are three major requirements for the successful use of immunotherapy in man. The first is that human tumors should have antigens on their surface which can elicit some sort of destructive response on the part of the host. As documented in Chapters 5 and 7, there is now ample evidence that tumor antigens do indeed exist in the human system. Whether these antigens can elicit a destructive response from the host is not yet clear. The second requirement is that immunocompetent cells be present in sufficient quantity to produce this appropriate destructive response. As pointed out also by others in this volume, the usual ratio of attacker to target cells in most in vitro assays involving cell destruction is of the order of 100 : 1. This means that immunotherapy may well be limited to situations where the residual tumor load is small. The third requirement is that there be no antagonistic effects—i.e., that the effective immune response not be blocked or impaired by some other product of the immune reaction, as discussed in Chapter 6.

This chapter will deal with attempts to increase the number of immunocompetent cells available in man for attack against tumor target cells. Where available, data relative to effects on antitumor immunity will also be presented.

Immunotherapy, like any other immunization procedure, can be categorized either as specific (directed against the tumor antigens themselves) or nonspecific (a general stimulation of the immune response). It can also be considered, by classical definitions again, to be active—effective via direct stimulation of the patient's own immune system; passive—stimulating the immune system of another individual and administering the products of that immune reaction to the patient; or adoptive—where there is transfer of the machinery for continuous

215

maintenance of specific immunity rather than a product of an immune reaction with a finite half-life (2).

This report will deal first with active immunotherapy. Much of the recent work in this area has been with adjuvants. The treatments have been specific, nonspecific, and combinations of the two. We will emphasize areas which are currently under active clinical investigation. The reader is referred to other recent reviews for further details in some areas (3–6).

NONSPECIFIC ACTIVE IMMUNOTHERAPY

Bacterial Cells and Their Products

There has been great interest through the years in the possibility of treating cancer patients with vaccines and bacterial products to inhibit tumor growth. Coley (7) in 1891 observed that patients who had erysipelas in an area of the skin which was involved with sarcoma might have regression of the sarcoma if they survived their erysipelas. He tried to extend these observations by administering Coley's toxins, mixtures of heat-killed streptococci and other organisms, such as *Serratia marcescens,* which did occasionally produce regression when injected directly into tumors. They have also been administered intramuscularly or intravenously with less dramatic but still objective responses.

In a retrospective analysis of what he termed a "natural" experiment, Ruckdeschel and colleagues (8) concluded that the occurrence of postoperative empyema improved survival in 18 patients with pulmonary resection for carcinoma of the lung when compared with 34 controls from the same institution. They felt that the protection conferred on the patients by postoperative empyema may have been mediated by the activation of regional cellular immune mechanisms. The beneficial effect of the intrapleural infection was found principally in patients with tumor limited to the lung and its draining regional lymph nodes. Six of seven patients in this group survived for five years. In an attempt to exploit this phenomenon a number of substances of bacterial origin have been studied for their activity against human tumors with special attention to their effect on the immunologic reaction to tumor antigens.

Bacillus Calmette-Guerin (BCG). Bacillus Calmette-Guerin (BCG) was first developed by Calmette and Guerin through progressive attenuation of the bovine tubercle bacillus through passage in medium containing beef bile. It was first used in 1921 as a vaccine against tuberculosis. Because of the initial successes, mass vaccination was encouraged. It was not until 30 years later that an adequately controlled trial in humans was started. As a result of the lack of firm evidence of efficacy many scientists opposed its use as a tuberculosis vaccine for many years (9). Perhaps there is a lesson for immunotherapists in this historical observation.

The antitumor effect of BCG was first demonstrated in a prophylactic system. Animals infected with viable organisms were resistant to the development of subsequently implanted tumors (10). It was thought that this antitumor effect was related to a generalized increase in the activity of the reticuloendothelial system, and it seemed possible that similar effects might be seen in man (11). In 1970 Davignon et al. (12–14) reported that the incidence of leukemia in children under

Table 1   "Prophylactic" Effect of BCG on the Development of Malignancy

Age BCG Given	Incidence of		Reference	No.
	Leukemia	Lymphoma		
?Neonate	Decreased	Not studied	Davignon (1970)	(12)
Neonate	Decreased	Not studied	Rosenthal (1972)	(15)
School children, approx. 13	Slight decrease	Slight decrease	BMRC (1972)	(22)
Older children, adults	No change	No change	Comstock (1971)	(23)
1–18	Slight decrease	Increase	Comstock (1975)	(24)

15 in Quebec who had received BCG was about half that in children who had not. Rosenthal et al. (15) obtained similar data in a retrospective study of neonates immunized with BCG in Chicago. However, certain methodological aspects of these studies have been criticized (16,17), and studies of statistics from different geographic areas with different policies of BCG administration have failed to demonstrate any statistically significant effect of BCG on the incidence of leukemia (18–22) or lymphoma and Hodgkin's disease in adults (23).

In one recent large controlled clinical trial of BCG vaccine the incidence of leukemia was slightly less in the vaccinated than in the control group, but the incidence of lymphoma was increased at a statistically significant level. Thus, at the moment, although there seems to be good evidence that prior infection with BCG inhibits the successful development of tumors in animals, the evidence that it affects the spontaneous development of tumors in man is conflicting and somewhat equivocal. Some of these studies are summarized in Table 1. This subject has recently been reviewed (24,25).

In addition to its prophylactic effect on tumor development, BCG has also been shown to have a therapeutic effect on established animal tumors. The requirements for this effect are that (1) the tumor be small, (2) the host animal have the ability to develop an immune response to mycobacterial antigens, (3) adequate viable organisms be injected, (4) the BCG and tumor cells be administered in close proximity to one another, and (5) the host be able to develop an immune response to tumor-associated antigens. These points have recently been reviewed (26).

Clinical therapeutic trials in man with BCG have been of two general types. First, cutaneous tumors have been treated by direct intralesional injection of BCG. Second, BCG has been used with or without tumor cells as an adjuvant after the main tumor burden has been decreased by chemotherapy, radiotherapy or surgery.

Morton and his co-workers first began giving intralesional injections of BCG to patients with dermal metastases of malignant melanoma in 1967. They have recently reviewed their data (27). In 36 patients with intracutaneous metastases they have seen regression in 684/754 (91%) of lesions which were directly injected and 6/36 (17%) of those uninjected. In 9 patients with subcutaneous and/or visceral metastases there was regression in only 8/26 (31%) of injected lesions and 0/9 uninjected nodules. These investigators are now attempting to reduce the tumor load surgically before immunotherapy in this latter group of patients. Bornstein et al. (28) also saw regression of injected nodules in 4/4 patients who had only intradermal disease and in only 1/10 with subcutaneous or visceral involvement. A number of other groups have confirmed this work by Morton (29–33). Table 2 cites seven recent studies and shows that regression of injected melanoma nodules can be expected in over half of the patients, particularly those who have only intradermal metastases. Indeed, regression of uninjected nodules was limited to this group of patients. One patient has now been reported (34) with 64 intracutaneous metastases of malignant melanoma. Over an eight-month period 17 lesions were inoculated with BCG. All injected lesions and 47 uninjected lesions regressed and a single pulmonary metastasis shrank over 50% in size. This is the first documented case of a pulmonary metastasis responding to this form of treatment. A number of trials have been recently reviewed (35,36).

In most of the reports where it has been studied, it appears that the immunocompetence of the patient is important for the response. Most patients were skin-tested with either dinitrochlorobenzene (DNCB) or purified protein derivative (PPD). Therapeutic responses were usually limited to those patients who either were reactive at the start of the study or became reactive during therapy (27,29,30), except in Balazarini's study (31), where this reactivity to PPD before therapy appeared to make no difference in response rate.

Attempts to increase tumor-specific immunity by addition of autologous lymphocytes sensitized to tumor antigen in vitro and neuraminidase-treated tumor cells to intralesional BCG injections has not as yet increased the response rate (37,38). Minton (39) adopted a different strategy in a study involving eight patients with metastatic malignant melanoma who had progressive disease. All had undergone surgical excision and four received chemotherapy as well. BCG

Table 2   Response of Melanoma to Direct Intralesional Injection BCG

Number of Patients	Regression of Injected Nodules	Regression of Uninjected Nodules	Site of Metastasis	Reference	No.
36	684/754 (91%)	6/36 (17%)	ID[a]	Morton (1974)	(27)
9	8/26 (31%)	0/9 (0%)	SQ/V[a]		
4	4	2	ID	Bornstein (1973)	(28)
11	1	0	SQ/V		
25	15	2[b]		Pinsky (1973)	(29)
9	7	2	ID	Nathanson (1972)	(30)
21	68/85 (80%)	0/21		Balzarini (1974)	(31)
7	3			Smith (1973)	(32)
2	1	0		Baker (1973)	(33)
TOTALS: 124	68%	10%			

[a] ID = intradermal
SQ = subcutaneous
V = visceral
[b] Both ID only.

was given to these patients in 10–15 separate intradermal or intratumor injections in the region of a metastasis. Mumps virus was injected into the tumor nodules. By the use of this combination of mumps and BCG inoculation, Minton achieved control of tumor growth in five patients, including three whose tumors were growing progressively with injections of BCG alone.

Klein (40) treated patients with epidermal cancers with a variety of local and systemic combinations of chemotherapy and immunotherapy. He found that the capacity of patients to show tumor regression after intratumoral injection of BCG or PPD was directly related to their immunocompetence. In some cases he administered either oral BCG or large doses of intradermal PPD in order to sensitize the patient prior to challenge of individual lesions. A total of 28 patients were studied (41). Regression of lesions directly injected with BCG occurred in 18 (78%) and regression of lesions at distant sites in 7 (30%). In addition, 11 patients (64%) had regression of lesions directly injected with PPD and 4 (24%) had regression of lesions at distant sites after PPD treatment. Diseases studied included epithelial skin cancers (7 patients), mycosis fungoides (6 patients), carcinoma of the breast (7 patients), reticulum cell sarcoma (2 patients), lymphangiosarcoma (1 patient), Kaposi's sarcoma (2 patients), and malignant melanoma (3 patients). The number of tumors or extent of tumor within the skin did not appear to be related to the possibility for response. Indeed, one response to PPD was seen in a woman with a squamous cell carcinoma developing in an area of lupus vulgaris which was so large that it was initially considered unamenable to either surgery or radiotherapy (41).

Smith (32) has also seen responses in a small group of patients with dermal metastases of breast cancer. Rosenberg and Powell (42) treated subcutaneous metastases in a patient with widely metastatic carcinoma of the breast. There was regression of injected nodules but not of any uninjected nodules, and the patient's overall clinical status was not improved.

In addition to the above studies, a number of investigators have attempted to use BCG as a systemic adjuvant agent.

Bluming et al. (43) treated 12 patients who were clinically tumor free after surgical excision of cutaneous melanomas and regional nodes with either a high dose of Pasteur BCG by scarification or a low dose of Glaxo BCG intradermally. This was not a randomized study. However, the group that received the higher dose of BCG had the best response. Ikonopisov (44) studied 33 patients with melanoma. Of these, 23 had disseminated disease, and there was no obvious effect of immunotherapy. Ten patients presented with localized disease which had been surgically resected. Two of three who had surgery alone are dead and the third has generalized disease. Both of two patients who received irradiated tumor cells alone are alive with no evidence of disease (NED), and 5/5 who received BCG alone are alive, one with local recurrence and four with NED. It was concluded that immunotherapy is a useful adjunct to surgery in melanoma.

Gutterman et al. have demonstrated an adjuvant effect of BCG in malignant melanoma under several different conditions. In an early report (45) they found no relapses in five patients with surgically resected malignant melanoma with regional lymph node involvement who had been treated by scarification with 6×10^8 viable Tice strain BCG organisms, compared to six relapses in 11 patients treated with lower doses of Pasteur liquid BCG. In a later report (46) they again emphasize the importance of the dose of BCG. Patients with disease which had spread to regional lymph nodes were treated after surgical removal of all known disease and BCG was applied by scarification until relapse. The disease-free interval and the survival of 52 patients were compared with historical controls treated with surgery alone from their institution. Patients treated with 6×10^8 viable units (VU) had significant prolongation of both parameters. The trend for patients with disseminated disease treated with 6×10^8 VU was similar. Patients treated with 6×10^7 VU did not show benefit from BCG. These authors also emphasize the importance of the primary site of tumor in response to immunotherapy. Patients with trunk and extremity primaries showed significant responses to BCG, but those with head and neck primaries did not, suggesting to them the importance of putting BCG into tumor-involved lymphatics. Only patients under 60 years of age had a response to BCG.

This same group of workers (47) have also studied 89 patients with disseminated malignant melanoma with a combination of dimethyltriazenoimidazole carboxamide (DTIC) administered intravenously and BCG administered by scarification. The results were compared to those in a retrospective group of 111 patients treated with DTIC alone. The duration of remission and survival was significantly longer for patients with both nonvisceral and visceral metastases treated with chemoimmunotherapy than for those treated with chemotherapy alone ($p = 0.05$ and 0.001, respectively). A good prognosis was associated with immunocompetence before treatment or an increase in immunocompetence during treatment.

In another study (48), 47 patients in all stages of melanoma were treated with BCG administered orally as an adjunct to standard treatment regimens. Oral BCG alone resulted in marked regression of measurable disease in two patients with disseminated melanoma. This material was given as 120 mg. lyophilyzed BCG orally at 1–2 week intervals. Although this study is preliminary, the authors conclude that orally administered BCG may delay the development of local recurrence and distant spread. It had no effect on the progress of disease in patients with intracranial metastases or hepatic metastases from ocular malignant melanoma.

Grooms and Morton (49) have reviewed their causes for failure with adjuvant immunotherapy in malignant melanoma in 144 patients treated with BCG alone or combined with tumor cell vaccine following surgical extirpation of tumor. When these patients were compared with patients treated with surgery alone, there was obvious improvement in recurrence and survival rates in both Stage II and Stage III patients. However, the failures in the immunotherapy treatment group were most frequently due to brain metastases, particularly in Stage II disease, where 14 deaths (79%) involved central nervous system (CNS) metastases, which sometimes represented the only site of metastasis. They feel this reemphasizes the concept that the brain is an immunologically privileged site.

Another category of neoplasm that has been extensively studied includes various lymphoproliferative disorders. Sokal et al. (50) reported that during 1965–67, 50 tuberculin-negative malignant lymphoma patients (both Hodgkin's and non-Hodgkin's) with Stages IB and IIA disease who had received primary radiotherapy or chemotherapy were randomly assigned to serve as controls or to receive BCG. BCG was given as one to three or more doses intradermally until conversion of the tuberculin skin test occurred. Among the 22 control patients, 17 (77%) relapsed in a mean of 10.6 months. In the 28 immunized patients, 17 or

61% relapsed in a mean of 25.9 months. These differences are significant ($p = 0.01$) and suggest that BCG delayed the appearance of new lesions in these patients.

Thomas and his colleagues (51) have been using oral BCG or intralesional BCG as the sole maintenance therapy in patients with non-Hodgkin's lymphoma and are sufficiently encouraged by their findings to have initiated a randomized clinical trial. However, Magrath and Ziegler (52) have studied BCG administered by scarification for its capacity to increase remission duration in patients with Burkitt's lymphoma in a controlled randomized trial. Eleven of 21 patients in the BCG-treated group and 11/19 controls have relapsed. BCG treatment increased the rate of recovery from tumor-induced immunosuppression, but within the BCG-treated group the patients who relapsed had the most rapid improvement in immunocompetence (53). Upon reevaluating their staging methods, it appeared to these researchers that patients in the BCG group should have had a better prognosis than the controls; therefore they were concerned that BCG in these patients may actually have been deleterious.

The initial report of successful immunotherapy in acute lymphatic leukemia (ALL) was that of Mathe et al. (54). These patients had received up to 18 months of cytoreductive chemotherapy before being randomized to no further maintenance or immunotherapy with BCG and allogeneic leukemia cells alone or in combination. All ten patients with no maintenance had relapsed within 200 days while 7/20 on immunotherapy were still in remission at over 2,000 days. These studies have been extended, and Mathe now feels that prognosis for response to both chemotherapy and immunotherapy can be correlated with morphologic subcategories of leukemia (55).

Other investigators have been unable to demonstrate a therapeutic effect of BCG in ALL. In two large studies children with previously untreated ALL were given chemotherapy and then randomized to receive either BCG alone, no further therapy, or twice-weekly methotrexate maintenance. In one study the initial maintenance chemotherapy was four or eight months of methotrexate (56); in the other, five months of a multiple drug combination (57). In both studies methotrexate led to significant prolongation of remission compared with no further treatment or BCG alone, which were not significantly different from one another. In a third study in adults with lymphatic leukemia, BCG given between courses of combination chemotherapy did not lead to significant prolongation of remission duration (58).

We have studied the effect of BCG in remission maintenance in ALL first in patients with prior therapy (59) and more recently in previously untreated patients with ALL (60), who were randomized to receive chemotherapy alone or with BCG plus allogeneic cells given as four weekly doses of 4×10^7 cells plus one vial of live Pasteur Institute BCG administered at the same intradermal site. These doses were pulsed in every six months during maintenance chemotherapy. There was no significant difference in remission duration between the different treatment arms, and we interpret these data as showing that the BCG added nothing to the effect that could be achieved with drugs alone in ALL.

In acute myelogenous leukemia (AML), on the other hand, several studies suggest that an immunotherapeutic effect from BCG is a possibility. Powles et al. (61) gave BCG plus irradiated leukemia cells to patients on maintenance chemotherapy. The total number of cells injected was about 1×10^9 in 5–10 ml doses in three sites with Glaxo BCG equivalent to about 1×10^6 live organisms at a fourth site. Injections were given weekly for three weeks with chemotherapy every fourth week. These investigators found that 14/19 patients relapsed in the group receiving chemotherapy alone compared with 15/23 patients who received additional immunotherapy. The median remission length for the chemotherapy group was 188 days compared with 312 for the immunotherapy patients. This prolongation of remission duration is not statistically significant; however, the difference in survival of 303 days for the chemotherapy group compared to 545 days for the immunotherapy group is significant with a $p < 0.003$. The authors feel that perhaps this increase in survival is due to the ability of the immunotherapy-treated patients to achieve second remissions. It was the impression of Freeman et al. (62) that patients with AML who had received BCG during maintenance therapy had a high rate of reinduction of remission. Vogler and Chan (63) reported patients with AML who had been induced into remission with cytosine arabinoside and thioguanine. Consolidation chemotherapy was given; then patients were randomized to receive maintenance therapy with either methotrexate alone at 30 mg/m twice weekly by mouth or BCG followed by methotrexate. The BCG was administered as approximately 3×10^8 organisms by the multiple Tine technique weekly for four weeks. Remission duration was prolonged from 26 weeks for the 23 patients receiving methotrexate alone to 39.4 weeks for the 18 patients receiving BCG plus methotrexate. This difference was significant at the $p < 0.002$ level. In a third study (58) BCG given between pulses of combination chemotherapy prolonged remission duration significantly in AML as well. At the time of the report 10/14 AML patients maintained on chemotherapy and immunotherapy were in remission (median duration 72+ weeks) compared with 9/21 patients maintained with chemotherapy alone (median 60 weeks). This difference is significant at the $p = 0.04$ level. Thus it appears that BCG may have a definite immunotherapeutic effect in remission maintenance in AML.

A number of similar studies have been performed in patients with chronic myelogenous leukemia (CML). For example, 32 patients with CML were treated with intradermal inoculations of BCG plus human tissue culture cells (64). The cells were originally thought to be of myeloid origin but later shown to have lymphoid characteristics. All patients continued to receive appropriate chemotherapy. Seventeen patients with Ph-positive CML in control at the time of initial inoculation were considered good risk patients. Their survival was compared with 28 nonimmunized Ph-positive patients treated at Roswell Park from 1960–1969 and was significantly better ($p < 0.01$). For the 15 poor risk patients immunotherapy was deemed "beneficial" in five, including three who had unusually prolonged survival after development of blast crisis, but no controls were available for comparison. In another uncontrolled study (65) BCG was given to CML patients on maintenance with myeleran. Allogeneic cells were also administered. Patients who successfully made antibody were felt by the authors to have a more stable course than those who did not.

A number of studies involving various solid tumors have also been performed. One example involves patients with lung cancer. Several small studies based on the use of BCG or a tuberculin extract such as Freund's adjuvant given intradermally, often with tumor extract as well, have been recently reviewed (66). No complete regressions were obtained in any patients, although some authors felt radiographic lesions occasionally improved and survival was sometimes increased in the immunotherapy-treated patients. If the requirements for BCG immunotherapy in man are similar to those in animal models, then close physical contact between tumor cells and BCG would seem to be important. In an attempt to achieve this type of contact, administration of BCG by aerosol to lung cancer patients has been attempted (67,68). Local and systemic reactions were frequent but none were fatal, and the authors felt this might be a feasible procedure in man. Intrapleural BCG (7.2×10^6 viable units) given to patients with malignant pleural effusion (69) resulted in better control of pleural disease, and a controlled trial of BCG postoperatively in lung cancer patients is now underway. All patients were given INH one to two weeks after BCG in this latter study, and reactions were limited to fever and malaise.

Donaldson (70) treated 16 patients with advanced or recurrent squamous cell carcinoma of the head and neck with a combination of methotrexate, isoniazid, and BCG. A greater than 50% decrease in size of the lesion was achieved in 13 of these (81%), with a mean duration in excess of 265 days (range 6–708+). He felt that remission duration with this combination was superior to the results achieved with methotrexate alone reported by other investigators. Donaldson also felt that the isoniazid was a critical element in this regimen for an adjuvant effect, not just for its antituberculous effect. Attempts by another group of workers to achieve remission in patients with squamous cell carcinoma of the head and neck, who were not eligible for further treatment with radiation or surgery, were unsuccessful when methotrexate, BCG, and an autologous tumor vaccine were used. No beneficial responses were seen in 13 patients (71).

Several studies are currently underway assessing the effect of BCG in gastrointestinal cancer. Patients with Duke's stage C carcinoma of the colon—i.e., those whose tumor has extended to the mesenteric lymph nodes but not beyond—are being randomized after surgery to receive maintenance therapy with either BCG alone or BCG plus 5-fluorouracil (5 FU) (72). Twenty patients have been entered on study, and after ten months all are clinically free of disease. These results are as yet too early to evaluate.

Sonkin (73) treated patients with a variety of gynecologic malignancies with BCG. These patients were also receiving concurrent chemotherapy. No benefit was seen in those patients with endometrial, cervical, or ovarian carcinomas; however, some was suggested in patients with choriocarcinoma. Bagshawe (74) has failed to see an effect of BCG in this disease, however.

Guinan (75) saw no change in clinical status in ten patients with Stage IV adenocarcinoma of the prostate treated with Tice BCG given by the multipuncture technique intradermally. He also discusses (76) the few other individual case reports of prostatic carcinoma where responses may have been seen to immunotherapy.

Townsend and Eilber (77) describe patients with osteogenic sarcoma who received adjuvant immunotherapy with BCG and allogeneic tumor cell vaccines after complete surgical resection. Three of 17 patients who received adjuvant immunotherapy are alive at the time of the report without disease compared to 0/12 patients who did not. In 80% of immunotherapy patients disease recurred rapidly, within three months of operation. This led the authors to postulate that subclinical disease was present when immunotherapy was begun. They now feel adjuvant chemotherapy should also be given to these patients. At the same institution soft-tissue sarcoma patients were treated with BCG and tumor cell vaccines (78). Of those treated with immunotherapy, 16/27 (59%) are alive without disease. These results are significantly better than those obtained without immunotherapy, as only 6/32 (21%) are free of disease.

Toxicity of BCG Therapy.   Intratumor injection with BCG frequently has resulted in fever, chills, localized abscess formation, and sinuses that drain for up to three months. In 25 patients Sparks and his colleagues (78) saw a flulike syndrome in 16, fever of 40°C or higher in 12, and reversible hepatic dysfunction in 6. Three patients in this group who became jaundiced all had liver biopsies, and granulomatous hepatitis was seen. No BCG organisms were recovered on culture. One patient recovered spontaneously; the other two responded rapidly to INH administration. In another series Pinsky et al. (29) described systemic side effects in 29 patients, which included fever in 26, a flulike syndrome in 12, and hepatic dysfunction in 14. These signs subsided after 8–9 weeks or more rapidly if isoniazid therapy was given. BCG bacteremia was demonstrable only during the first half hour after BCG administration. Two other patients with a clinical picture of hepatitis and granulomata on liver biopsy have been described, one of whom responded rapidly to INH (79) and another who had BCG demonstrated on culture from the biopsy specimen (80). The combination of culture evidence and clinical response to INH seems to prove that, in some patients at least, the hepatic granulomata are due to disseminated infection with BCG. Indeed, one patient has been reported with widespread systemic tuberculosis at post mortem after treatment with intratumor inoculation of BCG for metastatic malignant melanoma (81).

In another series (82) 12 of 21 patients treated with BCG immunotherapy developed hepatic abnormalities and all were biopsied. Six of them showed hepatic granulomas on biopsy. The indication for biopsy in five of these was an abnormal scan, the other was biopsied because of progressive hepatomegaly. No patient showed significant clinical or biochemical evidence of deteriorating liver function. The development of hepatic granulomas was not related to the total amount of BCG administered, duration of therapy, or immunologic status of the patients. Acid-fast organisms were not present in the granulomata, and these authors felt this syndrome represented a hypersensitivity reaction to antigens present in the BCG vaccine. Thus it is not clear how much of the hepatic reaction represents direct infection and how much represents hypersensitivity.

It is also not clear how much of the flulike syndrome represents hypersensitivity. In general, those patients who have best responded to BCG administration have included those who have had the most vigorous febrile responses. Pretreatment with benadryl and aspirin prior to and for several days following intralesional injection can reduce this toxicity (78).

Severe hypersensitivity reactions have been seen after repeated injections. Anaphylactic shock was seen in one patient by Morton (83). One patient who recovered suffered shock, oliguria, and gangrene of the fingers (29). Two fatalities in elderly patients with shock, oliguria, and laboratory evidence of a consumption coagulopathy have been seen (84,85).

Direct intradermal injection of BCG results in shallow ulcers up to 2 cm. in diameter, which heal after 4–6 weeks (86). Two deaths from disseminated tuberculosis have been reported in a series of over 300 patients treated in this fashion, and in one there was culture evidence that the responsible organism was BCG (86). In this same series two individuals developed erythema nodosum, associated in one with pancytopenia and purpura. One patient also showed reactivation of a dormant tuberculous infection with *Mycobacterium terrae* after a severe febrile reaction to the tenth BCG inoculation.

Much less toxicity has been reported after intradermal administration of BCG by multiple puncture or scarification, although itching and ulceration are common. Superinfection of an ulcer with *Staph. aureus* has been reported in one patient (63). A generalized skin rash occurred in 15/23 patients in one series (78). Hepatic dysfunction had a low incidence occurring in 2/18 patients (63), 2/23 patients (78), and 0/16 (45) in three different series. Ten to 25% of patients have experienced low-grade fever and malaise. One patient is reported to have developed an immune thrombocytopenia (87). Some patients have developed hyperplasia of regional lymph nodes after intradermal injection by multiple puncture (61) as well as intralesional injection (27), which may require biopsy to differentiate hyperplasia from recurrent malignant disease. [With oral administration most patients develop gastrointestinal symptoms, such as nausea and diarrhea, which do not prohibit further therapy, and a few have fever (48,51).]

Systemic toxicity, then, particularly after intratumoral injection, can be serious and even fatal, with both infection and hypersensitivity contributing to produce symptoms in most patients. With intradermal injection toxicity is less, although certainly not negligible. Considering the heroic doses of BCG which have been employed and the immunosuppressed state of many of the recipients with disseminated cancer, it is remarkable that more toxicity has not been seen.

Effect of BCG Immunotherapy on the Immune Response in Man.   Studies in human patients receiving BCG have generally shown an increase in nonspecific immune responses to a variety of delayed hypersensitivity antigens following intradermal BCG administration (43,45,53,88). Although some authors have shown only an increase in response to PPD (59,60), in one study there was an increase in absolute lymphocyte count in the BCG-treated group compared with untreated controls, but there was no effect on the lymphocyte response to PHA (57). Repeated administration of BCG has now been reported to depress cellular immunity in animals (89), and this may be expected to be seen in man as well. In general, immunoglobulin levels have not been affected by BCG (38,59).

The evidence for a specific cellular immune response to tumor during BCG immunotherapy has been best studied in melanoma; it includes the lymphocytic and histiocytic character of the granulomatous response demonstrated with serial biopsies at the site of regressing lesions (30,90,91) and the halo of inflammation around noninjected regressing lesions, which on biopsy show a cellular response of a similar character (90). Similar cellular reactions have been seen in patients with spontaneous tumor regression (92).

In vitro responses to tumor antigen have also been seen. Lymphocytes which are cytotoxic to melanoma cells in culture have been demonstrated in patients prior to therapy (28,30,93). Two patients who had no cytotoxic reaction before therapy showed progressively cytotoxic lymphocytes after BCG with regression of injected and noninjected nodules. One patient whose reactivity had not changed showed clinical progression of tumor (94). An increase in in vitro blastogenic response to melanoma antigen was shown in 3/4 patients who responded to direct intratumor inoculation of BCG (91). In one study (93) incubation of lymphocytes cytotoxic to melanoma cell lines with melanoma antigen decreased their antimelanoma cytotoxic activity, suggesting specificity of the response. Thus in some patients a change in in vitro cellular reactivity to tumor accompanied a good therapeutic response.

Complement-dependent cytotoxic antibodies to melanoma-associated antigens have been reported, and an increase in titer with successful immunotherapy has been seen (90,95). BCG therapy also decreased the level of a circulating inhibitor, which abrogated the response of sensitized lymphocytes to melanoma in one patient (91). However, in another patient (96), who had lymphocytes highly cytotoxic to autogenous tumor cells, BCG injection into a tumor nodule was associated with accelerated clinical deterioration, and his serum after BCG injection was found to completely block the tumor-specific lymphocyte reactivity.

Specific immune responses in leukemia have not been demonstrated to change dramatically with BCG. Antibody-dependent lymphocyte cytotoxicity (LDA) was demonstrated in the serum of 10/11 patients (97). Of these sera six were from patients who had received immunotherapy and four from those who had not. During immunotherapy 9/16 patients studied developed or showed a significant rise in the LDA activity, four showed a decrease, while the remainder showed a constant level of activity. It is too early to correlate these changes with response to therapy, although in at least one patient there was a suggestive rise in antibody titers during immunotherapy with a fall prior to recrudescence of disease. Until the clinical significance of these laboratory assays is more clearly understood, it is difficult to know what might be considered the desired in vitro effect of immunotherapy.

Methanol Extraction Residue of BCG (MER).   The methanol extraction residue of phenol-killed acetone-washed BCG organisms has been found to be a potent modulator of some immune responses and has been shown to have a therapeutic effect in some model tumor systems (98). This material has several theoretical advantages over BCG as a potential immunotherapeutic agent in man. MER is a nonliving entity and cannot, therefore, induce a progressive infectious disease. It is a stable agent and need not be administered directly into a tumor focus in order to elicit heightened tumor resistance (99).

This material is now being used in several clinical trials. Three trials were designed merely to discover whether it could be given in man and what a tolerated dose might be. In the first (100), MER was administered in doses of 0.25 to 1 mg per meter squared on a weekly or monthly basis to 47 patients. Sterile abscesses occurred in 55% of patients given 0.2 mg/site and 16% at 0.1 mg/site, local pain in 19%, and fever in 22%. PPD conversions from negative to positive occurred in 3/16 patients. Before MER, 33 delayed hypersensitivity responses to a variety of antigens were positive compared to 45 post MER. These authors concluded that MER caused mild toxicity and appeared to have an immunostimulatory effect.

Moertel et al. (101) gave 1 mg of MER in 5 divided monthly doses to patients with advanced gastrointestinal carcinoma. This was well tolerated. Three objective responses were seen in the 35 patients studied. The only significant side effects were local skin reactions. There did appear to be a stimulatory effect on delayed hypersensitivity responses or in vitro responses to PHA.

In a third study (102) 27 patients with advanced cancer were treated with intradermal MER, given as 0.1 mg per site in ten injections for a total dose of 1.0 mg/patient either monthly or every other week. All patients had a local inflammatory reaction that progressed to necrosis and sometimes contained caseous material. In 3 of 27 patients regional lymph nodes became palpable and tender. Four patients had fever up to 39°C which lasted 24–72 hours after injection. One patient had a generalized eruption 10 days after the second course of MER, with a rash resembling the reaction in the MER injection sites. Improvement of skin reactivity occurred in 9/18 patients tested with recall antigens.

Two pilot therapeutic trials have been performed. In one ongoing study (103) patients with AML in remission are randomized to receive chemotherapy alone or in combination with MER. Twenty-six patients are entered to date and the remission duration and survival in the MER group is longer, though not statistically significantly so, than that in the chemotherapy alone group. Patients receiving MER in this study have been reported (104) to have a more vigorous antibody response to KLH and blastogenic response to PHA in vitro than those not receiving MER.

In another pilot study (105) six AML patients treated with chemotherapy alone relapsed in from 63–162 days. Five later patients treated with identical drugs plus MER have remissions ranging from 92+ to 193+ days. These promising early studies suggest that more controlled clinical trials with this material are indicated.

Corynebacterium Parvum. *Corynebacterium parvum* is a gram-positive anaerobic organism which has been shown to be a typical adjuvant in that it boosts the antibody response to a variety of antigens. It appears to stimulate the reticuloendothelial system in experimental animals, with the consequent emergence of large numbers of activated macrophages. Some responses, however, particularly those of T cells, have been depressed by this agent, and the stimulation of a population of suppressor cells has been postulated. This agent has antitumor activity in some animal systems. However, the timing of administration with respect to other chemotherapeutic agents is critical, and enhancement has sometimes been seen. The experimental work with this material has been recently reviewed (106).

Israel and his colleagues in France have performed several clinical trials with *C. parvum*. In their first report (107) they describe patients with a variety of metastatic cancers divided into two groups: control (71 patients) and experimental (70 patients). All patients received identical chemotherapy with a combination of cyclophosphamide 15 mg/kg, 5 fluorouracil 15 mg/kg, methotrexate 0.5 mg/kg, vinblastine 0.1 mg/kg, and rufocromomycine 0.003 mg/kg every 8 to 15 days. *C. parvum* was administered as a heat-killed, formalinized suspension with 2 mg/ml of bacterial material. Injections were given once or twice a week subcutaneously in the arm with 2–4 mg per injection. Patients experienced local pain. If this was severe, 2% Xylocaine was added to the bacterial suspension. Occasional fatigue and fever were seen. Mean survival for the treated group was 10.5 months compared to 6.1 months for the control patients. This difference was statistically significant. Patients in both the treated and the control group who were tuberculin-positive had significantly better responses than those who were not.

These same investigators (108) continued their study in patients with epidermoid bronchogenic carcinoma until they had a control group of 75 and a *C. parvum* treated group of 68 patients. Chemotherapy was given, as above, to all patients. *C. parvum* was given as 4 mg in 2 cc subcutaneously once a week mixed with 0.5 mg 1% lignocaine. The mean survival was 5.6 months for the control and 9.8 months for the treated group. The rate of tumor regression was the same in both groups of patients. The difference in survival was due to the duration of response and a better ratio of "no change" versus "progression" in the *C. parvum* treated group than in the controls. Similar increases in survival were seen for patients with oat cell bronchogenic carcinoma, advanced breast carcinoma, and advanced nonlymphomatous sarcomas. Again the patients tuberculin-positive in both the control and treated groups had better survivals.

Several Phase I studies with *C. parvum* have been recently reported. With subcutaneous administration, all patients had local soreness with an occasional febrile reaction (109). During intralesional injection of *C. parvum* (110) into dermal metastases to maximum tolerated doses (up to 18 mg.) there was a much higher incidence of toxicity, with 100% of patients showing chills and fever, 33% nausea, and 30% transient hepatic dysfunction. Three of 14 patients in this study showed regression of injected lesions.

Recently, interest has also arisen in the intravenous administration of *C. parvum*. During Phase I trials (109) this route of administration was found to produce considerably more systemic toxicity than subcutaneous administration, with 78% of patients experiencing chills and fever, 55% nausea and vomiting, and 24% headache and/or malaise. Dyspnea, wheezing, and hypertension with vasospasm were also observed. In three patients who received over 10 mg/m² a syndrome resembling thrombotic thrombocytopenic purpura was seen.

Similar results including blood pressure changes were reported in another study (111). Here reactions were noted to be more intense at initial doses above 1 mg/m², were maximal during the first three days, and decreased or disappeared in subsequent days. This increased tolerance with repeated doses appears to be a consistent finding. In another study (112) febrile reactions were seen in all patients given 4 mg of *C. parvum* intravenously, but tolerance developed after 6–8 days to a maximum tolerated intravenous dose of 10 mg. A recent therapeutic trial of intravenous *C. parvum* has also been reported (113). In 20 patients with disseminated carcinoma, daily infusions of *C. parvum* were given alone at doses of 4 mg/day 5 days per week for 4–16 weeks. All patients had fever and 20% had nausea, vomiting, and headache as well. In eight patients the lesions regressed to less than 50% of their original size. The authors feel that this shows that nonspecific immune stimulation after repeated intravenous infusions of an immunostimulant can by itself induce regression in disseminated disease. This does not agree with the current concept that immunotherapy can be effective only against minimal residual disease.

Doubtless many other clinical studies with this adjuvant will soon be reported. Experimental models would suggest that *C. granulosum* may also prove to be a useful antitumor agent (108).

Viruses and Related Compounds

In addition to bacterial cells and their products, there has been some interest in the use of viruses for nonspecific immunotherapy. Spontaneous regression in a patient with biopsy-proven Burkitt's lymphoma has been observed after measles infection (114). A few patients with myelogenous leukemia have shown a fall in peripheral blast counts after intentional infection with virus (115), and one patient even showed repeated regression after several infections (116). An occasional patient has also been reported who has shown regression of solid tumors after intentional systemic viral infection (117).

Vaccinia virus has been used as a therapeutic agent by direct intratumor inoculation in patients with disseminated malignant melanoma. Regression of established disease has been seen in a number of patients (118–121), although in one study (122) it was noted that no tumor regression was obtained in any patient who had been vaccinated within the preceding five years and all patients who had a satisfactory response had a severe systemic and local reaction to the virus. It has recently been suggested that inoculation of vaccinia virus into melanoma lesions 14 days prior to excisional surgery improves prognosis and survival (123). The authors believe that this is due to a cytopathic effect of the virus on melanoma cells as well as a possible stimulation of antitumor cell-mediated immunity. Similar regressions have been reported (124) in patients with a variety of solid tumors after local and systemic administration of infectious mumps virus.

Tumor tissue culture cells, modified by virus and reinfused in an attempt to produce concomitant reactions to both viral and tumor antigens, have produced regressions in animal tumor models. Clinical studies employing this theoretical approach are underway (125), and patients can be shown to have developed antiviral antibody during treatment.

Antiviral Agents

In laboratory animals, both endogenously induced and passively administered interferon have antiviral effects against a variety of infections including those caused by oncogenic viruses. In addition to possible prevention of recruitment of new cells into the transformed state, interferon might possess direct oncoloytic activity. Interferon may also potentiate cytotoxicity of sensitized lymphocytes and enhance the phagocytic activity of unsensitized macrophages so that it might in fact increase antitumor immunity as well. Interferon itself can be administered to man either intravenously, intramuscularly, or by topical application, e.g., to the nasal mucosa. Measurable levels of circulating interferon can be achieved, and toxicity is minimal. These studies are early, and clinical results are not yet interpretable (126).

Interferon inducers are also being studied for their antitumor effect in man. In one study (127) it was felt that Poly I:C had an antileukemic effect, although the simultaneous administration of other agents made interpretation of the data difficult. Poly A:U has also been found safe to administer to man (128). Further studies with these compounds are awaited with great interest.

Chemical Sensitizers

Klein (129) sensitized patients with skin cancer to dinitrochlorobenzene (DNCB). He then tested the patients in a quantitative fashion and applied DNCB to areas involved with carcinoma in the lowest concentration which would cause erythema in the normal skin. The tumor sites had more intense inflammatory responses than the intervening normal skin and often regressed. Klein reported regressions in over 95% of treated superficial basal cell carcinomas. Fifty patients with superficial basal cell carcinomas and squamous cell carcinomas in situ have been followed for up to 5 years without recurrence. Levis et al. (130), using similar techniques, treated 113 tumors in 5 DNCB-sensitized patients with multiple basal cell carcinomas with topical DNCB. Thirty-six out of 113 (23%) of the lesions showed complete clinical regression for periods of 5 to 18 months. An additional 29% showed partial regression. There was variation in response from patient to patient, and there was also variation in response of different tumors in the same patient. The authors felt that size might be a factor in the response, since none of the 9 nodular tumors greater than 5 mm in diameter showed complete regression. They also treated 26 lesions with the primary irritant, croton oil, and caused complete regression in 6 (23%) of treated tumors. Stjernsward and Levin (131) sensitized 21 patients to DNCB and noted regression of tumor nodules in 13 patients, including those with basal cell carcinoma, mycosis fungoides, lymphoma metastatic to the skin, and carcinoma of the breast metastatic to the skin.

It is unclear whether the mechanism of the DNCB effect in these situations involves tumor immunity or is a more nonspecific response to immunologically induced inflammation. It does appear, however, that topical application of DNCB is of value in the treatment of individuals with numerous small basal cell carcinomata. Other skin tumors may also respond to such therapy.

SPECIFIC ACTIVE IMMUNOTHERAPY

The modicum of success with nonspecific active immunotherapy, particularly that which involves direct injection into tumor nodules of infectious material, is encouraging, although the immune basis of these responses has yet to be firmly established. Experience with what might be termed true immunotherapy—i.e., that involving tumor-associated or tumor-specific antigens—has been much less positive. A summary of early trials (6) leads to the conclusion that specific active immunotherapy with tumor cells or extracts thereof is unlikely to be of benefit to patients with advanced disease.

Recent attempts at specific immunotherapy have involved immunization of patients with tumor cells that have altered in some manner, such as by passage in tissue culture. In these studies the tumor tissue cultured is either autologous or of similar type. The earliest trials to be reported involved sarcomas. Patients with a variety of soft tissue sarcomas were treated by Morton and his colleagues (90) with cell vaccines. Increases in cytotoxic antibody against tumor occurred in these patients, but no clinical effect on the disease itself was noted. Sinkovics et al. (132) described one patient with rhabdomyosarcoma who showed cellular and serum factors reactive to a rhabdomyosarcoma cell line in tissue culture. These changed markedly with the amount of tumor load; they increased with initial successful chemotherapy, fell again with relapse, and increased again with resection of metastasis. This patient is now being treated with a viral lysate of a rhabdomyosarcoma cell line.

Antisera raised in rabbits after injection of a Burkitt lymphoma tissue culture cell line (RAJI) have been found to cross-react with acute leukemia blast cells in a complement-dependent system in vitro (133). For this reason it seemed logical to

treat patients with acute leukemia with RAJI cells in an attempt to induce formation of such a cytotoxic antibody in the hopes that it might have therapeutic benefit
for the patient (134). Patients with late stage acute lymphatic leukemia were
randomized to receive 5-day combination chemotherapy (cyclophosphamide,
oncovin, arabinosyl cytosine, and prednisone, COAP), either alone or in combination with injections of RAJI cells interspersed between courses of chemotherapy
given as 1×10^8 cells on days 15, 17, and 19 of each treatment cycle. Remission
duration in both treatment groups was identical; however, complement-
dependent cytotoxic antibody was seen in 5/8 immunized patients and 0/8 controls. This antibody reacted with RAJI and both allogeneic and autologous acute
leukemia cells. It seems, then, in these studies with tissue culture cells alone, that
there is evidence for increased immune reactivity to tumor cells in terms of
increased titers of cytotoxic antibody or numbers of cytotoxic lymphocytes, but
the clinical course of the patients is as yet unaffected. The treatment of patients
with chronic myelogenous leukemia with cell vaccines and BCG has already been
described (64,65).

Other investigators, on the basis of animal models, have been attempting to
immunize patients with cells modified by neuraminidase treatment, which, it was
hoped, would remove sialic acid and expose antigen sites. Patients with acute
myelogenous leukemia (135) were given chemotherapy either alone or in combination with 10^{10} vibrio cholera neuraminidase-treated allogeneic myeloblasts
injected in approximately 50 separate sites in different node drainage areas. Of
ten patients who had received previous antileukemic therapy, six immunized
patients had more than twice the remission duration of controls. In previously
untreated patients the median remission duration on chemotherapy alone was 20
weeks for seven patients, while 5/7 patients receiving immunotherapy remained
in remission from 56–97 weeks.

PASSIVE IMMUNOTHERAPY

Of the various types of immunotherapy, passive immunotherapy with serum
seems the least likely to be successful (3). It is difficult to produce high-titer
antisera reactive only with tumor antigens and not normal antigens from the host.
Tumor enhancement occurs more often with serotherapy than with cellular
therapy in animal models. Finally, immunoglobulin molecules, being large, tend
to enter and leave the circulation slowly, Therefore, only very small tumor cell
deposits or those within the circulation, such as in leukemia, would be likely to be
affected.

Xenogeneic Sera

Trials with xenogeneic sera have been difficult to perform. In addition to the
difficulties noted above, such trials also require the administration of foreign
protein for a prolonged period with the resultant risk of allergic reactions.
Nevertheless, in an early trial Lindstrom (136) saw some clinical response upon
administration of sera prepared in rabbits after immunization with myeloid
leukemia cells. De Carvalho (137) prepared hyperimmune gamma globulin in

horses against antigens separated from normal antigens in tumor tissue by pre-cipitation of the latter by antibodies against normal tissues. Thirteen of 15 leukemia patients had remissions on immune gamma globulin lasting from 4 weeks to 29 months. Sekla and colleagues (138) were unable to produce remission in five patients with heterologous immune globulins prepared in a slightly differ-ent fashion. Tsirimbas et al. (139) treated five patients with chronic lymphatic leukemia with horse antilymphocyte serum. In 3/5 patients the peripheral counts fell to around 40% of their initial value.

As might be expected, serotherapy of solid tumors has been less rewarding than in the leukemias. De Carvalho (137) saw few objective evidences of response in solid tumor patients with globulins prepared as for the leukemias. Marsh et al. (140) administered a rabbit antitumor serum to patients with a variety of solid tumors. They saw no clinical effect, although at autopsy, in some patients, anti-body was selectively localized in areas of sarcomatous cells. In a recent trial (141) using serum prepared from melanoma-immunized chimpanzees, Parks et al. noted acute necrosis of visceral disease in two of three patients, although the regressions were incomplete and were complicated by fatal thrombocytopenia in one patient.

Allogeneic Sera

Allogeneic sera have been studied for their therapeutic effect in leukemia as well. Several investigators have attempted to treat leukemias and lymphomas with serums containing antibodies against human lymphocytes. In a study by Laszlo et al. (142) antilymphocyte plasma was prepared by immunizing normal subjects against normal lymphocytes. IgG globulin was then separated from this plasma and administered to three patients with chronic lymphocytic leukemia. In each patient there was a transient lymphopenia and decrease in lymph node size after infusion. Djerassi (143) treated four patients with acute lymphocytic leukemia with serum with a high titer against leukocytes from a patient with thalassemia major who had been sensitized against both granulocytes and lymphocytes of many individuals. In all four patients there was a fall in peripheral white count. Herberman et al. (144) administered serum with cytotoxic antibodies from a multigravid female to seven patients with lymphoproliferative disorders. His patients responded with falls in lymphocyte and platelet counts averaging 48.8% and 25.5% of pretreatment values. Effects lasted one day. Two of five patients had shrinkage of peripheral lymphatic tissue. Four patients had minor side effects such as fever and chills and two had respiratory distress.

Allogeneic sera in which the donors have been purposely immunized against tumor cells have also been studied. Brittingham and Chaplin (145) immunized a normal donor with leukocytes from a patient with chronic myelocytic leukemia. The normal subject was then reimmunized three years later with whole blood from a second patient with chronic myelocytic leukemia. An antileukocyte anti-body active against donor cells appeared in the normal subject. Gamma globulin was obtained from this donor's plasma and administered to the leukemic patients whose cells had been used for reimmunization. There was no apparent beneficial effect on the patient's illness. Skurkovich and co-workers (146) immunized pa-tients with leukemia with leukemia cells from other patients. Eight to fifteen days after immunization, plasma was exchanged 2–3 times between donor pairs of patients. Six pairs of children were treated, and three complete and five partial hematologic remissions were observed. Seven of these responding patients had received steroid and cytotostatic therapy as well, but one complete remission was achieved with immunotherapy alone.

Remission plasma has also been given in attempt at passive therapy. Skurkovich and co-workers (147) collected autologous plasma and leukocytes early in remission and administered these to patients in later states of remission. They felt that remission duration was prolonged by this maneuver. Ngu (148), using late remission sera from patients with Burkitt's lymphoma, felt that he produced regressions in patients with active disease, but these results were not confirmed by Fass et al. (149) in studies in five patients. Serum from patients with spontaneous regressions of malignant melanoma has occasionally induced regression when administered to other patients (150).

Conjugated Antibody

Since the direct effect of antibody has been disappointing in the treatment of tumors, investigators are now trying to take advantage of the specificity of antibody to deliver other cytotoxic materials directly to the tumor cells. In animal models, antitumor drugs have been bound to a variety of substances including alkylating agents such as chlorambucil (151) and antitumor antibiotics such as daunomycin (152). Antibodies have also been tagged with radioactive isotopes such as I^{131}, but early clinical trial with this material in patients with melanoblastoma were disappointing (153). They have also been conjugated to toxins such as diphtheria (154) and enzymes with cytotoxic potential (155).

Another possible synergistic effect between antibody and chemotherapy has been described by Segerling et al. (156), who showed that guinea pig hepatoma cells normally resistant to killing by antibody and complement are rendered sensitive after treatment with chemotherapeutic agents. Thus it appears that the most useful application of serotherapy may be in the creative use of this modality in conjunction with more conventional types of therapy.

ADOPTIVE IMMUNOTHERAPY

Adoptive immunotherapy with whole cells carries with it the significant risk of graft-versus-host disease if the recipient is immunoincompetent. This fact makes clinical trials difficult to perform and to evaluate. In addition, if the recipient is immunocompetent, it is likely that there will be rapid rejection of donor material after several allogeneic transfusions or immunizations. Thus, if the antitumor effect requires viable whole cells, it would be best to give the potential effective dose over a short period of time.

If one desires to do specific immunotherapy, there is the added difficulty of selecting an individual whom it is appropriate to immunize with tumor material. In general this has been felt to be another patient with a tumor. These individuals are, of course, likely to have some degree of immunoincompetence themselves, which means that they may not have an adequate response, even to the transplanted tumor. In addition, it is of interest to consider a study by Nadler and Moore (157) in which a series of patients with disseminated malignancy had autotransplantation of tumor performed surgically. "Takes" occurred in only 11 of 72, implying that metastatic disease either is successful in establishing itself only part of the time, or that metastases are subject to different growth controls than is transplanted autologous tumor. Since most donors for specific immunotherapy are sensitized by transplantation or by immunization, there may be some practical reasons to consider these potential differences in antigen presentation.

Therapy with Nonactivated Cells

Patients have been treated in a nonspecific fashion with allogeneic whole cells from spleen (158) or from spleen and later xenogeneic (pig) lymph node cells from an animal sensitized to tumor (159). In both situations temporary regressions and relief of pain were seen in some patients. Three patients with ovarian cancer (158) with ascites had complete regression of ascites after spleen cell infusion.

Bone marrow has been used in an attempt to produce a graft-versus-tumor response that would be more vigorous than the graft-versus-host response. A number of patients with acute leukemia have been treated in this fashion after ablative chemotherapy or whole-body radiotherapy to eradicate the patient's own normal and malignant bone marrow cells. Some long-term remissions have been seen, and this mode of therapy, which has been recently reviewed (160), is still under active investigation.

Therapy with Cells Activated in vitro

Frenster and co-workers (161) have infused autologous lymphocytes which were cultured for 1–2 days with PHA. They obtained a regression of pulmonary metastases in 8/10 patients after this procedure, but no regressions were observed at extrapulmonary sites. Cheema and Hersh (162) injected PHA-activated lymphocytes around local metastatic lesions and saw regressions in injected lesions, although no systemic benefit was seen.

Therapy with Tissue Culture Cells

Moore and co-workers (163) established a lymphoid line from a patient with malignant melanoma and transfused large quantities of cultured cells back into the patient. During the first course of therapy 344 grams of cells were given, and some metastatic nodules shrank measurably in size. The remainder were surgically excised after the 45th day. The cultured cells were labeled and after infusion were found to be rapidly sequestered in the lung with only small numbers localized around the neoplastic nodules. One week later, lymphocytotherapy was continued with another 180 g of cultivated lymphocytes. Three months later recurrent nodules were found. Another 250 g of cells were given with no effect on the tumor growth. The infusions were complicated by daily chills and fever. At post mortem (164) the recurrent lesions of this patient's tumor were characterized by an unusual stromal reaction involving lymphoblasts and plasma cells, which the authors felt might represent a cellular immune response to tumor.

Therapy with Specific Cells

Therapy with Cells Sensitized in vivo.   Nadler and Moore (165) took 118 paired patients and transplanted tumors from patients in Group A subcutaneously into patients in Group B. All except two patients in Group B rejected the tumor transplants, so it was assumed they were sensitized. Lymphocytes were transferred from Group B to Group A patients and 23/118 had a positive response, including three with complete remissions of which two lasted over two years, one in a patient with disseminated malignant melanoma, and one in a patient with pulmonary metastases from osteogenic sarcoma.

Marsh and his co-workers (140) studied 19 patients with osteosarcoma. Seven patients served as implant donors, five as both donors and recipients, and seven as recipients only. Tumor tissue from each donor, obtained at amputation, was implanted in a recipient, and then after 14 days sensitized lymphocytes from the respective recipients were given to the donors. The tumor implants were rejected without apparent harm to the recipients. There was no apparent benefit in any patient who had obvious pulmonary metastatic disease at the onset of therapy; however, the authors felt the course of a few of the other patients might have stabilized after infusion of lymphocytes and feel that this type of investigation is worth pursuing.

Humphrey et al. (166) studied 135 patients, of whom 54 were available for objective evaluation. Patients were paired by diagnosis, and these patients were given an extract of tumor cells as a vaccine for 4–8 weeks. After this period most patients received from 5–8 exchanges of plasma and leukocytes. Thirteen patients of the 54 had some evidence of response with decrease in size of measurable tumor masses. Of these, two had a response before transfusion was begun and two more had a response early in the course of the exchanges, suggesting a response to vaccine alone. There is no discussion of toxicity in this report.

Krementz et al. (167) have employed similar procedures, using either tumor extracts or tumor cells in tissue culture to sensitize the donors. Five complete and five partial remissions were seen in 58 treated patients.

Therapy with Cells Sensitized in vitro.   In a number of animal models, exposure of subject's lymphocytes to his own or similar tumor cells growing in vitro results in increased cytotoxic activity of the lymphocytes against cultured tumor cells (2). This type of in vitro immunization would circumvent the theoretical difficulties involved in in vivo immunization.

Three patients (168) with widespread metastatic malignant melanoma were treated by having their white blood cells sensitized to their tumor during culture in vitro for a period of ten days. These white cells were then injected intravenously into the original patient, either daily or every other day. The dose depended upon the numbers of cells available, but it was attempted to inoculate a minimum of one billion cells each time. The only toxicity was chills and a brief period of fever between 38.3 and 38.9°C. No objective responses were observed in any of these three patients. This approach apparently is also underway in other laboratories (2).

IMMUNOTHERAPY WITH SUBCELLULAR MATERIALS

The difficulties of graft-versus-host disease and donor rejection of whole cells could both be obviated if the active principle could be extracted from cells and administered in a subcellular form. The immunocompetence of the immunized host is, of course, still a matter of concern. The material of this sort which has undergone the widest clinical trial is transfer factor.

Transfer Factor

This material was first described by H. S. Lawrence in 1954 (169), when he reported the transfer of tuberculin skin test reactivity from a tuberculin-positive donor to a tuberculin-negative recipient using a cell-free leukocyte lysate extract. Since then transfer factor (TF) activity has continued to be defined by the ability of this purified material to transfer delayed hypersensitivity responses when prepared from skin-test-positive donors and given to skin-test-negative recipients. The ability to mount an accelerated allograft rejection can also be transferred (170). Subsequent studies have shown that this activity resides in lymphocytes, not granulocytes (171,172). TF is dialyzable, of low molecular weight (less than 10,000 daltons), and resistant to DNase, RNase, and trypsin (173) as well as to endogenous lysosomal hydrolases (174). Further purification of dialyzable transfer factor (TFd) with chromatographic techniques has separated a material (TFc) with increased biologic activity (175). Further studies by Crawford et al. (176), although preliminary, suggest that TFc is an adenine-containing single-stranded ribonucleotide associated with at least one amino acid.

Characterization of TF has been hampered by the lack of an animal model or standard in vitro system. Biological activities have suggested to some that TF is a replicating informational or derepressor molecule. The action of TF does not appear to involve passive transfer, because the effects last longer in most normal recipients than would be expected from such transfer alone (174).

The clinical trials with TF reported in the recent literature are described in Table 3. There are significant variables in each of these trials. The methods of preparation of TF have varied to some degree from one institution to another. This subject is reviewed by Neidhart and LoBuglio (177). In the majority of studies the individual doses of TF were prepared from preparations containing 1 × 10^8 to 1 × 10^9 or more lymphocytes.

Another variable in these studies is the rationale used for donor selection. Some investigators have used a protocol similar to that used for whole cell preparations described above, namely the immunization of the donor (usually another patient) with tumor cells or cell extracts prior to the harvesting of TF. Brandes (178) and Krementz (179) used paired patients with similar tumors. Krementz (179) administered a tumor vaccine as well as TF and saw regression of soft tissue but not bone metastases in 1/5 patients. In the Brandes study (178) both injected and uninjected nodules regressed in one patient. Smith (32) and Thompson (180) also

Table 3   Clinical Trials with Transfer Factor

Malignancy	Response[a]	Concurrent Therapy	Reference	No.
Malignant melanoma	5/10	BCG	Smith (1973)	(32)
	1/2		Brandes (1971)	(178)
	1/9	Unknown	Spitler (1973)	(181)
	1/5	Cell vaccine	Krementz (1974)	(179)
	0/6		Bukowski (1975)	(182)
	2/7		Silva (1975)	(185)
	3/11		Vetto (1975)	(186)
Breast carcinoma	1/5		Oettgen (1971)	(187,188)
	1/6	BCG	Smith (1973)	(32)
	1/1		Silva (1975)	(185)
Renal cell carcinoma	0/1	BCG	Smith (1973)	(32)
	2/3	Unknown	Fudenberg (1974)	(195)
Nasopharyngeal carcinoma	1/2		Goldenberg (1972)	(189)
Adenocarcinoma of colon	1/1		Vetta (1975)	(186)
Vaginal carcinoma	1/1		Silva (1975)	(185)
Ovarian carcinoma	0/1		Silva (1975)	(185)
Lung carcinoma	0/1		Silva (1975)	(185)
Alveolar soft part sarcoma	1/1		Neidhart (1972)	(184)
Fibrosarcoma	1/1		Neidhart (1974)	(177)
Rhabdomyosarcoma	1/2	Radiation	Vetto (1975)	(186)
Osteogenic sarcoma	0/1	Cell vaccine	Krementz (1974)	(179)
	1/1		Neidhart (1974)	(177)
	9/13	BCG	Levin (1975)	(183)
Hodgkin's disease	1/1	BCG	McIlvanie (1973)	(190)
Acute lymphatic leukemia	0/5	Drugs	Neidhart (1974)	(177)
Thymoma	0/1		Silva (1975)	(185)
Miscellaneous tumors	12/40		Thompson (1971)	(180)
	1/6	BCG	Smith (1974)	(32)
	5/20		Vetto (1975)	(186)

[a] Criteria for response vary with different investigators. In some instances lack of progression and in other instances failure of recurrence on postoperative adjuvant therapy are considered a "response."

used paired patients but with dissimilar tumors. Smith, who gave BCG concurrently with TF, saw responses ranging from cessation of growth to complete regression of melanoma nodules lasting more than two years in one patient. Thompson (180) treated 40 patients with a variety of tumors. TF was injected subcutaneously around visible tumor or on the extremities. Seven of 19 patients with extensive metastatic disease had greater than 50% regression in measurable tumor with clinical responses lasting up to 17 months.

Other investigators have attempted to select normal donors who have shown in vitro evidence of response to tumor cells. Spitler et al. (181) found family members of patients had immunity to tumor antigens, demonstrated either by increased DNA synthesis or by MIF production by lymphocytes in response to in vitro exposure to soluble melanoma antigen. Nine patients with widely disseminated disease were treated with TF from such donors. Eight had no clinical response and no conversion of in vitro assays; one patient had clinical regression of disease and conversion of lymphocyte transformation in vitro to melanoma antigens.

Bukowski et al. (182) treated 6 patients with stages III and IV malignant melanoma with TF from donors whose lymphocytes were highly cytotoxic to cultured melanoma cells. Skin test reactivity to recall antigens was transferred in 3/6 patients, but there were no clinical responses.

Levin et al. (183), using TF from donors who were household contacts and who had positive in vitro assay for tumor-specific cell-mediated cytotoxicity, treated 13 patients with osteogenic sarcoma. In five patients TF was begun after surgery while patients had no evidence of disease. All are alive and tumor-free for 7+ to 24+ months. Of five patients with metastatic disease at the time TF was begun, the investigators felt that there was significant stabilization of disease in four. Cell-mediated cytotoxicity to their tumor increased in all patients with osteogenic sarcoma after therapy with tumor-specific TF, with no increase in cell-mediated cytotoxicity against control tumor lines. Therapy with non-tumor-specific TF caused a decrease in cell-mediated cytotoxicity in all patients to whom it was given. Reinstitution of tumor-specific transfer factor (TS-TF) in each case was accompanied by an increase in cell-mediated cytotoxicity, suggesting that the use of non-tumor-specific TF may be undesirable.

Neidhart et al. (177) treated one patient by systemic and intralesional injection with fibrosarcoma and skin nodules with TFd from a family member who had positive in vitro activity against tumor cells. The disease remained stable for six months; then the patient deteriorated and died. Neidhart et al. (177,184) also treated a patient with a soft part sarcoma with TF prepared from lymphocytes from an identical twin which produced MIF in response to purified tumor antigen. The patient's MIF response to tumor antigen became transiently positive after the second dose and his disease remained stable for 12 months, after which there was rapid deterioration and death.

Neidhart et al. (177) treated five patients with ALL using TF from family donors who had positive in vitro MIF assays to leukemia cells. There was some evidence of effect on skin test reactivity to nontumor antigens but no effect on the clinical course of the disease. Other workers have used various donors on the assumption that antitumor activity might exist, although there was no direct demonstration of this. Silva et al. (185) treated seven patients with melanoma with TF from family members, normal black donors, or donors with halo or multiple nevi. He saw stabilization of disease in two patients and no response in five. Vetto et al. (186) treated 35 patients with advanced recurrent cancer with TF from cohabitants of patients in doses equivalent to 10^9 lymphocytes at two-week intervals. There were 11/35 responses, including three complete regressions, lasting from 1 to 13 months. While TF donor lymphocytes were not tested for in vitro activity against the recipient tumors, clinical responsiveness correlated with the patients' conversion to dermal reactivity to specific tumor antigens, and loss of reactivity heralded relapse.

Oettgen et al. (187,188), working on the hypothesis that breast cancer might well be caused by a ubiquitous agent that would have clinical expression only in individuals whose reaction to this agent was deficient in some sense, used pooled TFd from healthy women over 40 to treat breast carcinoma. They successfully transferred delayed hypersensitivity to tuberculin and/or streptococcal antigens in 3/5. One patient who received a total dose of TF equivalent to 205×10^9 lymphocytes had partial tumor regression after direct tumor inoculation which lasted six months.

Goldenberg et al. (189) treated patients with nasopharyngeal carcinoma with TFd from pooled donors who had had mononucleosis, thinking that perhaps EBV was an etiologic agent in both. Of the two patients treated, one had a definite but temporary tumor regression and one an apparent slowing of tumor growth along with intense lymphocytic infiltration of the tumor.

Another potentially attractive source of TF would be that prepared from patients in remission. Neidhart et al. (178) treated one patient with osteogenic sarcoma with TF from the patient's father who was a ten-year "cure" of rhabdomyosarcoma and showed positive MIF response to the patient's tumor. The patient initially had pulmonary metastases which resolved after four months' treatment with chemotherapy. The patient remained disease-free 17+ months and had changes in general cellular immune responses consistent with a TF effect.

Silva (185) saw local inflammation following administration of TF obtained from patients with similar neoplasms in remission and disease stabilization for four months in one breast carcinoma patient and regression for six months in one vaginal carcinoma patient.

The final rationale we will discuss for donor selection is that TF might act to stimulate the immune system in some nonspecific fashion which would be beneficial to the patient. McIlvanie (190) treated one patient with Hodgkin's disease with BCG and TF from tuberculin-positive and negative donors in an attempt to get a therapeutic response to the BCG. Temporary regression of disease was reported. Smith et al. (191) have reported that it is impossible to transfer delayed hypersensitivity to patients with Hodgkin's disease unless the TF donors are themselves Hodgkin's disease patients. Positive transfer of delayed hypersensitivity to Stage IV Hodgkin's disease patients in remission was confirmed by Ng et al. (192). This may imply that TF used in Hodgkin's disease studies must be collected from Hodgkin's disease patients.

An interesting potential use of TF as an immune regulator is being investigated by Silverman and co-workers (193), who are administering TF from normal donors to patients with Waldenstrom's macroglobulinemia and multiple myeloma. They have postulated that many of the manifestations of these diseases may reflect faulty T-B cell interactions which might be normalized with TF. One patient with macroglobulinemia and two with multiple myeloma have each received TF from a total of 12×10^8 lymphocytes intramuscularly over a two-month period in combination with standard chemotherapeutic regimens. In the macroglobulinemia patient there was an initial decrease in IgM levels by greater than 40%. In the two patients with IgG myeloma there was an increase in in vitro response of lymphocytes to PHA and a decrease in response to pokeweed mitogen. It is too early to evaluate any long-term clinical response in these patients.

Hayes et al. (194) demonstrated that TF could transfer skin test reactivity in children with leukemia receiving immunosuppressive chemotherapy. TF induced positive skin test reactivity in 7/7 and increased T lymphocytes in 5/7 patients treated with MTX and 6 MP only, but induced reactivity in only 2/8 and in fact decreased T lymphocytes in 6/8 treated with MTX, 6 MP, CTX, and Ara-C. Thus, the response to TF was influenced by the drug combination used.

Transfer Factor Toxicity.   Local reactions to TF injection are common, with immediate pain and erythema at the site of injection. Pain at the site of the tumor is also reported, which at times may be so severe that the patient elects to discontinue treatment (195). However, major systemic complications are rare. TFd is nonimmunogenic and there have been no allergic reactions reported, nor any reports of acceleration of tumor growth in patients treated with TF.

One child (196) with severe combined immunodeficiency disease developed a malignant B cell lymphoproliferative disorder and polyclonal gammopathy three weeks after receiving one injection of TF in a dose of 1×10^9 lymphocytes. Another patient (197) with Wiskott-Aldrich syndrome developed hemolytic anemia. Although these were temporally related to TF administration, the markedly increased incidence of malignancy and autoimmune hemolytic anemia in primary immunodeficiency diseases is well known, and the occurrence may be coincidental.

Inflammatory response at the site of tumor, with edema, may be confused with disease progression. Fudenberg et al. (195) reported a patient with multiple lung metastases. Three weeks after TF therapy the lung lesions appeared increased and he developed pleural effusions. The effusions turned out to be sterile and free of tumor cells, but did contain many lymphocytes, monocytes, and few polys. Levin et al. (184) reported a group of five patients with osteogenic sarcoma with inoperable primary or metastatic lesions who, when treated with TF, experienced pain and inflammation in the area of the tumor with transient febrile episodes 18–36 hours after TF was injected subcutaneously in the deltoid region. From three of these patients tumor was obtained by biopsy or surgical resection, and it was found that after TF there was significant new infiltration with lymphocytes.

Hackett et al. (198) did electron microscopy of osteogenic sarcoma tissue from patients treated and not treated with TF. In patients where TF had been given, lymphocytic infiltration was present in the tumor. In patients who had not received TF, no lymphocytes were present in comparable areas, nor were lymphocytes seen in areas of tumor from the same patient which had been removed prior to TF therapy. Many areas of tumor examined after TF administration had disoriented collagen matrix, indicating it was laid down by tumor cells, but no tumor cells and few lymphocytes were seen in these areas.

Another factor which must be considered in these studies is the effect of leukophoresis for large numbers of lymphocytes on the TF donor. Fudenberg et al. (195) reported eight TF donors with strong tumor-specific cell-mediated cytotoxicity who, after repeatedly being used as donors (one at least twice weekly for 9 months), completely lost all cytotoxicity to osteogenic sarcoma antigens. After 3 to 4 months without use as donors, the tumor-specific cytotoxicity was restored to previous levels in all cases.

Waldman et al. (199) evaluated the effects of leukophoresis of 10^{10} lymphocytes on six melanoma patients receiving BCG and on six normal volunteers. Measuring MIF release, blastogenic response to mitogens, MLC responsiveness, and percent T and B lymphocytes, he found that there was, in the normal group, a

42% decrease in peripheral lymphocytes which returned to normal within three days, and in the melanoma group a 34% increase in peripheral lymphocytes which had not completely returned to normal at seven days. Both groups showed no change in skin reactivity to DNCB or recall antigens and significant but transient decreases in MIF production and blastogenic response which returned to normal within 24 hours. All other immunologic parameters were either increased or unchanged. Thus it appears that transient decreases in immune reactivity may occur in the donor.

"Immune" RNA

"Immune" RNA is a large molecular weight substance ($1-3 \times 10^5$ daltons) which can transfer both cellular and humoral immunity (200). It is sensitive to RNase but not to DNase or pronase, is derived from macrophages and lymphocytes, and is capable of interspecies transfer. This material, if active, would have the advantage that the donor could be an animal of another species immunized with tumor rather than a normal human or patient donor.

Two types of "immune" RNA are currently under investigation. One is an RNA-antigen complex described by Fishman (201), which may behave as a "superantigen" and which is partially pronase-sensitive. The other, composed of RNA alone, free of detectable antigen moieties, may in fact be a true informative type of RNA. Transfer of antitumor activity has been attempted with this latter type of "immune" RNA (202).

Alexander (203) reported the first successful transfer of antitumor immunity by "immune" RNA in rat sarcoma using xenogeneic RNA extracted from lymphoid cells of sheep which had been immunized with the specific rat tumor. Ramming and Pilch (204,205) demonstrated mediation of immune responses against chemically induced murine sarcomas by xenogeneic "immune" RNA. Induction of immune responses in human lymphoid cells by xenogeneic immune RNA derived from specifically sensitized animal lymphoid cells was first demonstrated by Paque and Dray (206). Han (207) was able to transfer skin test reactivity to recall antigens to 9/10 patients with Hodgkin's disease using "immune" RNA obtained from one normal and one Hodgkin's disease donor sensitive to these antigens. The "immune" RNA was effective when injected near the skin test site or on the opposite forearm, suggesting that systemic transfer occurred.

Mediation of immune responses to human tumors with "immune" RNA was first reported by Pilch et al. (202). Nonimmune human lymphocytes from normal donors were converted to effector cells specifically cytotoxic to human tumor cells in vitro by incubation with xenogeneic immune RNA extracted from lymphoid organs of animals that had previously been immunized to human tumors. Specific cytotoxicity was induced to four human melanomas, a human gastric adenocarcinoma, and a human adenocarcinoma of the breast.

"Immune" RNA (I-RNA) is under investigation for therapeutic efficacy in man. Pilch et al. (208) treated 20 patients with xenogeneic "immune" RNA extracted from lymphoid organs of sheep immunized with autologous or allogeneic tumor tissue, using an intradermal dose of 1–4 mg weekly. The patients included 9 with renal carcinoma, 7 with melanoma, 1 with gastric carcinoma, 1 with breast carcinoma, 1 with sarcoma, and 1 with bladder carcinoma. Of the 9 patients with renal carcinoma, one, whose large recurrent tumor was excised with positive margins, remained free of disease after 12+ months, four patients with large primary tumors and multiple metastases showed decrease in growth curves of rapidly progressing metastases, and two patients exhibited slow regression of metastases. One patient with alveolar sarcoma with pulmonary metastases had a decrease in the size of nodules. The one patient with gastric carcinoma (202), who underwent surgical resection with no gross disease remaining but with 15/17 positive nodes, was begun on I-RNA therapy postoperatively and remained asymptomatic and free of detectable disease many months later. Only 1/20 treated patients developed new lesions or continued growth of old lesions. Eleven of 13 patients receiving I-RNA from sheep immunized with KLH as well as tumor tissue developed skin test reactivity to KLH after 6–8 weeks of therapy. No local or systemic toxicity was noted in any of the patients (208).

Thymosin

Thymosin is a small molecular weight polypeptide, derived from the thymus of animals, which can improve general cellular immune reactivity in animals (209).

Costanzi and co-workers (210) administered thymosin intramuscularly to five patients with disseminated neoplasms at doses of 50–250 mg/m daily for seven days. Four of five patients demonstrated an increase in delayed hypersensitivity responses and increased E rosette forming cells. There was no evidence of cardiopulmonary, hepatic, renal, or hematopoietic toxicity. One patient developed a transient urticarial rash on the seventh day, which resolved spontaneously. Schafer and co-workers (211) administered thymosin to seven immunodeficient patients with advanced malignancy in intramuscular or subcutaneous doses of 1, 10 or 30 mg/m daily for seven days. Immunologic reactivity as measured by skin test reactivity, "active" and "total" E rosette formation, and in vitro lymphocyte blastogenesis, increased in 5/7 patients and was stable in the other two. During therapy one patient exhibited disease progression while 6/7 remained stable. Although one patient developed local erythema, no other side effects were noted. It would seem, thus far, that thymosin may be safely administered to patients.

SUMMARY AND CONCLUSIONS

Tumor immunologists are aware of the many problems that may arise in trying to apply animal models to human tumor immunology (212). One that is of prime importance involves enhancement or increase of tumor growth with immune reactivity to tumor. The critical factor in enhancement appears to be the relative ratio of immune material to tumor. Small quantities of immunoreactive substances may enhance tumor growth while large quantities may be toxic or inhibitory. This enhancing effect can be seen with antibody as reviewed by the Hellströms (213), or can be produced by a small number of immune lymphocytes as described by Prehn (214), or macrophages as noted by Fidler (215,216). There are no totally convincing data that enhancement has occurred in man, although a few individual cases where this has been suspected (93) have been reported. However, it remains a potential complication of immunotherapy, and protocols should be designed to detect it if it occurs.

Regardless of the theoretical limitations of immunotherapy, one should look at the practical results achieved in man and see whether any trends that would indicate directions for immunotherapy in the future can be detected. First, active nonspecific immunotherapy appears to be effective, particularly in situations where the primary or metastatic tumor lesions involve the skin and are therefore accessible for direct intralesional injection. Nonimmune mechanisms associated with infection or inflammation might, of course, be responsible for tumor lysis under these circumstances, as was shown by the response of melanoma to croton oil in the study by Levis et al. (130). Responses might also be due to the hyperthemia elicited during this type of therapy (217), since hyperthemia alone has been shown to have antitumor activity. Nevertheless, tumor nodules may be made to disappear from the skin by these techniques, and this lead should be followed.

On the other hand, when we try to produce a "specific" effect, it becomes obvious that the desired immune response, i.e., that which might be therapeutically effective, is often elusive. In fact, although there appears to be a good correlation between the ability to mount nonspecific cellular immune reactions and prognosis (218), the correlation between specific reactivity to tumor antigens and prognosis is less clear (219,220). Recent trials using tumor tissue culture cells as immunogens have tended to show that the patients' immune reactivity against tumor target cells in vitro may be increased during immunotherapy, but there has been to date no striking clinical benefit for the patients. Adoptive immunotherapy, using transfer factor or perhaps some similar material, may avoid some of the dangers of infusing whole, immunogenic and/or immunocompetent cells into patients and may be of some benefit, particularly in patients with sarcomas, as was seen in Table 3. It is also interesting that no form of immunotherapy appears as yet to have been consistently useful in tumors of the lymphoid system, implying perhaps that patients who are immunoincompetent may be incapable of mounting an appropriate response to immunotherapy.

There is currently a great deal of interest in the potential of immunotherapy in the treatment of cancer in man. Many basic and clinical studies are underway. It is our hope that these studies will be conducted in a careful enough fashion so that the results obtained will lead to a better understanding of the underlying mechanisms of tumor immunity, even in situations where the specific therapeutic effect may be disappointing.

REFERENCES

1. Hellström, I., and Hellström, K. E., *Cancer* **34,** 1461 (1974).
2. McKhann, C. F., and Gunnarsson, A., *Cancer* **34,** 1521 (1974).
3. Hersh, E. M., Gutterman, J. U., and Mavligit, G., *Immunotherapy of Cancer in Man: Scientific Basis and Current Status,* Charles C Thomas, Springfield, Ill., 1973.
4. Henderson, E. S., and Leventhal, B. G., *Immunotherapy of Leukemia,* Cancer Chemotherapy II, The Twenty-Second Hahnemann Symposium (Isadore Brodsky, S. Benham Kahn, and J. H. Moyer, eds.), Grune and Stratton, New York, 1972, p. 327.
5. Baker, M. A., and Taub, R. N., *Allergy* **17,** 227 (1973).
6. Currie, G. A., *Brit. J. Cancer* **26,** 141 (1972).
7. Nauts, H. C., Fowler, G. A. A., and Bogatko, F. H., *Acta Med. Scand. Suppl.* **145,** 5 (1953).
8. Ruckdeschel, J. C., Codish, S. D., Stranahan, A., and McKneally, M. F., *N. Engl. J. Med.* **287,** 1013 (1972).

9. Crispen, R. G., *Seminars in Oncology* **1,** 311 (1974).

10. Halpern, B. N., Biozzi, G., Stiffel, C., et al., *Compt. Rend. Soc. Biol.* **153,** 919 (1959).

11. Old, L. J., Benacerraf, B., Clarke, D. A., et al., *Cancer Res.* **21,** 1281 (1961).

12. Davignon, L., Lemonde, P., Robillar, P., et al., *Lancet* **2,** 638 (1970).

13. Davignon, L., Lemonde, P., St. Pierre, J., et al., *Lancet* **1,** 80 (1971).

14. Davignon, L., Lemonde, P., St. Pierre, J., et al., *Lancet* **1,** 799 (1971).

15. Rosenthal, S. R., Crispen, R. G., Thorne, M. G., Plekarski, N., Raisys, N., and Rettig, P., *J. Am. Med. Assoc.* **222,** 1543 (1972).

16. Kinlen, O. A., and Pike, M. C., *Lancet* **2,** 398 (1971).

17. Schneiderman, M. A., and Levin, D. L., *Cancer Res.* **33,** 1498 (1973).

18. Waaler, H. T., *Lancet* **2,** 1314 (1970).

19. Heins, G., and Stuart, A., *Lancet* **1,** 183 (1971).

20. Berkeley, J. S., *Lancet* **1,** 183 (1971).

21. Clark, J., *Lancet* **1,** 751 (1971).

22. British Medical Research Council, *Bull. WHO* **46,** 371 (1972).

23. Comstock, G. W., Livesay, V. T., and Webster, R. G., *Lancet* **2,** 1062 (1971).

24. Comstock, G. W., Martinez, I., and Livesay, V. T., *J. Nat. Cancer Inst.* **54,** 835 (1975).

25. Hoover, R. N., *Cancer Res.* **36,** 652 (1976).

26. Bast, R. C., Jr., Zbar, B., Borsos, T., and Rapp, H. J., *N. Engl. J. Med.* **290,** 1413 (1974).

27. Morton, D. L., Eilber, F. R., Holmes, E. C., Hunt, J. S., Ketcham, A. S., Silverstein, M. J., and Sparks, F. C. *Ann. Surgery* **180,** 635 (1974).

28. Bornstein, R., Mastrangelo, M. J., Sulit, H., Chee, D., Yarbro, J. W., Prehn, L. M., and Prehn, R. T., *National Cancer Institute Monograph* **39,** 213 (1973).

29. Pinksy, C. A., Hirshaut, Y., and Oettgen, H. F., *National Cancer Institute Monograph* **39,** 225 (1973).

30. Nathanson, L., *Cancer Chemotherapy Reports* **56,** 659 (1972).

31. Balzarini, G. P., Cascinelli, N., Fontana, V., and Veronesi, U., *Tumori* **60,** 345 (1974).

32. Smith, G. V., Morse, P. A., Deraps, G. D., Raju, S., and Hardy, J. D., *Surgery* **74,** 59 (1973).

33. Baker, M. A., and Taub, R., *Lancet* **1,** 1117 (1973).

34. Mastrangelo, M. J., Bellett, R. E., Berkelhammer, J., and Clark, W. H., Jr., *Cancer* **36,** 1305 (1975).

35. Bast, R. C., Jr., Zbar, B., Borsos, T., and Rapp, H. J., *N. Engl. J. Med.* **290,** 1458 (1974).

36. Nathanson, L., *Seminars in Oncology* **1,** 337 (1974).

37. Seigler, H. F., Shingleton, W. W., Metzgar, R. S., Buckley, C. E., III, Bergoc, P. M., Miller, D. S., Fetter, B. F., and Phaup, M. B., *Surgery* **72,** 162 (1972).

38. Seigler, H. F., Shingleton, W. W., Metzgar, R. S., Buckley, C. E., and Bergoc, P. M., *Ann. Surgery* **178,** 352 (1973).

39. Minton, J. P., *Arch. Surgery* **106,** 503 (1973).

40. Klein, E., *National Cancer Institute Monograph* **39,** 139 (1973).

41. Klein, E., Holtermann, O. A., Papermaster, B., Milgrom, H., Rosner, D., Klein, L., Walker, M. J., and Zbar, B., *National Cancer Institute Monograph* **39,** 229 (1973).

42. Rosenberg, E., and Powell, R., *South. Med. J.* **66,** 1359 (1973).

43. Bluming, A. Z., Vogel, C. L., Ziegler, J. L., Mody, N., and Kamya, G., *Ann. Intern. Med.* **76,** 405 (1972).

44. Ikonopisov, R. L., *Tumori* **58,** 121 (1972).

45. Gutterman, J. U., Mavligit, G., McBride, C., Frei, E., III, Freireich, E. J., and Hersh, E. M., *Lancet* **1,** 1208 (1973).

46. Gutterman, J., Mavligit, G., Kennedy, A., and Hersh, E., *Proc. Amer. Assoc. Cancer Res. and Amer. Soc. Clin. Oncology* **16,** 245 (1975).

47. Gutterman, J. U., Mavligit, G., Gottlieb, J. A., Burgess, M. A., McBride, C. E., Einhorn, L., Freireich, E. J., and Hersh, E. M., *N. Engl. J. Med.* **291,** 592 (1974).

48. MacGregor, A. B., Falk, R. E., Landi, S., Ambus, U., and Langer, B., *Surg. Gyn. Obst.* **141,** 747 (1975).

49. Grooms, G. A., and Morton, D. L., *Proc. Amer. Assoc. Cancer Res. and Amer. Soc. Clin. Oncology* **16,** 261 (1975).

50. Sokal, J. E., Aungst, C. W., and Snyderman, M., *N. Engl. J. Med* **291,** 1226 (1974).

51. Thomas, J. W., Plenderleith, I. H., Clements, D. V., and Landi, S., *Clin. Exp. Immunol.* **21,** 82 (1975).

52. Ziegler, J. L., and Magrath, I. T., *National Cancer Institute Monograph* **39,** 199 (1973).

53. Magrath, I. T., and Ziegler, J. L., *Brit. Med. J.* (in press).

54. Mathe, G., Amiel, J. L., Schwarzenberg, L., Schneider, M., Cattan, A., Schlumberger, J. R., Hayat, M., and DeVassal, F., *Lancet* **1,** 697 (1969).

55. Mathe, G., Weiner, R., Pouillart, P., Schwarzenberg, L., Jasmin, C., Schneider, M., Hayat, M., Amiel, J. L., DeVassal, F., and Rosenfeld, C., *National Cancer Institute Monograph* **39,** 165 (1973).

56. Heyn, R. M., Joo, P., Karon, M., Nesbit, M., Shore, N., Breslow, N., Weiner, J., Reed, A., and Hammond, D., *Blood* **46,** 431 (1975).

57. British Medical Research Council Working Party of Leukemia in Childhood, *Brit. Med. J.* **4,** 189 (1971).

58. Gutterman, J. U., Hersh, E. M., Rodriguez, V., McCredie, K. B., Mavligit, G., Reed, R., Burgess, M. A., Smith, T., Gehan, E., Bodey, G. P., Sr., and Freireich, E. J., *Lancet* **2,** 1405 (1974).

59. Leventhal, B. G., Le Pourhiet, A., Halterman, R. H., Henderson, E. S., and Herberman, R. B., *National Cancer Institute Monograph* **39,** 177 (1973).

60. Poplack, D. G., Graw, R. G., Pomeroy, T. C., Henderson, F. S., and Leventhal, B. G., *Proc. Amer. Assoc. Cancer Res. and Amer. Soc. Clin. Oncology* **16,** 230 (1975).

61. Powles, R. L., Crowther, D., Bateman, C. J. T., Meard, M. E. J., McElwain, T. C., Russell, J., Lister, T. A., Whitehouse, J. M. A., Wrigley, P. F. M., Pike, M., Alexander, P., and Fairley, G. Hamilton, *Brit. Med. J.* **2,** 571 (1973).

62. Freeman, C. B., Harris, R., Geary, C. G., Leyland, M. J., MacIver, J. E., and Delamore, I. W., *Brit. Med. J.* **2,** 571 (1973).

63. Vogler, W. R., and Chan, Y. K., *Lancet* **2,** 128 (1974).

64. Sokal, J. E., Aungst, C. W., and Grace, J. T., Jr., *National Cancer Institute Monograph* **39,** 195 (1973).

65. Ramachandar K., Baker, M. A. and Taub, R. N., *Blood* **46,** 845 (1975).

66. Hersh, E. M., Mavligit, G. M., and Gutterman, J. U., *Seminars in Oncology* **1,** 273 (1974).

67. Cusumano, C. L., Jernigan, J. A., and Waldman, R. H., *J. Nat. Cancer Inst.* **55,** 275 (1975).

68. Garner, F. B., Meyer, C. A., White, D. S., and Lipton, A., *Cancer* **35,** 1088 (1975).

69. McKneally, M. F., Maver, C., Civerchia, L., Codish, S., Kausel, H. W., and Alley, R. D., "Regional Immunotherapy for Lung Cancer Using Intrapleural BCG," in *Neoplasm Immunity: Theory and Application* (Ray G. Crispen, ed.), ITR, Chicago, 1975, p. 153.

70. Donaldson, R. C., *Amer. J. Surgery* **124,** 527 (1972).

71. Richter, P., Chakravorty, R. C., King, R. F., and Terz, J. J., *Clin. Res.* **23,** 342A (1975).

72. Mavligit, G. M., Gutterman, J. U., Burgess, M. A., Speer, J. F., Reed, R. C., Martin, R. C., McBride, C. M., Copeland, E. M., Gehan, E. A., and Hersh, E. M., *Digestive Diseases* **19,** 1047 (1974).

73. Sonkin, R., Condeyras, M., and Blondon, J., *J. Gyn Obst. Biol. Reprod.* **1,** 61 (1972).

74. Bagshawe, K., *Proc. Roy. Soc. Med.* **64,** 1043 (1971).

75. Guinan, P., Bush, I. M., John, T., Sadoughi, N., and Ablin, R. J., *Lancet* **2,** 443 (1973).

76. Guinan, P., John, T., Crispen, R. G., Ablin, R. J., and Bush, I., in *Neoplasma Immunity: BCG Vaccination,* Schori Press, Illinois, 1974.

77. Townsend, C. M., and Eilber, F. R., *Proc. Amer. Assoc. Cancer Res. and Amer. Soc. Clin. Oncology* **16,** 261 (1975).

78. Sparks, F. C., Silverstein, M. J., Hunt, J. S., Haskell, C. M., Pilch, H. Y., and Morton, D. L., *N. Engl. J. Med.* **289,** 827 (1973).

79. Rosenberg, E. B., Karmen, S. P., Schwartzman, R. J., and Colsky, J., *Arch. Int. Med.* **134,** 796 (1974).

80. Case Records of the Massachusetts General Hospital, *N. Engl. J. Med.* **293,** 443 (1975).

81. Gerner, R. E., and Moore, G. E., *N. Engl. J. Med.* **290,** 343 (1973).

82. Bodurtha, A., Kim, Y. H., Laucius, J. F., Donaton, R. A., and Mastrangelo, M. J., *Amer. J. Clin. Pathol.* **61,** 747 (1974).

83. Morton, D. L., Eilber, F. R., Malmgren, R. A., et al., *Surgery* **68,** 158 (1970).

84. McKhann, C., and Gunnarsson, A., in *Neoplasm Immunity: BCG Vaccination,* Institute for Tuberculosis Research, Schori Press, Illinois, 1974, pp. 31–44.

85. Spitler, L., Wybran, J., Lieberman, R., Levinson, D., Epstein, W., and Hendrickson, C., in *Malignant Melanoma: Clinical and Immunologic Evaluation and Complications,* Institute for Tuberculosis Research, Schori Press, Illinois, 1974, pp. 45–48.

86. Aungst, C. W., Sokal, J. E., and Jager, B. V., *Ann. Intern. Med.* **82,** 666 (1975).

87. Kwaan, H., *Neoplasm Immunity: BCG Vaccination,* Institute for Tuberculosis Research, Schori Press, Illinois, 1974, pp. 25–30.

88. Chess, L., Bock, G. N., Ungaro, P. C., Buchholz, D. H., and Mardiney, M. R., *J. Nat. Cancer Inst.* **51,** 57 (1973).

89. Lamoureux, G., and Poisson, R., *Lancet* **1,** 989 (1974).

90. Morton, D. L., Holmes, E. C., Eilber, F. R., and Wood, W. C., *Ann. Intern. Med.* **74,** 587 (1971).

91. Lieberman, R., Epstein, W., and Fudenberg, H. H., *Brit. J. Cancer* **14,** 401 (1974).

92. Bulkley, G. B., Cohen, M., Banks, P. M., Char, D. H., and Ketcham, A. S., *Cancer* **36,** 485 (1975).

93. Levy, N., Seigler, H., Shingleton, W. W., *Cancer* **34,** 1548 (1974).

94. Sulit, H., Chee, D., Mastrangelo, M., Bornstein, R., Prehn, R. T., and Yarbro, J., *Proc. Amer. Assoc. Cancer Res.* **13,** 74 (1972).

95. Morton, D. L., *National Cancer Institute Monograph* **35,** 375 (1972).

96. Levy, N. L., Mahaley, M. S., Jr., and Day, E. D., *Int. J. Cancer* **10,** 244 (1972).

97. Hersey, P., MacLennan, I. C., Campbell, A. C., Harris, R., and Freeman, C. B., *Clin. Exp. Immunol.* **14,** 159 (1973).

98. Weiss, D. W., and Yashphe, D. J., "Nonspecific Stimulation of Antimicrobial and Antitumor Resistance and of Immunological Responsiveness by the MER Fraction of Tubercle Bacilli," in *Dynamic Aspects of Host-Parasite Relationships, Vol. 1, Academic Press, New York, 1973, pp. 133–223.*

99. Yron, I., Weiss, D. W., Robinson, E., Cohen, D., Adelberg, M. G., Mekori, T., and Haber, M., *National Cancer Institute Monograph* **39,** 33 (1973).

100. Richman, S. P., *Proc. Amer. Assoc. Cancer Res. and Amer. Soc. Clin. Oncology* **16,** 227 (1975).

101. Moertel, C. G., Ritts, R. E., Schuttand, A. J., Hahn, R. G., *Cancer Res* **35,** 3075 (1975).

102. Robinson, E., Bartal, A., Cohen, Y., and Haasz, R., *Brit. J. Cancer* **32,** 1 (1975).

103. Weiss, D. W., Stupp, Y., Manny, N., and Izak, G., *Transplantation Proc.* (in press, 1975).

104. Stupp, Y., Manny, N., Weiss, D. W., and Izak, G., *Proceedings of the International Society of Haematology, European and African Division* (in press, 1975).

105. Cuttner, J., Holland, J. F., Bekesi, J. G., Ramachandar, K., and Donovan, O., *Proc. Amer. Assoc. Cancer Res. and Amer. Soc. Clin. Oncology* **16,** 264 (1975).

106. Scott, M. T., *Seminars in Oncology* **1,** 367 (1974).

107. Israel, L., and Halpern, B., *La Nouvelle Press Medicale* **1,** 19 (1972).

108. Israel, L., and Edelstein, R., "Nonspecific Immunostimulation with *Corynebacterium Parvum* in Human Cancer," in *Immunological Aspects of Neoplasia,* M. D. Anderson Hospital and Tumor Institute at Houston, Williams & Wilkins, Baltimore, 1974.

109. Reed, R. C., Gutterman, J. U., Mavligit, G. M., and Hersh, E. M., *Proc. Amer. Assoc. Cancer Res. and Amer. Soc. Clin. Oncology* **16,** 228 (1975).

110. Cunningham-Rundles, W. F., Hirshaut, Y., Pinsky, C. M., and Oettgen, H. F., *Clin. Res* **23,** 337A (1975).

111. Band, P. R., Jao-King, C., Urtasun, R., and Haraphongse, M., *Proc. Amer. Assoc. Cancer Res. and Amer. Soc. Clin. Oncology* **16,** 9 (1975).

112. Hirshaut, Y., Pinsky, C., Cunningham-Rundles, W., Rao, B., Fried, J., and Oettgen, H., *Proc. Amer. Cancer Res. and Amer. Soc. Clin. Oncology* **16,** 181 (1975).

113. Israel, L., Edelstein, R., Depierre, A., and Dimitrov, N., *J. Nat. Cancer Inst.* **55,** 29 (1975).

114. Bluming, A. Z., and Ziegler, J., *Lancet* **2,** 105 (1971).

115. Sauter, C., Gerber, A., Lindenmann, J., and Martz, G., *Schweiz Med. Wschr.* **102,** 285 (1972).

116. Wheelock, E. F., and Dingle, J. H., *N. Engl. J. Med.* **271,** 645 (1964).

117. Webb, H. E., Wetherley-Mein, G., Gordon-Smith, C. E., and McMahon, D., *Brit. J. Med.* **1,** 258 (1966).

118. Burdick, K. H., *Arch. Dermatol.* **82,** 438 (1960).

119. Belisario, J. C., and Milton, G. W., *Australasian J. Haematol.* **6,** 113 (1961).

120. Hunter, J. I., Newton, K. A., Westbery, S., Lacey, B. W., *Brit. Med. J.* **2,** 512 (1970).

121. Roenigk, H. H., Deodhar, S., St. Jacques, R., and Burdick, K., *Arch. Dermatol.* **109,** 668 (1974).

122. Milton, G. W., and Brown, M. M. L., *NZ Aust. J. Surgery* **35,** 286 (1970).

123. Everall, J. D., Doherty, C. J., Wand, J., and Dowd, P. M., *Lancet* **2,** 583 (1975).

124. Asada, T., *Cancer* **34,** 1907 (1974).

125. Green, A. A., Webster, R. G., and Smith, K., *Proc. Amer. Assoc. Cancer Res. and Amer. Soc. Clin. Oncology* **16,** 271 (1975).

126. Merigan, T. C., *Cancer Chemotherapy Reports Part I* **58,** 571 (1974).

127. Mathe, G., Amiel, J. L., Schwarzenberg, L., et al., *Eur. J. Clin. Biol. Res.* **15,** 671 (1970).

128. Wanebo, H. J., Oettgen, H. F., Lundy, J., Stock, C. C., and Old, L. J., *Proc. Amer. Assoc. Cancer Res. and Amer. Soc. Clin. Oncology* **16,** 179 (1975).

129. Klein, E., *Cancer Res.* **29,** 2351 (1969).

130. Levis, W. R., Kraemer, K. H., Klingler, W. G., Peck, G. L., and Terry, W. D., *Cancer Res.* **33,** 3036 (1973).

131. Stjernsward, J., and Levin, A., *Cancer* **28,** 628 (1971).

132. Sinkovics, J. G., Williams, D. E., Campos, L. T., Kay, H. D., and Romero, J. G., *Seminars in Oncology* **1,** 351 (1974).

133. Mann, D. L., Halterman, R., and Leventhal, B., *Cancer* **34,** 1446 (1974).

134. Sacks, K. L., Olweny, C., Mann, D. L., Simon, R., Johnson, G. E., Poplack, D. G., and Leventhal, B., *Cancer Res.* **35,** 3715 (1975).

135. Bekesi, J. G., Holland, J. F., Yates, J. W., Henderson, E., and Fleminger, R., *Proc. Amer. Assoc. Cancer Res. and Amer. Soc. Clin. Oncology* **16,** 121 (1975).

136. Lindstrom, G. A., *Acta Med. Scand. Suppl.* **22,** 1 (1927).

137. de Carvalho, S., *Cancer* **16,** 306 (1963).

138. Sekla, B., Holeckova, E., Janele, J., Libansky, J., Hnevkovsky, O., *Neoplasma* **14,** 641 (1967).

139. Tsirimbas, A. D., Pichlmayr, R., Horninung, B., Pfisterer, H., Thierfelder, S., Brendel, W., and Stich, W., *Klin. Wschr.* **46,** 583 (1968).

140. Marsh, B., Flynn, L., and Enneking, W., *J. Bone and Joint Surgery* **54A,** 1367 (1972).

141. Parks, L. C., Smith, W. J., Beebe, B., Winn, L., Rafajko, R., Rolley, R., and Williams, G. Melville, *Proc. Amer. Assoc. Cancer Res. and Amer. Soc. Clin. Oncology* **16,** 134 (1975).

142. Laszlo, J., Buckley, C. E., and Amos, D. B., *Blood* **31,** 104 (1968).

143. Djerassi, I., *Clinical Pediatrics* **7,** 272 (1968).

144. Herberman, R. B., Oren, M. E., Rogentine, G. N., and Fahey, J. L., *Cancer* **28,** 365 (1971).

145. Brittingham, T. E., and Chaplin, H., *Cancer* **13,** 412 (1960).

146. Skurkovich, S. V., Kisljak, N. S., Machonkova, L. A., and Begunenko, S.-A., *Nature* **223,** 509 (1969).

147. Skurkovich, S. V., Makhaonova, L. A., Reznichenko, F. M., and Chervonskiy, G. I., *Blood* **33,** 186 (1969).

148. Ngu, V., *Brit. Med. J.* **1,** 345 (1967).

149. Fass, L., Herberman, R. B., Ziegler, J., and Morrow, R. H., *J. Nat. Cancer Inst.* **44,** 145 (1970).

150. Sumner, W. C., and Foraker, A. G., *Cancer* **13,** 79 (1960).

151. Ghose, T., and Nigam, S. P., *Cancer* **29,** 1398 (1972).

152. Levy, R., Hurwitz, E., Maron, R., Arnon, R., and Sela, M., *Cancer Res.* **35,** 1182 (1975).

153. Vial, A. B., and Callahan, W., *Cancer* **10,** 999 (1957).

154. Moolton, F. L., and Cooperband, S. R., *Science* **169,** 68 (1970).

155. Parker, C. W., *Pharmacol. Rev.* **25,** 325 (1973).

156. Segerling, M., Ohanian, S. H., and Borsos, T., *Cancer Res.* **35,** 3195 (1975).

157. Nadler, S. H., and Moore, G. E., *J. Amer. Med. Assoc.* **191,** 105 (1965).

158. Woodruff, M. F. A., and Noland, B., *Lancet* **2,** 426 (1963).

159. Symes, M. O., and Riddell, A. G., *Lancet* **1,** 1054 (1968).

160. Thomas, E. D., Storb, R., Clift, R. A., Fefer, A., Johnson, F. L., Neiman, P. E., Lerner, K. G., Glucksberg, H., and Buckner, C. G., *N. Engl. J. Med.* **292,** 832 and 895 (1975).

161. Frenster, J., and Rogoway, W. M., *Yearbook of Oncology,* 1970, Abstract 327.

162. Cheema, A. R., and Hersh, E. M., *Cancer* **29,** 982 (1972).

163. Moore, G. E., and Moore, M. D., *N.Y. State J. Med.* **69,** 460 (1969).

164. Suk, D., Pickren, M., and Moore, G. E., *N.Y. State J. Med.* 2479 (Oct. 15, 1973).

165. Nadler, S. H., and Moore, G. E., *Arch. Surg.* **99,** 376 (1969).

166. Humphrey, L. J., Murray, D. R., and Boehm, O. R., *Surg. Gyn. Obst.* **132,** 437 (1971).

167. Krementz, E. T., Samuels, M. S., Wallace, J. H., and Benes, E. N., *Surg. Gyn. Obst.* **133,** 209 (1971).

168. Nadler, S. H., and Moore, G. E., *Ann. Surg.* **164,** 482 (1966).

169. Lawrence, H. S., *J. Clin. Invest.* **34,** 219 (1954).

170. Lawrence, H. S., *Trans. Assoc. Amer. Physicians* **76,** 84 (1963).

171. Hattler, B. G., and Amos, D. B., *J. Nat. Cancer Inst.* **35,** 927 (1965).

172. Wybran, J., and Fudenberg, H. A., *J. Clin. Invest.* **52,** 1026 (1973).

173. Lawrence, H. S., and Pappenheimer, A. M., *J. Exp. Med.* **104,** 321 (1956).

174. Lawrence, H. S., *Adv. Immunology* **11,** 195 (1969).

175. Neidhart, J. A., Schwartz, R. S., Hurtubise, P. E., Murphy, S. G., Metz, E. N., Balcerzak, S. P., and LoBuglio, A. F., *Cellular Immunol.* **9,** 319 (1973).

176. Crawford, J., Neidhart, J., Hurtubise, P., Murphy, S., Metz, E., Balcerzak, S. P., and LoBuglio, A. F., *Clin. Res.* **21,** 836A (1973).

177. Neidhart, J. A., and LoBuglio, A. F., *Seminars in Oncology* **1,** 379 (1974).

178. Brandes, L. M., Galton, D. A. G., and Wiltshaw, E., *Lancet* **2,** 294 (1971).

179. Krementz, E. T., Mansell, P. W. A., Hornung, M. O., Samuels, M. S., Sutherland, C. A., and Benes, E. N., *Cancer* **33,** 394 (1974).

180. Thompson, R. B., *Rev. Europ. Etudes Clin. et Biol.* **16,** 201 (1971).

181. Spitler, L. E., Wybran, J., Fudenberg, H. H., and Levin, A. S., *Clin. Res.* **21,** 221 (1973).

182. Bukowski, R. M., Deodhar, S., and Hewlett, J. S., *Proc. Second Workshop on Transfer Factor* (in press, 1975).

183. Levin, A. S., Byers, V. S., Fudenberg, H. H., Wybran, J., Hackett, A. J., Johnston, J. O., and Spitler, L. E., *J. Clin. Invest.* **55,** 487 (1975).

184. Neidhart, J., Hilberg, J., Allen, E., Metz, E., Balcerzak, S. S., and LoBuglio, A., *Clin. Res.* **20,** 748 (1972).

185. Silva, J., Allen, J., Wheeler, R., Bull, F., and Morley, G., *Proc. Second Workshop on Transfer Factor* (in press, 1975).

186. Vetto, R. M., Burger, D. R., Nolte, J., and Vandenbark, A. A., *Proc. Second Workshop on Transfer Factor* (in press, 1975).

187. Oettgen, H., Old, L., Farrow, J., Valentine, F., Lawrence, S., and Thomas, L., *Clin. Res.* **50,** 71a (1971).

188. Oettgen, H. F., Old, L. J., Farrow, J. H., Valentine, F., Lawrence, H. S., and Thomas, L., *Proc. Nat. Acad. Sci.* **71,** 2319 (1974).

189. Goldenberg, G. J., and Brandes, L. J., *Clin. Res.* **20,** 947 (1972).

190. McIlvanie, S. K., Abstract #47, Amer. Soc. Hematology (1973).

191. Smith, R. A., Ezdinli, E., Bigley, N. J., and Han, T., *Lancet* **I,** 434 (1973).

192. Ng, R. P., Moran, C. J., Alexopoulos, C. G., and Bellingham, A. J., *Lancet* **II,** 901 (1975).

193. Silverman, M. A., Meltz, S., Sorokin, C., and Glade, P. R., *Proc. Second Workshop on Transfer Factor* (in press, 1975).

194. Hayes, A., Borella, L., and Mauer, A. M., *Proc. Amer. Assoc. Cancer Res. and Amer. Soc. Clin. Oncology* **16,** 108 (1975).

195. Fudenberg, H. H., Levin, A. S., Spitler, L. E., Wybran, J., and Byers, V., *Hosp. Pract. JAN,* 95 (1974).

196. Gelfand, E. W., Baumal, R., Huber, J., Brookston, M. C., and Shumak, K. H., *N. Engl. J. Med.* **289,** 1385 (1973).

197. Ballow, M., DuPont, B., and Good, R. A., *J. Pediatrics* **83,** 772 (1973).

198. Hackett, A. J., Springer, E. L., Levin, A. S., and Fink, M. A., *Proc. Amer. Assoc. Cancer Res. and Amer. Soc. Clin. Oncology* **16,** 193 (1975).

199. Waldman, S. R., Roth, J., Silverstein, M., Veltman, L., and Pilch, Y. H., *Proc. Amer. Assoc. Cancer Res. and Amer. Soc. Clin. Oncol.* **15,** 184 (1974).

200. Deckers, P. J., and Pilch, Y. H., *Cancer* **28,** 1219 (1971).

201. Fishman, J., and Adler, F. L., *J. Exp. Med.* **117,** 595 (1963).

202. Pilch, Y. H., and deKernion, J. B., *Seminars in Oncology* **1,** 387 (1974).

203. Alexander, P., Delorme, E. J., Hamilton, L. D. G., et al., *Nature* **213,** 569 (1967).

204. Ramming, K. P., and Pilch, Y. H., *Science* **168,** 492 (1970).

205. Ramming, K. P., and Pilch, Y. H., *J. Nat. Cancer Inst.* **46,** 735 (1971).

206. Paque, R. E., and Dray, S., *Cell Immunol.* **5,** 30 (1972).

207. Han, T., *Clin. Exp. Immunol.* **14,** 213 (1973).

208. Pilch, Y. H., Fritze, D., Kern, D. H., and deKernion, J. B., *Proc. Amer. Assoc. Cancer Res. and Amer. Soc. Clin. Oncology* **16,** 258 (1975).

209. Goldstein, A. L., Guha, A., Zatz, M. M., Hardy, M. A., and White, A., *Proc. Natl. Acad. Sci. USA* **69,** 800 (1972).

210. Costanzi, J., Gagliano, R., Loukas, D., Sakai, H., Thurman, G., Harris, N., and Goldstein, A., *Proc. Amer. Assoc. Cancer Res. and Amer. Soc. Clin. Oncology* **16,** 135 (1975).

211. Schafer, L. A., Washington, M. L., and Goldstein, A. L., *Proc. Amer. Assoc. Cancer Res. and Amer. Soc. Clin. Oncology* **16,** 233 (1975).

212. Fink, M. A., *Seminars in Oncology* **1,** 425 (1974).

213. Hellström, K. E., and Hellström, I., *Ann. Rev. Microbiol.* **24,** 343 (1970).

214. Prehn, R. T., *Science* **176,** 170 (1972).

215. Fidler, I. J., *Cancer Res.* **34,** 491 (1974).

216. Fidler, I. J., *Cancer Res.* **34,** 1074 (1974).

217. Norman, R. L., *Lancet* **ii,** 867 (1975).

218. Hersh, E. M., Whitecar, J., and McCredie, K., *N. Engl. J. Med.* **285,** 1211, 1971.

219. Leventhal, B. G., Halterman, R. H., Rosenberg, E. B., and Herberman, R. B., *Cancer Res.* **32,** 1820 (1972).

220. Heppner, G., Henry, E., Stolbach, L., Cummings, F., McDonough, E., and Calabresi, P., *Cancer Res.* **35,** 1931 (1975).

Chapter Ten

Neoplasms of
the Immune System

ELAINE S. JAFFE AND IRA GREEN

Hematopathology Section, Laboratory of Pathology, National Cancer Institute, National Institutes of Health, and Laboratory of Immunology, National Institute of Allergy and Infectious Disease, National Institutes of Health, Bethesda, Maryland

During the past few years an intense and concentrated effort has been made to analyze the workings of the immune system. In the course of these studies it has been established that a number of different mononuclear cell types with various functions collaborate to execute different aspects of the immune response. Some of the immunologic functions can be ascribed to the large number of soluble mediators or lymphokines which are produced by each cell type. In addition, lymphoid cells have several immunologic functions that can be examined in vitro, such as lymphocyte-mediated cytotoxicity or proliferation in response to antigen, that are not known to be associated with the production of lymphokines. Furthermore, each of these mononuclear cell types has different types of receptors, special differentiation antigens, and other membrane properties which allow for identification of each cell type.

At the same time these activities were proceeding in the immunologic sphere, great advances were being made by chemotherapists and radiotherapists in the clinical evaluation and treatment of patients with lymphoreticular malignancies (LRM). Detailed staging procedures both by invasive and noninvasive modalities were introduced which brought greater attention to the way in which these diseases presented and spread. Advances in therapy, including modern combination chemotherapy, high-voltage radiotherapy, and modern clinical support measures, permitted longer survivals for these patients and permitted greater differences between these diseases to be appreciated. Contributions by pathologists included improved classification schemes which could relate significantly to these clinical differences, e.g., age, sex, symptoms, anatomic distribution of disease, risk of leukemia, and prognosis (1,2). These classification schemes were based primarily on conventional morphologic techniques including histology, histochemistry, and electron microscopy.

Within recent years the interests of the chemotherapist, radiotherapist, pathologist, and basic immunologist have begun to merge. As the malignant lymphomas are diseases of the immune system, an understanding of this system is basic to an understanding of the pathophysiology of these diseases. The concepts of homing and "traffic" of lymphocytes relate directly to the ways in which these diseases spread. The immunologic deficits manifested by these patients relate to which component of the immune system is affected by neoplasia. Furthermore, any classification scheme must recognize and relate to the functional and ontogenetic heterogeneity of the immune system.

The collaboration of scientists and subsequent integration of knowledge in these two spheres has proceeded in several areas. The first studies in which immunologic methodology, techniques, and thinking were brought to bear on clinical problems of patients dealt with the ability of these patients to respond with antigen in vivo. Next, a large variety of in vitro immunologic studies were performed with the mononuclear cells of these patients in an attempt to correlate the in vivo defects with the results of in vitro immunologic tests. Most recently, direct immunologic studies of the malignant cells themselves have been undertaken, including functional studies of these malignant cells as well as the identification of specific receptors and antigens on the malignant cells which allow these cells to be classified in terms of their normal cell of origin.

The first part of the review will deal with this latter subject—the immunologic classification of LRM and how these findings integrate into the morphological classification; in the second part we will review some of the correlations between the functional in vivo disorders of these patients and the results of in vitro tests as well as studies of the functions of the malignant lymphoid cells themselves.

IMMUNOLOGIC CHARACTERIZATION OF LYMPHORETICULAR MALIGNANCY

Two basic observations made in recent years have caused pathologists to reexamine conventional classification schemes for LRM. The first was that the small lymphocyte as seen in peripheral blood and lymphoid tissue is not an end-stage cell. The approach to classification of LRM had been to regard the small peripheral blood lymphocyte as the final product of a differentiation process. Neoplastic lymphocytes were graded as well differentiated or poorly differentiated based on the degree to which they resembled this cell. Larger cells with more abundant cytoplasm and less nuclear chromatin condensation were regarded as precursors of small lymphocytes or "poorly differentiated." The observation that the small lymphocytes upon exposure to the proper stimulus could transform into larger cells capable of high proliferative activity which, in turn, could generate more small lymphocytes made many of these assumptions invalid (3,4).

The second basic observation was, of course, that the morphologically homogeneous population of small lymphocytes represented at least two distinct cell types with different origins, functions, and sites of differentiation and localization (5,6)—i.e., thymus-dependent and thymus-independent lymphocytes. Although all lymphocytes probably derive from bone marrow precursors (7), thymus-dependent lymphocytes or T cells undergo final differentiation in the thymus before lodging in peripheral lymphoid organs. Thymus-independent or B lymphocytes undergo final differentiation in birds in the bursa of Fabricius and in mammals in a bursa-equivalent, perhaps the liver (8). These cells have different distributions in peripheral lymphoid organs. T cells are located primarily in the paracortex of lymph nodes and periarteriolar lymphoid sheaths of the splenic white pulp. B lymphocytes are distributed in the follicles of both lymph nodes and spleen and the medullary cords of lymph nodes. However, lymphocytes are not at all fixed at these sites. There is a normal "traffic" of lymphocytes, especially well demonstrated for T cells, by which they leave the blood stream, enter the lymph nodes via postcapillary venules, leave via efferent lymphatics to the thoracic duct lymph, and then enter the blood stream again (9). The normal traffic of B lymphocytes is not as yet established. However, it should be noted the patterns of spread of many malignant lymphomas can be related to the normal migration pathways of B and T cells and therefore the patterns of tumor cell distribution in LRM are quite distinct from those of nonhematopoietic malignancies. T and B lymphocytes are also characterized by different functions; B cells are involved in humoral immunity whereas T cells are generally involved in cell-mediated immunity. Of course, different subclasses of both these cell types have many distinct and specialized functions.

Presently used classification schemes for LRM were proposed at a time when the functional heterogeneity of the immune system was not appreciated. The methodology developed by modern immunology has only recently been applied to the study of these diseases. This immunologic characterization of LRM has relied heavily on the investigation of neoplastic cells for the presence of cell surface markers normally present on cells of the immune system, the T and B lymphocytes, and the mononuclear phagocytes. Our purpose is to review these investigations and relate the findings to current clinical and pathological understanding of lymphoreticular malignancies. For the purpose of these discussions we will employ the classification of non-Hodgkin's lymphomas proposed by Rappaport (10), which today remains the one most widely used within the United States. The Rappaport classification given in Table 1 describes malignant lymphomas in terms of both their cytologic composition and their pattern of growth, whether nodular or diffuse. Its clinical applicability has been demonstrated in a number of clinicopathologic studies (11,12,13).

Cell Surface Markers

We will first review the markers used to characterize normal and neoplastic cells of the immune system (Table 2). These markers are usually identified on cells in suspension. The techniques used can be applied to cells isolated from peripheral blood or solid tissues. In considering any data obtained from such studies it is important to consider the cellular composition of the cell suspension. If the population is not homogeneous, then auxiliary techniques, usually morphologic, must be introduced to identify the cells bearing a particular marker. Some of the markers can also be identified on cells in frozen tissue sections. Such a technique,

Table 1   Classification of Non-Hodgkin's Lymphomas (10)

Nodular (Follicular) Lymphomas
  Lymphocytic, poorly differentiated
  Mixed lymphocytic-histiocytic
  Histiocytic

Diffuse Lymphomas
  Lymphocytic, well differentiated
  Lymphocytic, intermediate differentiation
  Lymphocytic, poorly differentiated
  Mixed lymphocytic-histiocytic
  Histiocytic
  Undifferentiated, Burkitt's type
  Undifferentiated, pleomorphic (non-Burkitt)

Unclassified

Table 2   Markers of Human Mononuclear Cells [a]

Cell Type	SIg	C3	Fc	E	Iso-Ag	Phagocytosis
T lymphocyte	−	−	(∓)a	+	+	−
B lymphocyte	+	+	+	−	+	−
Mononuclear phagocyte	(+) [b]	(−) [c]				
	−	+	+	−	−	+

[a] *Abbreviations:*
  SIg: surface immunoglobulins
  C3: receptors for third component of complement
  Fc: receptors for Fc portion of IgG
  E: spontaneous rosette formation with sheep red blood cells
  Iso-Ag: presence of specific isoantigens
  Phagocytosis: easily demonstrable phagocytosis of particulate matter
[b] Receptor present on some activated T lymphocytes.
[c] Ig nonspecifically bound and not a product of cell synthesis.
[d] Receptors present on peripheral blood monocytes but not demonstrated on all tissue macrophages.

of course, has the advantage that the location within the intact tissue of cells bearing a particular marker can be determined. This is especially important if the population being studied is heterogeneous or if the tissue, e.g., lymph node, is only focally replaced by the neoplastic infiltrate. Such occurrences are not infrequent in the malignant lymphomas.

Surface Immunoglobulin (SIg).   Easily detectable membrane-bound immunoglobulin is considered the hallmark of a B lymphocyte (5,6). The immunoglobulin is synthesized by the cell and is usually restricted to one type of light chain and one class of heavy chain per lymphocyte at any given time (14). An exception to this generalization is the frequent simultaneous presence of the IgM and IgD heavy chains (15,16). The μ and δ chains present simultaneously share the same variable regions and are therefore of the same idiotype. It has been speculated that IgD is present as an antigen receptor (15). Cultured lymphoblastoid cells can also be found to synthesize immunoglobulins of multiple heavy chain classes (17). However, an individual lymphocyte or cells of a single clone have never been demonstrated to synthesize more than one light chain. Mononuclear phagocytes may also carry SIg, but the immunoglobulin is not a product of cell synthesis and is usually nonspecifically bound via Fc receptors or complement receptors on the cell membrane.

Several methods have been used to demonstrate that the immunoglobulin present on the membrane is a product of cell synthesis and thus demonstrate that the cell is a B lymphocyte. One method is enzymatic digestion by trypsin to remove the SIg and then short term culture to allow for resynthesis (18). A second method is to allow the cells to remain in short term culture in serum-free media and examine them for the presence of SIg at the end of this time (19). Within 12 hours most nonspecifically bound SIg will be spontaneously shed and only endogenous SIg will be present. Multiple washings at 37°C can also be used to remove adsorbed immune complexes (20). Another approach has been to combine immunofluorescence for SIg with cytochemical techniques for the identification of monocytes or histiocytes; the demonstration of peroxidase activity in an Ig-bearing cell eliminates that cell as a B lymphocyte (21).

Although monocytes, histiocytes, and granulocytes are the cell types most frequently encountered with receptors for immune complexes, activated T cells (22) as well as malignant cells of varied origins (23) also have been demonstrated to bear Fc receptors and thus to be capable of carrying nonspecifically bound SIg. Finally, a cell may carry SIg by virtue of an antibody directed against a constituent in the cell membrane. This can occur with normal lymphocytes in autoimmune disorders (19,24) or can occur with malignant cells as a consequence of antitumor antibodies.

Immunofluorescence is the most widely used technique for detecting SIg and is most reliable when applied to living cells in suspension. The use of fluorescein-conjugated antisera to detect cell-membrane-bound Ig in frozen tissue sections is not generally reliable because of immunoglobulin present in the interstitial lymph surrounding each cell. However, one study has reported success with this technique in rodents (25,26). These reagents can be used in frozen sections to detect cytoplasmic immunoglobulin, as would be found in plasma cells and cells actively secreting Ig. Antisera can be prepared against individual heavy or light chains (18), and such reagents are useful in evaluating the clonicity of lymphoid populations. Antisera can also be conjugated to peroxidase or ferritin for the identification of immunoglobulin at the ultrastructural level (27,28).

Complement Receptor.   Most B lymphocytes bear receptors for activated C3. The most widely used technique for identifying cells bearing complement receptors is a rosette technique in which an erythrocyte (E) is used as an antigen coated with antibody (A) and complement (C) (29). Cells in suspension bearing complement receptors will bind these complexes (EAC), producing a rosette. These rosettes can be quantitated as well as characterized morphologically. One can prepare an air-dried smear of them which can subsequently be stained, or the rosettes can be fixed and even examined ultrastructurally (30). Complement receptors can also be detected on cells in frozen tissue sections using the EAC reagent (31,32). It is important that the antibody used in preparation of the EAC complex be of the IgM class, since an IgGEAC reagent may also bind via IgG sites within the complex to cells bearing Fc receptors. Antigens other than erythrocytes (E) can be used in the complex, or a particle that will activate the alternate complement pathway can serve as both antigen and antibody. Bacteria (33,34) and zymosan (35) have both been used in this regard.

In humans, cells of bone marrow origin other than B lymphocytes also bear complement receptors. Granulocytes (36), erythrocytes, and peripheral blood monocytes (37) all have complement receptors, although differences occur in the nature of the receptors among these cell types (30). Recently an entirely nonhematopoietic location of a C3 receptor has been detected in the human renal glomerulus (38). The detailed specificity of C3 receptors on all these cell types can be more precisely characterized. C3b is cleaved by a serum enzyme, C3 inactivator, into the fragments C3c and C3d. C3c is released into the serum, whereas C3d remains attached to the complex (39). Thus, EAC prepared with whole serum contains a mixture of EAC3b and EAC3d. Whereas normal human lymphocytes have receptors for both C3b and C3d (40), granulocytes (36) and mononuclear phagocytes (41) may only have receptors for C3b. The immune adherence receptor on primate erythrocytes is also specific for C3b (42). Abnormal lymphocytes may also be deficient in some of these receptors (40). However, most EAC reagents used will bind to human granulocytes, monocytes, and erythrocytes. Thus, in quantitating the complement receptor lymphocytes (CRL) in a population, care must be taken to eliminate or identify these other cell types.

Fc Receptor.   B lymphocytes (43) and mononuclear phagocytes (44,45) bear receptors for the Fc fragment of IgG immunoglobulin, although again there are differences between the receptors of these two cell types. The Fc receptor of monocytes and histiocytes, initially described as a receptor for cytophilic antibody (44), demonstrates a much greater avidity and sensitivity for antigen-antibody complexes than that present on B lymphocytes. A reagent which readily binds to the Fc receptor of mononuclear phagocytes is IgGEA, an erythrocyte sensitized with subagglutinating concentrations of IgG (45). Mononuclear phagocytes both in suspension (32) and in frozen tissue sections (46) will bind IgGEA. With conventional techniques B lymphocytes do not readily recognize this complex (32,46). However, if the white cells and reagent red cells are centrifuged together to produce conditions of close contact, binding of IgGEA by B lymphocytes can occur (47). In frozen tissue sections if agglutinating levels of antibody are used to sensitize the red cells and if special washing procedures are used, again some binding by B cells will occur (23). Currently the Fc receptor on B lymphocytes is best demonstrated with radiolabeled soluble antigen-antibody complexes (43) or fluorescein-tagged aggregated human IgG (48). Recently Fc receptors have been demonstrated on activated T cells both in animals (49,50) and humans (22) as well as on virally infected cells (51,52) and malignant cells of varied origins (23). Thus one must use caution in categorizing a cell as a B lymphocyte or a mononuclear phagocyte based solely on the presence of an Fc receptor.

Receptors for Unsensitized Sheep Erythrocytes.   Under certain conditions living human T lymphocytes bind unsensitized sheep erythrocytes (53,54). Repeated studies have demonstrated the specificity of the reaction, although the mechanism of binding is as yet unclear. A charge pattern recognition has been speculated as being involved (55). The binding is extremely weak but may be stabilized and strengthened by prolonged incubation in the cold in the presence of serum (56) or by neuraminidase treatment of the sheep erythrocytes (57). Because of the tenuous binding, the application of this technique to frozen tissue sections is difficult; however, some groups have reported success with various methods (23,58). The E rosette phenomenon is retained by mitogen-transformed human T lymphocytes (59) as well as by T lymphocytic cell lines (60). Thus it is felt that the marker can also be used to identify neoplastic T lymphocytes.

Spontaneous rosette formation is not a phenomenon limited to human T cells and sheep erythrocytes. Mammalian lymphocytes from a variety of species will form rosettes with heterologous erythrocytes, and this rosette formation can be used as a marker for both B and T lymphocytes (56).

Human Lymphocytic Antigens. Human T lymphocytic differentiation antigens can be detected using heterologous antisera rendered specific by prior absorptions with B cell populations (61). Such antisera have been shown in cytotoxicity assays to lyse T lymphocytes selectively but have been less reliable in immunofluorescent assays. Some success has been reported with a sandwich or indirect technique (62). A human B lymphocyte antigen has also been identified (63), but anti-B antisera are not widely available.

Phagocytic Assays. The ability to phagocytose particulate matter is a characteristic feature of monocytes and macrophages, one which has been used to recognize them in in vitro assays (64). Peripheral blood monocytes and B lymphocytes share many surface features—e.g., the presence of receptors for complement and IgG. Thus in studying lymphocytic populations, whether benign or malignant, it is crucial to identify or eliminate mononuclear phagocytes. Phagocytosis can be used to accomplish both of these ends. Mononuclear phagocytes can be identified by the phagocytosis of latex particles, neutral red, or other available markers. These cells will also engulf adherent erythrocytes if incubated at 37°C after rosette formation with either EAC or IgGEA, whereas B lymphocytes will not. Monocytes can be depleted by incubation with iron particles and then sedimentation in a Ficoll-hypaque gradient or passage through a magnetic coil. However, it should be noted that immature monocytes may lack some of these properties, and that mononuclear phagocytes in other sites may differ in the nature of their membrane markers (41,46).

Surface Markers on Lymphoreticular Malignancies

The recognition of the above surface markers on lymphocytes and mononuclear phagocytes and the demonstration of these markers on the neoplastic counterparts of these cells have prompted an increasing number of investigations of lymphomas and leukemias. In examining results obtained by different investigators, one should bear in mind that the pathological and clinical criteria used to categorize these diseases as well as the methodologies employed may vary among laboratories. Nevertheless, the markers in many well-defined clinicopathological entities have been repeatedly shown to demonstrate consistent patterns.

Our approach to reviewing the surface marker studies of the lymphoreticular malignancies is to relate the neoplastic proliferations to the normal cells of the immune system and to relate observed structural and morphologic features to the function of these cells. If one recognizes that the structural compartments of a normal lymph node (Fig. 1) represent as well the functional components of the immune system, and if one views the malignant lymphomas as neoplastic counterparts of these compartments, then much of the pathophysiology of the malignant lymphomas is readily understandable. The malignant cells commonly mirror the growth pattern and function of their benign progenitors, and in many instances it is possible to relate the immunologic data to the histopathology and clinical pattern of disease.

Nodular (Follicular) Lymphoma.   Lymphomas demonstrating a nodular or follicular growth pattern comprise a major subdivision of malignant lymphoma with clinically and pathologically distinctive features (65). In the United States they represent approximately 50 percent of all non-Hodgkin's lymphomas, occurring with equal frequency in males and females, and affecting predominantly older age groups.

The relationship between normal lymphoid follicles and the nodular proliferations seen pathologically in this disease has been the subject of long-standing controversy. Rappaport subclassified the nodular lymphomas based on the cytologic composition of the neoplastic nodules (Table 1) (10). The smaller cells

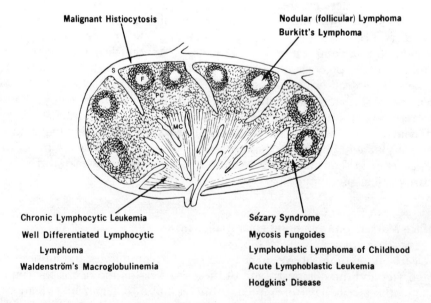

Figure 1. Schematic representation of a normal lymph node illustrating anatomic and functional compartments. The malignant lymphomas are conceptually and functionally related to the above compartments. *Abbreviations:* S = sinuses, F = follicles, PC = paracortex, MC = medullary cords.

with condensed nuclear chromatin and sparse cytoplasm were termed poorly differentiated lymphocytes because of their irregular nuclear features yet obvious morphologic similarity to normal lymphocytes. The larger cells with vesicular nuclei, prominent nucleoli, and more abundant cytoplasm were termed histiocytic, again because of their morphologic resemblance to normal histiocytes. A tumor was subclassified as poorly differentiated lymphocytic if the small cells predominated, histiocytic if the large cells predominated, and mixed if there was a mixture of the two cell types without a preponderance of either one. Rappaport felt that there was no evidence linking these proliferations to follicles; he felt that the nodular pattern was an architectural variant that could be seen in any of the histologic types of non-Hodgkin's lymphoma (1). Although the Rappaport classification has been shown to have clinical and prognostic significance, recent evidence proves that these tumors are derived from the lymphoid follicles (Fig. 1). Both cell types are in fact follicular B lymphocytes exhibiting different degrees of transformation and different kinetic states.

The first strong evidence linking nodular lymphoma to the lymphoid follicle came from the cytochemical (66,67) and ultrastructural (68,69) studies of Lennert and others. Lennert characterized the cells in normal germinal centers, terming them germinocytes and germinoblasts, and viewed the nodular lymphomas as neoplastic expansions of one or more of these normal cell types (70). Thus the neoplastic germinocyte was the morphologic equivalent of the "poorly differentiated lymphocyte" of Rappaport and the germinoblast was equivalent to the "histiocyte" seen in these tumors. An additional cell type was identified, the "dendritic reticulum cell," its processes connected by desmosomal attachments (71,72). This cell, as well, was identified in nodular lymphomas and was considered to be a marker indicating their follicular origin (73,74).

Recent immunologic evidence further establishes that nodular lymphomas are germinal center neoplasms. Regardless of the cytologic subtype, the neoplastic cells can be demonstrated to be B lymphocytes by virtue of the presence of monoclonal SIg (62,75) and abundant C3 receptors (76). This latter marker may be of particular significance, since it is present on only a portion of the B cell population, and in our studies it appears to be characteristic of cells of the lymphoid follicle (76). Because of the focal way in which nodular lymphoma infiltrates a lymph node, the proportion of T lymphocytes identified in a suspension from such a node may be high, often greater than 50 percent (62,76). This observation has led some authors to interpret these nodular lymphomas as being of T cell type (77). However, there is no evidence that the T lymphocytes identified in such cases are in fact the neoplastic population, and there is ample evidence to suggest that they are not. The monoclonal nature of the B cell population in *all* cases studied suggests strongly that they represent a neoplastic expansion of this cell type (62,75). Furthermore, when morphologic techniques have been coupled with quantitative analysis, the cytologically atypical cells have been of B cell origin, whereas the cells of T cell origin appear cytologically normal (76). In addition, when EAC binding was performed on frozen tissue sections, the cells within the proliferating nodules could be demonstrated to bear complement receptors (76). Finally, it was observed that in nodes showing extensive replacement by tumor histologically, the proportion of T cells identified in suspension was low (76).

Additional evidence for the B cell nature of nodular lymphomas is seen in partially involved lymph nodes and spleens, usually obtained at staging laparotomies. The neoplastic cells often populate selectively and multifocally the B cell areas of these tissues, i.e., the eccentric lymphoid follicles of the splenic white pulp and the lymphoid follicles of nodes (78). In contrast, thymic-dependent zones are populated by cytologically normal lymphocytes and often appear atrophic. In rare instances when multiple biopsy specimens from a patient with nodular lymphoma have been evaluated with monospecific fluoresceinated antisera, the neoplastic cells in suspension isolated from multiple sites have all exhibited the same light chain and the same heavy chain (75). This finding could indicate in situ neoplastic transformation of multiple follicle; i.e., either triggering by a stimulus which could direct all the cells within the follicle to synthesize the same immunoglobulin moiety, or selective proliferation of a population already committed to synthesize that immunoglobulin. An alternate possibility is that this phenomenon is a manifestation of migration and homing of the neoplastic cells selectively to the B cell zones. Of great interest is the observed simultaneous presence of IgM and IgD of the same light chain type on the surface of nodular lymphoma cells (75). As mentioned above, IgM and IgD are also found together on the majority of normal peripheral blood B lymphocytes (15,16) and in other B cell neoplasias, e.g., chronic lymphocytic leukemia (79,80).

Although nodular lymphomas are B cell neoplasms, the incidence of serum immunoglobulin abnormalities, either monoclonal gammopathy (81) or hypogammaglobulinemia, in this disease is low. This is readily understandable when one recognizes that the germinal center is not part of the secretory B cell system. Although plasma cells can occasionally be identified within germinal centers, secretion of antibody is not a function of germinal center cells. Rather, the germinal center is thought to play a role in antigen trapping (82) and subsequent B lymphocyte proliferation (83,84).

The cytologic spectrum of nodular lymphomas reflects the cytologic spectrum of the normal lymphoid follicle. Both cell types, i.e., the poorly differentiated cleaved lymphocytes and the larger cells which had been termed "histiocytes," are in fact B lymphocytes with identical patterns of immunologic markers. However, although these cells are identical immunologically, they are vastly different kinetically. The large cells (histiocytes) appear to represent the proliferative element within the tumor; as these cells increase in number, the tumor tends to have a more aggressive clinical course (11–13, 85). Thus, a great contribution of the Rappaport classification is the recognition of different clinical and prognostic groups within this disease. However, although the large cells are highly proliferative, for reasons not entirely understood they rarely gain access to the peripheral blood. The small cells (poorly differentiated lymphocytes) better express the migratory capacity of a normal lymphocyte with a great tendency to disseminate to involve bone marrow, liver, and peripheral blood. Patients with nodular lymphoma of the poorly differentiated lymphocytic type often present with generalized adenopathy and widely disseminated disease. However, the cells in this disease are not highly aggressive in terms of either an ability to infiltrate and destroy tissue or a tendency to proliferate rapidly. Thus, nodular lymphoma of this cell type is a disease in which the patient, although presenting with widespread disease, feels well and has a long clinical course.

As we have mentioned, when the cells of nodular lymphoma disseminate, they retain their immunologic markers. Thus, patients with nodular lymphoma and a leukemic blood picture have circulating cells that demonstrate abundant SIg and numerous complement receptors. The disease clinically at this point has been termed lymphosarcoma cell leukemia (86,87) and the cells termed "buttock" cells because of their prominent nuclear indentations. The above pattern of immunologic markers differs from that seen on another B cell malignancy, chronic lymphocytic leukemia (see below), and can be used to distinguish these different cell types in the peripheral blood.

Chronic Lymphocytic Leukemia (CLL) and Diffuse Well-Differentiated Lymphocytic Lymphoma (WDL).   In any clinicopathologic or immunologic review of lymphoreticular malignancy, chronic lymphocytic leukemia (CLL) and diffuse well-differentiated lymphocytic lymphoma (WDL) should be considered together. In fact, these diseases simply represent different clinical presentations and anatomic distributions of the same neoplastic population. In both diseases one sees a proliferation of small, uniform, mature-appearing lymphocytes that infiltrate bone marrow and lymph nodes in a diffuse fashion. Well-differentiated lymphocytic lymphomas with a nodular growth pattern are extremely rare, if they exist at all. These cells, like their normal counterparts, the small lymphocytes, are highly motile and readily gain access to peripheral blood. Thus, the high incidence of CLL in patients with WDL is readily understandable. Likewise, in patients with CLL a blind lymph node biopsy may often show replacement by a monotonous population of small lymphocytes, even though gross adenopathy is not appreciated. It is not understood why these different clinical patterns are present—why in some patients adenopathy is a prominent feature whereas in others peripheral blood and bone marrow involvement predominate. Nevertheless, both diseases have a similar clinical course, which is characteristically indolent with minimal symptomatology.

To date, the immunologic markers expressed on the cells of CLL and WDL are identical (78,88). Nevertheless, at some future time it can be expected that a fine difference in surface structure will be identified that will correlate with the different distributions of the cells of these two related diseases. Nearly all cases studied have been shown to be of B lymphocytic origin. The cells are characterized by the presence of monoclonal SIg, with all cells bearing a single light chain (18,89–96). Although some cases of CLL had been reported as polyclonal (97,98), it is likely that this apparent polyclonality was a spurious result secondary to the adsorption of circulating immune complexes and/or immunoglobulin aggregates via Fc receptors present on the neoplastic cells (99). As stated previously, IgM and IgD coexist on most normal immunoglobulin-bearing peripheral blood lymphocytes (15,16). Similarly, the cells of CLL in most cases also bear both IgM and IgD (79,80,100–102). When these immunoglobulins appear together on either normal or leukemic lymphocytes, they have been shown to be associated with the same light chain. It is speculated that IgD is present as an antigen receptor and is not an immunoglobulin product intended for secretion (15).

The simultaneous presence of IgM and IgD does not contradict the monoclonal nature of the proliferation in CLL. In fact, in those cases so studied, the IgM and IgD proteins were demonstrated to be of the same idiotype and in some cases had the same antibody specificity (80,100,103). In these patients the serum demonstrated an M component (IgM) which permitted the preparation of an antiidiotypic antibody. It is only in these rare cases that the idiotypic specificity of the immunoglobulin can be investigated. However, in other cases of CLL the cell surface immunoglobulins have been demonstrated to be not only of the same class (IgM, IgA or IgG) but also of the same allotype (96). Thus, all evidence points to a monoclonal proliferation of B lymphocytes in CLL and WDL.

As mentioned above, although both CLL and nodular lymphomas are B cell malignancies, the markers found on these cells differ in some respects. The nature and distribution of the SIg identified in CLL and WDL differ from that present in nodular lymphoma. When examined by immunofluorescent techniques, the cells of nodular lymphoma demonstrate abundant immunoglobulin with bright fluorescent spots, "chunks," and frequent spontaneous capping. In contrast, the cells of CLL and WDL consistently demonstrate a very faint staining, and many cells may appear negative, depending on the sensitivity of the technique used (62,78,88).

In addition to the presence of SIg, the cells of CLL and WDL also demonstrate other B cell markers. The cells have receptors for both aggregated IgG (99,104) and C3 (94,105,106). However, the cells of CLL and nodular lymphoma again appear to differ in the nature of their complement receptors. Whereas the cells of nodular lymphoma appear to have abundant complement receptors and will bind EAC readily both in suspension and in tissue sections, the cells of CLL demonstrate an apparent reduction in C3 receptors. In suspension CLL cells form "weak" rosettes with EAC, binding relatively few red cells, and in frozen tissue sections, again because of an apparent deficiency in C3 receptors, binding of EAC does not occur (88). This contrast between these two neoplastic B cell populations can be compared to the cells of normal lymph nodes. When studied by the frozen section rosette technique, the cells of nodular lymphoma resemble follicular B lymphocytes in having strong C3 receptors, whereas the cells of WDL and CLL resemble medullary cord B cells in that only weak or no binding of EAC is observed (76).

There is some evidence that this apparent deficiency of complement receptors on CLL cells is a qualitative rather than a quantitative one. One study has shown that whereas normal peripheral blood B cells have receptors for both EAC43b and EAC43d, lymphocytes from some patients with CLL bind only EAC43d (40). In an EAC reagent prepared with whole mouse serum containing C3 inactivator, the reagent will be a mixture of EAC43b and EAC43d. Thus, it is understandable that this reagent would be bound better by normal lymphocytes with both receptors than by CLL cells with only one. Whether quantitative differences in these receptors also exist remains to be determined. Furthermore, the nature of the specific complement receptors on different subpopulations of normal B lymphocytes or on nodular lymphoma cells is not yet elucidated. It is known that as a B lymphocyte differentiates towards a plasma cell and acquires the ability to secrete immunoglobulin, there is a loss of the complement receptor such that at the plasma cell stage no complement receptors are demonstrable (29). However, whether receptors for EAC43b are lost before receptors for EAC43d in this differentiation process is not known. Such information would, of course, be valuable in identifying precisely the normal equivalent of the CLL cell.

It has been speculated that CLL and WDL represent a block in the maturation of B lymphocytes. According to this hypothesis, these diseases represent more an accumulation of cells than an active neoplastic proliferation. Evidence in support of this hypothesis is the low proliferation of these cells both in vivo and in vitro (107–108). Salmon and Seligmann have speculated that CLL and WDL represent an expansion of the "virgin" B lymphocyte, untouched by antigen (109). Such a cell is immunologically committed and has a specific antigenic receptor on its cell membrane. This specificity would account for the observed monoclonal nature of the cell surface immunoglobulin on CLL cells. However, an alternate and equally acceptable hypothesis is that CLL and WDL represent an expansion of the memory B cell. Information as to the nature of the complement receptors on these different B cell populations might help to pinpoint the normal cell of origin for CLL and WDL. Of course, alternatively, the absence of receptors for EAC43b on CLL cells might merely be a consequence of neoplastic transformation.

Although one can view CLL and WDL as diseases of the secretory arm of the B cell system, the neoplastic equivalent of the medullary cord B lymphocyte (Fig. 1), the capacity for immunosecretion exhibited by most cases is relatively limited. The immunoglobulin determinants are expressed only on the cell membrane, and secretion of Ig into the serum does not occur (110). In fact, most patients with CLL exhibit abnormally low serum immunoglobulin levels, perhaps because there are reduced numbers of normal B cells, or perhaps because of the secretion of suppressor substances or chalones. These patients also commonly exhibit some degree of clinical immunodeficiency when exposed to antigens requiring an antibody response, such as *Pneumococcus* (111). In contrast, patients with nodular or follicular lymphomas, felt to be diseases of the proliferative arm of the B cell system (Fig. 1), do not exhibit serum immunoglobulin abnormalities with any greater frequency than the normal population and do not manifest clinical immunodeficiency.

However, in a low percentage of patients with CLL a small monoclonal serum immunoglobulin spike can be identified (112), and in all cases thus far studied the serum Ig is of the same class and even the same idiotype as the surface Ig. Waldenstrom's macroglobulinemia represents one further step in the differentiation of the medullary cord B lymphocyte toward a plasma cell. In these patients immunosecretion is a more conspicuous phenomenon and the serum demonstrates a large monoclonal spike, again most commonly IgM. In these well-differentiated lymphocytic lymphomas the cells frequently show some plasmacytoid features cytologically and, like normal plasma cells, have less of a tendency than nonsecretory lymphocytes to involve the peripheral blood and produce a frankly leukemic state. Although monoclonal SIg has been identified on the surface of lymphocytes in Waldenstrom's macroglobulinemia (103,113), the presence or absence of complement receptors on these cells has not been determined. C3 receptors have been shown to be absent on myeloma cells (114) and one would predict them to be absent in Waldenstrom's cells as well.

Burkitt's Lymphoma. Burkitt's lymphoma is a tumor with distinctive cytologic and clinical features (115–117).Although the tumor was initially described among African children in Uganda, sporadic cases occur in nonendemic areas, such as the United States, with identical pathologic features. Both clinical differences and similarities exist in the disease as it occurs in African and American patients (116,117). Although Burkitt's lymphoma has been classified cytologically as an undifferentiated lymphoma, in vitro studies have shown the cells to be monoclonal B lymphocytes in a majority of cases (118–121). Receptors for complement have also been demonstrated on tumor cells obtained from the tumor (118). Although the number of American cases studied is relatively small, there has been no difference between the markers present on African and American cases. However, as with other primitive or undifferentiated neoplasms, some cases have demonstrated no surface markers.

It has been suggested that Burkitt's lymphoma is derived from the lymphoid follicle (Fig. 1) (78,122). Although the tumor does not have a nodular growth pattern, in rare instances selective involvement of germinal centers has been seen (118). Furthermore, it seems reasonable to propose an origin from the proliferative arm of the B cell system, since this tumor is recognized to be the most rapidly replicating of all the lymphomas (123).

Acute Lymphoblastic Leukemia (ALL) and Lymphosarcoma of Childhood. The application of membrane surface marker studies to acute lymphoblastic leukemia (ALL) has contributed greatly to our understanding of this disease. Most cases of childhood ALL when examined with an anti-T antiserum can be demonstrated to be antigenically related to T cells (124–127). However, in a majority of such cases the cells do not form E rosettes (128–131); only in about 20 percent can E-rosetting be demonstrated (130,132). Of great interest is that fact that these "E-positive" cases seem consistently to have certain clinical features in common (132,133). These patients are generally older than children with classical ALL and show a preponderance of males. An anterior mediastinal mass can frequently be seen on chest roentgenograms at diagnosis, and these patients tend to present with higher white blood cell counts, often greater than $100,000/mm^3$. These E-positive cases also have been said to have a poorer prognosis, with earlier relapse and a high incidence of meningeal leukemia. Thus the surface marker studies have helped to define a particular subgroup of ALL with unique clinical and prognostic features. It may be that E-positive ALL represents T cell neoplasia at a different stage of differentiation than the more common E-negative cases. It may be appropriate to try different therapeutic approaches in these patients or to investigate different etiologies.

In a very small number of patients with ALL the cells have demonstrated B cell markers (134,135). In one particular series from France (135) the B cell cases also had distinguishing cytologic characteristics. When examined with the May-Grunwald-Giemsa stain the cells had uniformly and deeply basophilic cytoplasm with prominent nucleoli. Small lipid vacuoles were present in the cytoplasm (oil red O-positive), and the cells were usually devoid of PAS-positive material. These cytologic features are all characteristic of Burkitt's lymphoma and are absent in classical ALL. These patients had been treated with the chemotherapeutic regimen used for ALL, as the clinical presentation was that of ALL, but, as one might expect, remission was not achieved. It is encouraging to note that the membrane markers seem to correlate consistently with conventional morphologic criteria and to have prognostic and clinical relevance.

Lymphosarcoma of childhood (LSA) or childhood lymphoblastic lymphoma is closely related clinically, cytologically, and immunologically to "E-positive" ALL. Like E-positive ALL, it occurs in older children and young adults and has a high male-to-female ratio. Such patients frequently have mediastinal masses. It further shares the poor prognosis and aggressive clinical course of E-positive

ALL. As expected, the majority of these cases have demonstrated T cell markers, including both E-rosetting and reactivity with anti-T antisera (136–139). These tumors are also seen to involve preferentially the thymic-dependent portions of the lymphoreticular system (Fig. 1) (78). It may be that E-positive ALL and LSA represent different clinical presentations of the same neoplastic population, a situation analogous to chronic lymphocytic leukemia and well-differentiated lymphocytic lymphoma.

However, the results in one series suggest that the markers in LSA may be more heterogeneous (140). In this series the cells from only one of six cases formed E rosettes exclusively. The cells from three of six patients had receptors for complement but lacked other B cell markers and in one instance also retained T cell markers. Complement receptors have also been demonstrated in other instances of T cell neoplasia (141,142), and it has been speculated that their occurrence may indicate derepression or abnormal differentiation. Of note is the fact that most cases of ALL studied have not been investigated for complement receptors, so that their presence or absence in E-positive ALL is undetermined.

Mycosis Fungoides and Sezary's Syndrome.   Mycosis fungoides and the closely related entity of Sezary's syndrome (SS) are lymphoreticular malignancies apparently primary in the skin (143). In both disorders the cells demonstrate an epidermotropism that is lacking in other lymphomas, even when they do involve the cutis. Although certain clinical and pathological differences exist between Sezary's syndrome and mycosis fungoides, they share many cytologic and immunologic properties. Both of these diseases represent further examples of T cell neoplasia, and in most cases investigated T cell markers, including reactivity with anti-T cell antisera and E rosette formation, have been found (144–146). However, as with many of the lymphoreticular malignancies, some cases exist in which the typical markers were not found (147,148). The neoplastic cells also have certain cytochemical features that appear to be present in normal T cells (149). In addition, Sezary cells seem to share certain of the functional properties of normal T cells, a topic discussed later in this review. As with other of the T cell lymphomas, when visceral involvement occurs, the cells may selectively populate the paracortical areas of lymph nodes and the periarteriolar lymphoid sheaths of the splenic white pulp (150).

There is one other variant of non-Hodgkin's lymphoma that is unclassifiable in the Rappaport scheme (Table 1) and appears to be of T cell type. Although only a limited number of cases have been studied, those examined all have had certain consistent histologic features (151). Normal nodal elements are replaced by a polymorphous diffuse infiltrate composed of atypical lymphocytes admixed with benign-appearing epithelioid histiocytes. Occasional atypical transformed lymphocytes with prominent nucleoli may simulate mononuclear variants of Reed-Sternberg cells, although classical binucleate cells are not observed. The polymorphous pattern may also suggest Hodgkin's disease at initial examination; however, the pronounced atypia of the lymphoid population rules out this diagnosis. The neoplastic lymphocytes consistently demonstrate T cell markers (151). It has been speculated that perhaps the accumulation of histiocytes in these lesions results from the production of macrophage migration inhibition factor by the neoplastic T cells (151).

Non-Hodgkin's lymphomas with a histologic pattern similar to that described above have been described by Lennert and further studied by Scheurlen (152,153), although none of these cases was studied for surface markers. These tumors were initially described as a variant of Hodgkin's disease but later appreciated to be non-Hodgkin's lymphomas. They occur in adults and involve sites unusual for Hodgkin's disease, such as Waldeyer's ring and epitrochlear lymph nodes. A conspicuous feature has been the presence of epithelioid histiocytes in cords and nests admixed with a population of atypical lymphocytes. The epithelioid cell component appears to be lost as the disease progresses. These patients frequently have hyperglobulinemia, the polyclonal nature of which suggests that it is reactive rather than a product of the neoplastic population.

Histiocytic Lymphoma (Reticulum Cell Sarcoma).   The term "histiocytic" lymphoma has been applied to a broad group of non-Hodgkin's lymphomas with certain clinical and pathological features in common (85). They usually grow in a diffuse fashion and are composed of large cells with abundant cytoplasm, vesicular nuclei, and prominent nucleoli. They were termed "histiocytic" because the neoplastic cells share certain morphologic features with benign histiocytes (10), although functional evidence that they are histiocytes is lacking. They are characterized by an aggressive clinical course, but morphologically as well as clinically they seem to be a heterogeneous group of neoplasms.

Very few tumors of this type have been investigated immunologically, but the existing data suggest that they represent a common morphologic end point for transformed cells of diverse origins. Transformed lymphocytes of either B or T cell type, termed "immunoblasts" by Dameshek in 1963 (154), greatly resemble the cells of histiocytic lymphoma. Furthermore, their morphologic counterparts are sometimes observed in lymphomas established to be of lymphoid origin, such as nodular lymphoma. However, most cases of histiocytic lymphoma occurring *de novo* when studied have had no surface markers (78,155). Most likely these very dedifferentiated neoplasias have lost the membrane characteristics as well as the functional properties of the cells of origin. For example, it is noted that these tumors fail to demonstrate the homing patterns seen with "better-differentiated" lymphomas (78). A B cell origin has been postulated for most histiocytic lymphomas or reticulum cell sarcomas on the basis of increased immunoglobulins found in tumor extracts (156), but immunoglobulin production has not been demonstrated by tumor cells, nor has cell-associated immunoglobulin been identified in the majority of cases (78,155).

An exception to the absence of markers on the cells of diffuse histiocytic lymphoma is those cases occurring as a progression of a malignant lymphoma which does bear surface markers. In those instances the histiocytic lymphoma usually retains the markers of the better-differentiated lesion. This phenomenon has been seen in nodular lymphoma (78) and in chronic lymphocytic leukemia (157), where it is known clinically as Richter's syndrome (158). Furthermore, in cases of CLL undergoing this "blastic transformation" the histiocytic lymphomas have retained the same heavy and light chain as the preexisting CLL, indicating that they are most likely of the same clone (159).

Leukemic Reticuloendotheliosis (Hairy Cell Leukemia).   Hairy cell leukemia is a disorder characterized by chronic course, marked splenomegaly at the time of presentation, and the proliferation of characteristic mononuclear cells in the spleen, lymph nodes, bone marrow, and peripheral blood (160). The cells were termed "hairy" because of prominent cytoplasmic projections seen on air-dried smear preparations (161). The term "leukemia" is something of a misnomer, since these patients usually do not demonstrate a leukocytosis, and only occasional abnormal cells are present in the peripheral blood, especially prior to splenectomy (162). The origin of abnormal cells has been in dispute, largely because of their apparent hybrid nature. They have some features suggestive of a B lymphocytic origin, such as the presence of surface immunoglobulin demonstrated to be monoclonal in some instances (93,163–167), and complement receptors in one series (163). However, other features suggest a monocytic or histiocytic origin, such as their preferential localization in the spleen to the cords of Billroth. The cells also resemble monocytes cytochemically (168) and in scanning electron micrographs (169). Additional histio/monocytic features in some reported cases include a strong receptor for cytophilic antibody (46) and demonstrated phagocytic capacity for small particulate material (170). They may originate from a cell type present normally in very low numbers and not yet identified, or they may represent a hybrid induced by neoplasia. Indeed, different patients with this clinical entity may have abnormal cells with different surface characteristics.

Malignant Histiocytosis (Histiocytic Medullary Reticulosis) (171).   The clinical aggressiveness of this generally rapidly fatal disorder is in part due to the retention of function by the neoplastic cells. These patients frequently manifest rapidly progressive pancytopenia and jaundice attributed to the phagocytosis of normal blood elements by the malignant cells. The neoplastic histiocytes also retain certain membrane markers characteristic of histiocytes, having strong receptors for cytophilic antibody (151). However, these cells apparently lack a complement receptor (151). As discussed above, although complement receptors are easily demonstrable on peripheral blood monocytes, their presence and/or nature is less well established on tissue mononuclear phagocytic cells (41,46). The cells are also seen to populate areas normally occupied by histiocytes, such as the splenic cords of Billroth, lymph node sinuses, and sinusoids of the liver (Fig. 1).

Hodgkin's Disease.   In all of the above LRM the study of membrane surface markers has been conducted on the neoplastic population directly. However, in the lesions of Hodgkin's disease (HD) one sees a mixture of cytologically abnormal cells (the Reed-Sternberg cells and their mononuclear variants) admixed with apparently normal reactive elements. This coexistence of a neoplastic and reactive population has been supported by DNA-content analysis of HD cells, in which both aneuploid and diploid populations are identified (172). As a consequence, numerical data with regard to the presence of surface membrane markers on the cells isolated from HD lesions do not give direct data as to the markers present on the neoplastic cells. One must combine morphological analysis with any marker studies to identify the characteristics of the atypical cells. Furthermore, it has been found that Reed-Sternberg cells are difficult to isolate from HD lesions (173,174), perhaps because of fragility of these cells as well as fibrosis within the lesions.

For all of the above reasons there are very few direct data regarding the markers on the abnormal cells of HD. Two observers using immunoperoxidase sandwich techniques (28,175) have reported immunoglobulin within the cytoplasm of Reed-Sternberg cells. In one instance the immunoglobulin was of the IgG class and could be demonstrated to be monoclonal (176). In a second report, however, although some cases did appear to be monoclonal, other cases were found in which cells apparently contained both kappa and lambda light chains (175). In both of the above studies the authors interpret their findings as indicating a B cell origin for Reed-Sternberg cells. Immunoglobulin bound to the surface of Reed-Sternberg cells has also been reported and interpreted as indicative of a B cell origin (173). However, the mere presence of membrane-associated Ig does not necessarily mean that the cell is a B lymphocyte. A variety of cell types, including mononuclear phagocytes (44), activated T lymphocytes (22), and malignant cells of both epithelial and mesodermal origin (23), have receptors for the Fc portion of IgG. Furthermore, binding of IgGEA by Reed-Sternberg cells has been demonstrated, suggesting the presence of an Fc receptor (177), and thus the observed immunoglobulin might be passively adsorbed in vivo or in vitro. Finally, in theory any neoplastic cell can bear surface immunoglobulin as a consequence of an autoantibody directed against tumor-associated antigens. Thus, to prove a B cell origin one must rule out passive binding of immunoglobulin and ideally must demonstrate synthesis of immunoglobulin.

Other studies performed on HD lesions have concerned themselves with the identification of the reactive elements associated with the malignant cells. All but one report found an increased number of T cells in cell suspensions prepared from tumorous lesions (174,178,179). In one study no such increase could be demonstrated when results were compared with results obtained on the patients' peripheral blood (180). However, it should be noted that peripheral blood normally contains a predominance of T cells (approx. 70%), whereas splenic suspensions usually contain an equal or greater number of B cells (76). Thus, the results of this latter study apparently do reflect an increase in splenic T cells in these HD patients. It also appears cytologically that there is an interaction between these T lymphocytes and the neoplastic cells. In suspensions prepared from HD lesions the lymphocytes have been observed to be tightly bound to the atypical cells (181), and these adherent cells have been shown to be T cells, as evidenced by their ability to form E rosettes (174,182). The significance of this observation will be discussed later.

It appears that the residual B cell population may also play a role in the host's reaction to the neoplastic process, and, as one would expect with a humoral immune process, the response is seen distant from and not within the HD lesions. The presence of follicular hyperplasia is a well-recognized phenomenon in lymph nodes adjacent to or partially involved by HD, as well as in spleens obtained from patients with HD. Furthermore, one study has demonstrated increased IgG synthesis in uninvolved splenic tissue from patients with HD (183). These findings are discussed in greater detail in the next section of this chapter, in which the functional studies of HD are reviewed.

Conclusion.   As one can discern from the above discussion, immunologic studies to date have answered many questions about the origin and function of neoplastic lymphoreticular cells. Some of these data have already been shown to be of clinical and prognostic relevance, as in the subclassification of acute lymphocytic leukemia based on E-rosetting. It is also anticipated that these studies of neoplastic lymphoid cells will reveal new information regarding the normal cells of the immune system. For example, although both chronic lymphocytic leukemia and nodular lymphoma are B cell neoplasms, they appear to represent proliferations of different subclasses of B cells. It is expected that observations made on the neoplastic cells may have relevance for their normal counterparts.

As a consequence of these preliminary studies some authors have offered new classification schemes based on functional and immunologic concepts (122,184,185). Although some of these concepts are certainly valid, there are insufficient data to subclassify all the lymphomas according to their origin and function. Areas in which surface marker studies are particularly needed include the diffuse lymphomas of both poorly differentiated lymphocytic and large-cell or histiocytic type. It is hoped that as more cases are studied consistent immunologic observations will be made which can be correlated with histology, clinical course, and response to therapy. Only at that point would revision of current clinical relevant classification schemes be appropriate.

Numerous other processes are examined by the pathologist in which the nature of the lymphoid proliferation is not fully understood. Examples are the recently described angioimmunoblastic lymphadenopathy (186,187), lymphoepithelioma of the nasopharynx, and numerous instances of "atypical" lymphoid hyperplasia. It is anticipated that the application of immunologic studies may delineate the nature of the immune response in these cases, as well as its benignancy or malignancy.

FUNCTIONAL STUDIES

During the past ten years a variety of different types of functional studies have been performed on the mononuclear cells of patients with a number of different types of lymphomas. These studies can be grouped in two general classes. In the first type of study peripheral blood mononuclear cells were examined in patients in whom these circulating mononuclear cell populations were composed of normal cells. Patients with Hodgkin's disease, for example, would fall into this category. The second type of functional studies were performed in patients in whom the great majority of the circulating cells were malignant. Patients with acute and chronic lymphatic leukemia and patients with the Sezary syndrome fall into this latter category. The interpretation of the results of such functional studies therefore depends on whether the cell populations being studied are nonmalignant, predominantly malignant, or, as quite often is the case, a mixture of malignant and nonmalignant cells.

The types of functional studies performed in patients mirror to some extent the currently fashionable immunologic studies being performed by immunologists studying the various activities of normal lymphocyte populations. Thus, for example, at a time when stimulation of normal lymphocytes by lectins such as phytohemagglutinin (PHA) was in the mode, such studies were soon after performed on the lymphocytes from patients with lymphomas. At a somewhat later time when determination of B and T cells or mixed lymphocyte reactivity became the rage, similar studies were soon undertaken with malignant lymphoid cell populations.

Functional studies of this type can answer a number of different questions. For example, patients with Hodgkin's disease and non-Hodgkin's lymphomas have clinically apparent immunologic deficits (188–190). It was therefore expected that such deficits could be explored by study of in vitro lymphocyte activation. Questions as to whether the lymphocytes of such patients have intrinsic defects or whether there are serum factors in these patients which inhibit lymphocyte activity could be expected to be answered by such in vitro studies.

Certain functions have been ascribed to certain types of normal lymphoid cells. The identification of such a function or its lack in a population of malignant lymphoid cells would thus serve as an independent parameter in the determination of the origin of a particular malignant cell population. For example, a type of in vitro lymphocyte-mediated cytotoxicity has been described in which normal, nonimmunized lymphoid cells can kill antibody-coated target cells. This functional test is named antibody-dependent cellular cytotoxicity (ADCC) (191,192). There is unanimous agreement that non-T cells mediate this in vitro cytotoxicity; many observations suggest that the cell responsible is a subclass of B cells (192,193). If, for example, a malignant cell population of unknown type were capable of displaying this in vitro capacity, this could be strong evidence that the malignant cells were of B cell origin.

Functional studies of lymphoid cells may also provide insights into the pathophysiology of a particular disease state. For example, patients with Hodgkin's disease often itch, patients with the Sezary syndrome have erythroderma. Can these clinical manifestations be explained by supernormal production by malignant cells of certain lymphokines?

Another facet of functional studies of the malignant cells of the lymphoid system is the fact that each malignant cell population may represent a clonal expansion of a particular class of lymphoid cells. That is, normal lymphoid cell populations perform a rather large number of immunologic functions. At present it is not certain that each function is performed by a single cell type at a particular stage of differentiation, whether the same lymphocyte can perform many different functions, or whether different sublines of lymphocytes each perform a separate function. In addition, the intimate molecular bases for these diverse functions are almost entirely unknown. The functions of T cells are at present the most mysterious of all (194). Each malignant population of cells, and especially T cells and their products, therefore represents a possible gold mine of information waiting to be harvested. In the same way, fifteen years ago, the harvesting and examination of the product of malignant plasma cells —immunoglobulin—led directly to our present understanding of immunoglobulin structure and function. Examination of the abnormal always reveals important truths concerning normal function. Finally, in this regard some aspect of the normal or abnormal functioning of lymphoid cells may provide clues as to the prognosis, therapy, and management of this class of disease.

In this short review it will not be possible to cover the entire literature on this subject. Rather, selected topics will be dealt with, and only certain examples of a particular type of study will be presented. Emphasis will be placed on newer developments, and only studies in humans will be discussed.

First, we will briefly discuss the immunologic deficits found in patients with Hodgkin's disease (HD). This disease has been the most extensively studied (195–199). One reason for the intense interest in HD is that certain of its clinical aspects suggest that autoimmune mechanisms and lymphocyte civil wars may be part of the disease process (200,201). Kaplan and Smithers (202) and Green et al. (203) pointed out a number of years ago the similarities between HD and experimentally induced graft-versus-host reactions in animals leading to the runting syndrome. These ideas have again become fashionable. In both Hodgkin's disease and the runting syndrome, wasting, fever, autoimmune hemolytic anemia, and leukopenia may be observed. Patients with HD also manifest certain immunologic deficits. It was noted first that patients with HD were susceptible to those infectious diseases related to cell-mediated immunity. The ability to produce antibody after immunization and the level of natural antibodies were found to be relatively normal (197). These patients, when tested for their ability to form delayed reactions to common bacterial antigens or contact sensitizers, were found deficient; their ability to reject skin allografts was also impaired. Attempts to passively transfer delayed sensitivity to these patients with lymphocytes from sensitized donors also failed (204). There is a rough correlation between the extent and duration of disease in these patients and the degree of impairment.

To further explore these immunologic deficits a large number of studies of the in vitro behavior of peripheral blood lymphocytes from patients with HD were undertaken. The first studies, started about ten years ago, used mitogens such as PHA or bacterial, viral, and fungal antigens to which natural exposure had occurred. It is now recognized that the T lymphocyte is the predominant cell type that proliferates in response to PHA and the above antigens. The general conclusion from these in vitro studies was that the degree of proliferation induced by these agents is impaired in patients with HD. These defects can be observed in patients with limited disease and prior to any therapy (199), a phenomenon not often observed in non-Hodgkin's lymphomas. Furthermore, there is rough correlation between the stage of disease and the degree of impairment of these in vitro functions (195). Cells taken from patients in remission often show some degree of reversal of the in vitro defect (195). In the majority of the cases studied, serum factors did not appear to be the reason for the in vitro deficit. That is, cells from HD patients grown in normal sera did not have a restoration to normal function, and cells from normal individuals grown in the presence of serum from patients with HD did not have an impairment of in vitro proliferation (189). However, such inhibitory factors have been described in some patients with HD (205); in other studies, antibodies to lymphocytes have also been detected in a large percentage of patients with HD (206). A related study by Longmire demonstrated increased IgG production in the spleens of patients with HD; furthermore, this IgG had an affinity for homologous lymphocytes (183). Of interest is a recent report that demonstrates that the response of splenic lymphocytes of patients with HD to PHA may be normal, despite the fact that the PHA responsiveness of the peripheral blood lymphocytes in the same patients is defective (207).

Recently other immunologic assays have been performed on lymphocytes from patients with HD. One example is the widely used mixed-leukocyte reaction (MLR), in which peripheral blood leukocytes are mixed with leukocytes from an allogeneic individual. Because of the differences between the cell-surface antigens, lymphocyte proliferation occurs. It is generally accepted that the proliferating cells are predominantly T lymphocytes. The nature of the stimulating cell is less well established. In the commonly performed one-way MLR the stimulating cells are blocked from proliferation by radiation or mitomycin-C. In studies on the peripheral blood cells of patients with HD there appears to be some impairment of MLR. In one report on one-way MLR, lymphocytes from patients with HD did not respond but acted normally as antigenic targets for normal allogeneic lymphocytes (208). In another study the lymphocytes from patients with HD failed to act as stimulator cells in MLR (209). Another example of appliction of newer immunologic techniques to these problems is a recent report in which the PB lymphocytes of patients with HD fail to cap normally with fluorescein-labeled Con A (210).

In addition, certain mediators have been studied in the sera and cell supernatants of patients with HD. The production of mononuclear cell chemotactic factor in response to PHA was found to be normal in the lymphocytes of patients with Hodgkin's disease, despite the fact that DNA incorporation was impaired (211). The exact reason for this dissociation is not known. It is also of interest in relationship to the above study that an inactivator of neutrophil and monocyte chemotactic factor has been found in the sera of patients with HD (212). Whether the presence of this material has the in vivo effect of inactivating chemotactic factor and thereby reducing the degree of inflammation to infectious agents remains to be determined. Finally, in this regard, elevated levels of MIF have been found in the sera of patients with HD as well as other LRM (213) and the Sezary syndrome (214). The presence of elevated levels of serum MIF would tend to destroy the gradient between MIF concentrations in the tissues and the blood and would theoretically also impair trapping of monocytes in tissues, with a resultant impairment of normal imflammatory mechanisms.

Since the cell chiefly responsible for the in vitro responses to mitogens and antigens studied above is the T lymphocyte, it is certainly possible that any decrease in the in vitro responses observed is due to a decreased frequency of these cells in the peripheral blood of patients with HD.

The number of B and T lymphocytes in the peripheral blood of patients with Hodgkin's disease has been the subject of several reports (126,215–219). The percentage of T cells has been reported to be decreased in several studies (215,216,219). The percentage of B cells has been found to be normal in one study (218) and increased in two studies (126,216).

It should be recognized that the presence of lymphocytotoxic antibodies (206) and other antibodies in the sera of patients with HD may interfere with some of the tests used for B and T cell enumeration. For example, the number of B cells may appear to be elevated because T lymphocytes could be coated with these antibodies and therefore appear positive when stained with antiimmunoglobulin antisera. Conversely, if the sheep cell rosette technique (E-rosette technique) is used to detect T cells, this test may be interfered with by antibodies coating the surface of these T cells. In such an example the number of T cells determined by the use of fluoresceinated heterologous anti-T cell antibodies may be considerably higher than the number of T cells as measured by the E rosette technique. As can be seen, a variety of techniques may have to be used simultaneously to arrive at a correct answer to these questions. In the great majority of the in vitro functional studies performed to date on the lymphocytes of patients with HD, no concomitant study was done on the absolute number of T cells present in these in vitro test systems. In the future this type of study should be performed.

There is a rough correlation between the in vivo defects in delayed hypersensitivity or contact reactivity in patients with HD and the in vitro defects in these patients. Since the weight of evidence favors a predominant role for the T lymphocyte in both the in vivo and the in vitro reactivities, this overall result is not surprising. However, since the full molecular details of mitogen and antigen interactions with normal immunologically competent cells is unknown, it would be presumptuous to make judgments as to the nature of the defect in the immunologic machinery of the HD patient. However, if one is forced to speculate, a number of suggestions can be made.

First, the normal immunologic interactions between T cells, B cells, and macrophages may be interfered with because of the disordered architecture within the organs in which these interactions normally occur—namely, the lymph nodes and spleens of these patients. Second, the T lymphocytes may be already stimulated by and precommitted to tumor-specific or viral antigens; therefore, such lymphocytes could not be further stimulated to proliferate in response to other antigens or mitogens in vitro, since they were already proliferating in vivo. Third, their function could be interfered with by virtue of their being infected by an unknown virus. It is well known that the lymphocytes of patients with measles are also incapable of displaying many in vitro functions (220). Finally, an increase in number of a class of T lymphocytes (suppressor cells) could be present which would interfere with normal T or B cell functions. Potential serum inhibitory factors, although present in the form of antibodies directed against lymphocytes (as mentioned above), do not appear to play the major role in the inhibition of in vitro functions observed in these lymphocyte populations. Certainly all of these defects are seen in other patients with malignancy (both LRM and LRM type) and also in patients with benign but widespread granulomatous involvement of lymph nodes (sarcoid) (221). Whether the defects in all these patients will be similar remains to be determined.

As mentioned in the introduction to this section, in vitro studies of lymphocytes from the peripheral blood of patients with HD are done primarily on nonneoplastic cells. In the next section we will discuss functional studies of the lymphocytes of patients in whom a large percentage of the peripheral blood cells being studied are malignant.

The in vivo immunologic defects in patients with CLL are different than in patients with HD (222–227). These patients have relatively intact capacity for the elicitation of delayed hypersensitivity reactions to naturally occurring bacterial, viral, and fungal antigens, as well as a relatively intact capacity to respond to contact reactivity induced by the chemically reactive hapten dinitrochlorobenzene. However, they have a marked impairment in their ability to form circulating antibody after injection of antigens. In contrast to the situation in HD, the in vitro studies of peripheral blood lymphocytes of patients with CLL (especially if the white blood cell counts are markedly elevated) are being performed on the malignant cells themselves.

These cells show a marked impairment of the proliferative response to the mitogen PHA and the antigen PPD (222,227–229). There has been some controversy as to whether the small residual, delayed-in-time proliferation observed in these studies is due to the minor contamination by normal lymphocytes or whether CLL lymphocytes have some small ability to respond (230–232). Since the results of experiments in which small numbers of normal lymphocytes in vitro are exposed to mitogens or antigens show the same type of delayed and low-level response as seen in the blood of patients with CLL, it is concluded by several investigators that the responses actually observed in CLL blood are due to the presence of small numbers of normal lymphocytes (231,233). The apparent inability of CLL cells themselves to respond in vitro is in keeping with the fact that they represent malignant populations of B cells, and, as will be discussed in more detail later, normal B cells also are deficient in their capacity to respond in vitro to PHA or antigens (234–237). Also of relevance in this regard are two recent reports demonstrating that CLL cells have fewer binding sites for PHA and Con A than do normal peripheral blood lymphocytes (238,239). Unfortunately, the number of Con A and PHA binding sites on normal human B cells was not examined; therefore, it is not known whether the decreased number of sites on CLL cells is a peculiar feature of these malignant cells or is also a feature of normal B cells. Another possible explanation for the inability of CLL cells to respond in vitro to mitogens is a recently described inhibitor of transformation in the sera and cells of patients with malignancies (240). Such a factor has also been reported to be present in the sera and cell extracts of patients with CLL (241).

More recently other functional tests of lymphocyte reactivity have been developed and applied to CLL cells. These include the ability of lymphocytes to produce lymphokines in vitro, to be stimulated to proliferate in response to foreign lymphoid cells or to act as an antigenic stimulant for the proliferation of allogeneic cells, and to circulate from the blood to the lymph. Finally, lymphoid cells in vitro can exert by several different mechanisms cytotoxic effects on various types of target cells (242).

The capacity of CLL cells to perform in the above assays will be briefly described. CLL cells have been demonstrated to be incapable of responding to allogeneic cells in MLR (227) and they have a diminished capacity to act as stimulator cells in MLR (233). CLL cells also show an inability to recirculate from the blood to the lymph (243), but whether this is specific for CLL cells, or whether normal B cells also recirculate poorly as compared to T cells, has not been established. This inability of CLL cells to circulate from the blood to the lymph may be due to the decreased deformability of B cells as compared to T cells (244).

A number of different in vitro models of lymphocyte-mediated cytotoxicity exist. In one model, normal lymphocytes (from unimmunized animals) can interact with and kill antibody-coated target cells. The effector lymphocyte in this particular in vitro model is a non-T cell, and there is considerable evidence that the effector cell is a subclass of B lymphocyte (192,193).

In one study in which CLL cells were tested for their ability to perform in this assay, they were found to be defective (245). Whether this defect reflects some disorder of function in these neoplastic cells or whether the CLL cells arose from a subclass of normal B cells which normally are incapable of mediating this reaction is still uncertain. A further study of additional patients with CLL may answer this question; if effector CLL cells are found and their function analyzed, this may greatly accelerate our understanding of normal lymphocyte-mediated cytotoxicity.

Other aspects of the function of CLL cells currently being explored in detail are the synthesis, assembly, and secretion of the surface immunoglobulin of these cells (246). The nature of the SIg on CLL cells as well as its idiotypic restrictions has been discussed above.

The cells of another lymphocytic malignancy that have been examined recently are those of patients with Sezary syndrome (SS) and mycosis fungoides. As discussed above, in contrast to the B cell origin of CLL, the Sezary cell is derived from thymus-derived or T cells. Normal T cells have a number of different functions, including the ability to produce a variety of lymphokines in vitro, to stimulate and be stimulated in MLR, to be stimulated by certain mitogens, to act as helper cells for antibody production, and to act as killer cells in certain in vitro models of lymphocyte-mediated cytotoxicity. The malignant T cells in this disease can also be examined for some of these same capabilities.

At the outset it can be said that the responses of the cells of individual patients with this disease are quite heterogeneous. Thus, in studies for mitogen responsiveness (PHA and Concanavalin A) the cells of some patients failed to respond, while the cells of other patients responded, although in some cases to a lesser degree (146,147). In one study the cells from seven patients were examined for both mitogen responsiveness and function in the MLR (146). Those patients whose cells responded to mitogens also responded to stimulation by allogeneic normal lymphocytes. Cells from two out of three of these patients could also act normally as stimulator cells in MLR; however, the cells of one patient failed to stimulate normal allogeneic cells in MLR. The failure of these particular cells to stimulate in MLR is of great interest, since these cells contained HL-A antigens, as judged by their ability to be lysed by HL-A typing sera. These results, therefore, independently confirm the ideas obtained from genetic studies in HL-A recombinant families, that the HL-A antigens are not themselves the cell surface antigens which are recognized and reacted to in MLR (247).

Lymphotoxin, thought to be produced by T cells, is a lymphokine which can cause damage to target cells in vitro (248). Cells of four patients with SS were studied for their ability to produce this lymphokine after mitogen stimulation, and in each case lymphokine production was very low as compared to control cells (249). Another lymphokine produced by normal lymphocytes in response to antigen is blastogenic factor. Normal lymphocytes exposed to this factor are stimulated to proliferate. The abnormal lymphocytes of three patients with the Sezary syndrome failed to be stimulated by blastogenic factor (249).

Both B and T lymphocytes can produce macrophage migration inhibition factor (MIF). The in vitro ability to produce this lymphokine has been extensively correlated with the in vivo state of delayed hypersensitivity both in animals and in man. Furthermore, injection of MIF into the skin of experimental animals can elicit a reaction with a time course and histology which are quite similar to delayed hypersensitivity reactions (250). MIF activity is also found in the sera of immunized mice and guinea pigs after intravenous challenge with antigens (251). It is, therefore, of great interest that in two separate studies MIF was found in all the sera of all patients with SS (214,249). Furthermore, MIF activity could be obtained from the supernatants of Sezary cells incubated in vitro (214). Whether the apparent increased MIF production by these cells is responsible for the erythroderma observed in these patients is uncertain. An increased number of macrophages in the skin of these patients, which might be expected if such a theory is correct, is not actually observed. Furthermore, MIF is found in the sera of patients with other lymphoproliferative diseases in which erythroderma is not a clinical feature (213).

Although it is well established that T cells cooperate with B cells and macrophages to allow for the differentiation of B cells to plasma cells and for antibody production, the precise mode of action of T cells is unknown. A recent experiment performed by Broder and Waldman is most provocative in this regard. The lymphoid cells of normal individuals can be stimulated in vitro by pokeweed mitogen (PWM) to produce immunoglobulin. In a similar system the cells of a patient with severe combined immunodeficiency disease failed to do so. However, when admixed in vitro with Sezary cells and PWM, a marked augmentation of immunoglobulin production was observed (252). Normal T cells also demonstrate this function, suggesting that a factor was produced in large amounts by the abnormal T cells which could restore normal function to defective B cells. These data suggest that these abnormal T cells can act as helper T cells in terms of immunoglobulin production.

Conversely, it has been demonstrated that the T cells of certain patients with hypogammaglobulinemia can interfere with the secretion of immunoglobulin by normal B cells in in vitro systems (253). It can be expected that future functional studies of cells of patients with certain T cell lymphomas may demonstrate the same type of suppressor function. It is obvious that further analysis of these factors may provide a clue as to the treatment of patients with hypogammaglobulinemia. Taken as a whole, these preliminary studies of the function of these malignant T cells are quite exciting; however, the precise basis for the failure of certain T cell functions in this disease is uncertain.

Also, the final interpretation and understanding of all the above facts regarding the functions of malignant lymphoid cells is beclouded by the fact that there is a mountain of sometimes conflicting data and no unanimous agreement among immunologists concerning the precise roles of the normal lymphocytes of different classes with regard to these functions.

Two brief examples in this regard can be given. First, although in MLR in humans and animals the T cell is regarded as the cell that responds, the cell type that acts as the stimulator is less clear. At first it was assumed that in humans the T cell also acted as the stimulator cell. However, as purer populations of cells were employed, it was found that macrophages or adherent cells were necessary for the reaction (254–258). In one study, macrophages were ten times more efficient than any other cell (258). It was also learned that B cells stimulate even better than T cells. Platelets and neutrophils appear to be ineffective stimulators (258). However, skin cells and sperm cells do appear to stimulate in human MLR (259).

The interpretation of some of the results of MLR is also made difficult because of the following. The target cells are often X-irradiated or treated with mitomycin so that they will not proliferate in such reactions. However, it was not always fully appreciated that such blocked target cells could under some circumstances recognize the responder cells and produce blastogenic factors that in turn stimulated the responder cells. Thus, the responder cells in these instances proliferated, but not necessarily because they recognized and responded to the target stimulator cells (260,261). The current feeling is that B cells and macrophages are better stimulators in human MLR than T cells. Among nonlymphoid cells only skin and sperm are effective stimulators. Investigations of which nonmalignant cells are most effective as stimulators in human MLR are still being actively pursued.

The second example of the current uncertainties besetting immunologists is the question of exactly which cells, and under what circumstances, are stimulated by the most commonly used mitogens, PHA, Concanavalin A (Con A), and PWM. Although a few years ago this matter appeared to be settled—i.e., PHA and Con A stimulated only T cells, and PWM could stimulate both types of cells (262)—it is again the subject for renewed controversy. In part the reason is that newer techniques are being applied to old problems. For example, it has been recently reported that pure human B cells, eluted from a column containing antihuman Fab antibodies, could be stimulated by both PHA and Con A (235). In contrast to these findings another study reported that when pure human B cells were obtained by removing E-rosetted T cells from a mixed population, these B cells failed to respond to PHA, Con A, and PWM (236).

Again the interpretation of results in such studies is rendered difficult by the problems in preparing ultrapure populations of either monocytes, B cells, or T cells; the manipulations used in the purification procedures may alter the function of the cells obtained. Also, when mixtures of cells are used, the mitogen-stimulated cells (even if present in very small numbers) can produce blastogenic factors that can induce stimulation of bystander cells. Finally, PWM is a complex mixture of materials, and it has been shown that separate fractions of PWM can affect different cell populations (263). One of the great possible advantages of studying malignant populations of cells for these functions is that a sufficient quantity of homogeneous cells can be obtained for a more definitive study of the receptors and surface components involved in some of these interactions.

Two additional aspects of lymphocyte function can be applied and are relevant to studies of human LRM. The first has to do with receptors for virus on lymphocytes of different classes. Two separate studies have now demonstrated that only B lymphocytes have receptors for Epstein-Barr virus (EBV) (264,265). This is of particular interest, since the malignant cell of Burkitt's lymphoma, a disease thought to be closely associated with EBV, is in fact a B lymphocyte. Whether this is a coincidence or whether there is an increased susceptibility for malignant transformation of those cells bearing these viral receptors remains to be seen. Also, in a recent study of latent infection of mice with murine cytomegalovirus, it was noted that this virus could only be reactivated in vitro from B lymphocytes but not from T lymphocytes (266). Other recent evidence including functional studies suggests that T lymphocytes may have receptors for certain strains of myxovirus (267) including measles virus (220,268).

The second aspect of lymphocyte function that is currently being actively pursued has to do with the relationship between the histocompatibility alloantigenic structures on the surface of lymphoid cells and the function of these cells in recognition of foreign antigens. A large amount of information indicates that in several animal species there are immune response genes (Ir genes) that control the responses to a large number of naturally occuring antigens as well as to synthetic polyamino acid antigens, (269–271). These Ir genes are genetically linked to genes that control the presence of alloantigens on the surface of cells. The two species that have been most intensively analyzed in this regard are the mouse (272) and the guinea pig (273).

In the mouse the genetic region concerned is the H2 histocompatibility complex in the IX linkage group on the 17 chromosome. Here a series of genes have been identified which control cell surface alloantigens. These alloantigens are grouped into two general kinds, called the K and D series. The antigens of this series have a molecular weight (MW) of 40,000 and are associated with a smaller 11,000 MW (B₂ microglobulin). These alloantigens are found on all the cells of any animal (272,274). The Ia antigens are another class of cell surface antigens closely linked genetically to the K and D antigens. These have a lower MW and are found in highest density on B lymphocytes and at a lower density on T lymphocytes; many other tissues have no detectable Ia antigens (274). Studies performed in congenic recombinant mice demonstrate that the Ir genes are most closely linked with the Ia antigens. Genes in these same region also determine mixed lymphocyte reactivities in the mouse. In the human, alloantigens equivalent to the K and D series of the mouse also exist. These determine cell surface histocompatibility antigens and are called the La and four series of antigens (275). In addition, another genetic locus exists in humans controlling MLR reactivities (247). Antisera to these MLR loci are now becoming available.

The connection between the above and the subject of human LRM is that it is highly likely that the uniform populations of malignant cells that can be obtained from these tumors may have a restricted number or type of such MLR-locus antigens. It is known, for example, that different Ia antigens may be expressed on B and T cells (274). The availability of such cell populations will thus become highly useful for a number of different types of study. For example, complex sera can be absorbed with such cells so as to produce sera of more limited specificity. The cell surface antigenic structure of these malignant cells can also be studied by surface radioiodination, solubilization of membrane proteins, reaction with specific antibodies, and polyacrylamide gel electrophoresis (PAGE).

A demonstration of the usefulness of these techniques is to be found in a paper by Wernet and Kunkel (276). In this study selected lupus sera were found to be powerful inhibitors of the MLR. When these sera were used to precipitate radioactive lymphocyte surface extracts, which were then separated by PAGE, a number of different peaks were seen, indicating the sera contained a number of different antibodies. When these sera were absorbed with B lymphocytes and platelets, the sera still inhibited the MLR, and when the separation was repeated, a single peak appeared on the PAGE of MW 15,000. This same peak was found on thymocytes but not on B lymphocytes. The authors conclude that the 15,000 MW component on the T cell is involved in the recognition phase of MLR.

It is possible that a combination of such functional studies and immunochemically analytic studies can be even more fruitfully performed on cell membrane antigens of selected malignant cell populations, with the expectation of the identification of the structures responsible for a variety of immunologic functions as well as the chemical identification and isolation of tumor-specific transplantation antigens.

ACKNOWLEDGMENTS

The authors wish to thank Dr. Costan Berard and Dr. Hartmut Ruhl for helpful discussions and comments concerning this manuscript.

REFERENCES

1. Rappaport, H., Winter, W. J., and Hicks, E. B., *Cancer* **9**, 792 (1956).
2. Lukes, R. J., Butler, J. J., and Hicks, E. B., *Cancer* **19**, 317 (1966).
3. Mellman, W. J., and Rawnsley, H. M., *Fed. Proc.* **25**, 1720 (1966).
4. Roitt, I. M., Greaves, M. F., Torrigiani, G., Brostoff, J., and Playfair, J. H. L., *Lancet* **2**, 367 (1969).
5. Raff, M. D., *Immunology* **19**, 637 (1970).
6. Unanue, E. R., Grey, H. M., Rabellino, E., Campbell, P., and Schmidtke, J., *J. Exp. Med.* **133**, 1188 (1971).
7. Raff, M. D., *Nature* **242**, 19 (1973).
8. Owen, J. J. T., Cooper, M. D., Raff, M. D., *Nature* **249**, 361 (1974).
9. Ford, W. L., and Gowans, J. L., *Semin. Hematol.* **6**, 67 (1969).
10. Rappaport, H., "Tumors of the Hematopoietic System," in *Atlas of Tumor Pathology*, Section III, Fascicle 8, Armed Forces Institute of Pathology, Washington, D.C., 1966.
11. Jones, S. E., Fuks, Z., Bull, M., Kadin, M. E., Dorfman, R. F., Kaplan, H. S., Rosenberg, S. A., and Kim, H., *Cancer* **31**, 806 (1973).
12. Schein, P. S., Chabner, B. A., Canellos, G. P., Young, R. C., Berard, C. W., and DeVita, V. T., *Blood* **43**, 181 (1974).
13. Schein, P. S., Chabner, B., Canellos, G., Young, R. C., Berard, C. W., and DeVita, V. T., *Brit. J. Cancer* **31** (Suppl. II), 107 (1975).
14. Froland, S. S., and Natvig, J. B., *J. Exp. Med.* **136**, 409 (1972).
15. Rowe, D. S., Hug, K., Forni, L., and Pernis, B., *J. Exp. Med.* **138**, 965 (1973).
16. Fu, S. M., Winchester, R. J., and Kunkel, H. G., *J. Exp. Med.* **139**, 451 (1974).
17. Van Boxel, J. A., and Buell, D. N., *Nature* **251**, 443–444 (1974).
18. Preud'homme, J. L., and Seligmann, M., *Blood* **40**, 777 (1972).
19. Winchester, R. J., Winfield, J. B., Siegal, F., Wernet, P., Bentwich, Z., and Kunkel, H. G., *J. Clin. Inves.* **54**, 1082–1092 (1974).
20. Lobo, P., Westervelt, F. B., and Horwitz, D. A., *J. Immunol.* **114**, 116 (1975).
21. Preud'homme, J. L., and Flandrin, G., *J. Immunol.* **113**, 1650–1653 (1974).
22. Greaves, M., Janossy, G., and Doenhoff, M., *J. Exp. Med.* **140**, 1 (1974).
23. Tønder, O., Morse, P. A., and Humphrey, L. J., *J. Immunol.* **113**, 1162 (1974).
24. Preud'homme, J. L., and Seligmann, M., *Proc. Nat. Acad. Sci. USA* **69**, 2132 (1972).
25. Gutman, G. A., and Weissman, I. L., *Immunology* **23**, 465 (1972).
26. Weissman, I. L., *Trans. Reviews* **24**, 159 (1975).
27. Antoine, J. C., Avrameas, S., Gonatas, N. K., Stieber, A., and Gonatas, J. O., *J. Cell Biol.* **63**, 12 (1974).
28. Garvin, A. J., Spicer, S. S., Parmley, R. T., and Munster, A. M., *J. Exp. Med.* **39**, 1077 (1974).
29. Bianco, C., Patrick, R., and Nussenzweig, V., *J. Exp. Med.* **132**, 702 (1970).
30. Nussenzweig, V., *Adv. Immunol.* **19**, 217–258 (1974).
31. Dukor, P., Bianco, C., and Nussenzweig, V., *Proc. Natl. Acad. Sci. USA* **67**, 991 (1970).
32. Shevach, E. M., Jaffe, E. S., and Green, I., *Transplant. Rev.* **16**, 3 (1973).
33. Gormus, B. J., Crandall, R. B., and Shands, J. W., Jr., *J. Immunol.* **112**, 770–775 (1974).
34. Gelfand, J., Fauci, A. S., Green, I., and Frank, M. M., *J. Immunol.* **116**, 595 (1976).
35. Mendes, N. F., Miki, S. S., and Peixinho, Z. F., *J. Immunol.* **113**, 536 (1974).
36. Eden, A., Miller, G. W., and Nussenzweig, V., *J. Clin. Invest* **52**, 3239 (1973).
37. Huber, H., Polley, M. J., Linscott, W. D., Fudenberg, H. H., and Mullen-Eberhard, H. J., *Science* **162**, 1281 (1968).
38. Gelfand, M. D., Frank, M. M., and Green, I., *J. Exp. Med.* **142**, 1029 (1975).
39. Lackman, P. J., and Muller-Eberhard, H. J., *J. Immunol.* **110**, 691 (1968).

40. Ross, G. D., Polley, M. J., Rabellino, E. M., and Grey, H. M., *J. Exp. Med.* **138,** 798–811 (1973).

41. Reynolds, H. Y., Atkinson, J. P., Newball, H. H., and Frank, M. M., *J. Immunol.* **114,** 1813 (1975).

42. Nelson, D. C., *Adv. Immunol.* **3,** 131 (1963).

43. Basten, A., Miller, J. F. A. P., Sprent, J., and Pye, J., *J. Exp. Med.* **135,** 610 (1972).

44. Berken, A., and Benacerraf, B., *J. Exp. Med.* **123,** 119 (1966).

45. Huber, H., Douglas, S. D., and Fudenberg, H. H., *Immunology* **17,** 7 (1969).

46. Jaffe, E. S., Shevach, E. M., Frank, M. M., and Green, I., *Am. J. Med.* **57,** 108 (1974).

47. Kedar, E., Ortiz de Landazuri, M., and Fahey, J., *J. Immunol.* **112,** 37–46 (1974).

48. Dickler, H. B., and Kunkel, H. G., *J. Exp. Med.* **136,** 191 (1972).

49. Anderson, C. L., and Grey, H. M., *J. Exp. Med.* **139,** 1175 (1974).

50. Van Boxel, J. A., and Rosenstreich, D. L., *J. Exp. Med.* **139,** 1002 (1974).

51. Yasuda, J., and Milgrom, F., *Intern. Arch. Allergy Appl. Immunol.* **33,** 151–170 (1968).

52. Westmorland, D., and Watkins, J. F., *J. Gen. Virol.* **24,** 167–178 (1974).

53. Lay, W. H., Mendes, N. F., Bianco, C., and Nussenzweig, V., *Nature,* **230,** 531 (1971).

54. Jondal, M., Holm, G., and Wigzell, H., *J. Exp. Med.* **136,** 207 (1972).

55. Lalezari, P., Nehlsen, S. L., Novodoff, S., and Lalezari, I., *Proc. Nat. Acad. Sci. USA* **72,** 697–700 (1975).

56. Braganza, C. M., Stathopoulos, G., Daules, A. J. S., Papamichail, M., and Holborow, E. J., *Cell* **4,** 103–106 (1975).

57. Weiner, M. S., Bianco, C., and Nussenzweig, V., *Blood* **42,** 939 (1973).

58. Silveira, N. P. A., Mendes, N. F., and Tolnai, M. E. A., *J. Immunol.* **108,** 1456 (1972).

59. Collins, R. D., Smith, J. L., Clein, G. P., and Barker, C. R., *Br. J. Haemat.* **26,** 615 (1974).

60. Minowda, J., Ohnuma, T., and Moore, G. E., *J. Natl. Cancer Inst.* **49,** 891 (1972).

61. Smith, R. W., Terry, W. D., Buell, D. N., and Sell, K. W., *J. Immunol.* **110,** 884 (1973).

62. Aisenberg, A. C., and Long, J. C., *Am. J. Med.* **58,** 300–306 (1975).

63. Greaves, M. F., and Brown, G., *Nat. New Biol.* **246,** 116–119 (1973).

64. Cohn, A. Z., *Adv. Immunol.* **9,** 163 (1968).

65. Berard, C. W., and Dorfman, R. F., "Histopathology of Malignant Lymphomas," in *Clinics in Haematology* **3,** 39 (1974).

66. Lennert, K., *Pathologie der Halslymphknoten,* Springer, Berlin, 1964.

67. Lennert, K., "Classification of the Malignant Lymphomas (European Concept)," in *Progress in Lymphology,* Proceedings of the International Symposium on Lymphology, Zurich, Switzerland, Georg Thieme Verlag, Stuttgart, 1967.

68. Lennert, K., Caesar, R., and Muller, K., *Exp. Hematol.* **11,** 6 (abst.), 1966.

69. Kojima, J., Imai, Y., and Mori, N., "A Concept of Follicular Lymphoma," in *Malignant Diseases of the Hematopoietic System,* Gann Monograph on Cancer Research 15, University of Tokyo Press, 1973, p. 195.

70. Lennert, K., "Follicular Lymphoma: A Tumor of the Germinal Centers," in *Malignant Diseases of the Hematopoietic System,* Gann Monograph on Cancer Research 15, University of Tokyo Press, 1973, p. 217.

71. Nossal, G. J. V., Abbot, A., Mitchell, J., and Lummus, Z., *J. Exp. Med.* **127,** 277 (1968).

72. Maruyama, K., and Masuda, T., *Ann. Rep. Inst. Virus Res., Kyotolenu* **7,** 149 (1964).

73. Lennert, K., and Niedorf, H. R., *Virch. Arch.* **4,** 148 (1969).

74. Levine, G. D., and Dorfman, R. F., *Cancer* **35,** 148 (1975).

75. Leech, J. H., Glick, A. D., Waldron, J. A., Flexner, J. M., Horm, R. G., and Collins, R. D., *J. Natl. Cancer Inst.* **54,** 11–22 (1975).

76. Jaffe, E. S., Shevach, E. M., Frank, M. M., Berard, C. W., and Green, I., *N. Eng. J. Med.* **290,** 813 (1974).

77. Peter, C. W., Mackenzie, M. R., and Glassy, F. J., *Lancet* **ii,** 686–689 (1974).

78. Braylan, R. C., Jaffe, E. S., Berard, C. W., "Malignant Lymphomas," in *Pathology Annual,* Vol. 10, Appleton-Century Crofts, New York, 1975.

79. Kube, R. T., Grey, H. M., and Pirofsky, B., *J. Immunol.* **112,** 1952 (1974).

80. Salsano, F., Frøland, S. S., Natvig, J. B., and Michaelsen, T. E., *Scand. J. Immunol.* **3,** 841–846 (1974).

81. Moore, D. F., Migliore, P. J., Shullenberger, C. C., and Alexanian, R., *Ann. Intern. Med.* **72,** 43 (1970).

82. Nossal, G. J. V., Ada, G. L., and Austin, C. M., *Austr. J. Exp. Biol. Med. Sci.* **42,** 311–330 (1964).

83. Koburg, E., "Cell Production and Migration in the Tonsil," in *Germinal Centers in Immune Responses* (H. Cottier, N. Odartchenko, R. Schindler, and C. C. Congdon, eds.), Springer-Verlag, New York, 1967, pp. 176–182.

84. Wakefield, J. D., Cohen, M. W., McCluskey, J., and Thorbecke, G. J., "The Fate of Lymphoid Cells from the White Pulp at the Peak of Germinal Center Formation," in *Germinal Centers in Immune Responses* (H. Cottier, N. Odartchenko, R. Schindler, and C. C. Congdon, eds.), Springer-Verlag, New York, 1967, pp. 183–188.

85. Berard, C. W., "Reticuloendothelial System: An Overview of Neoplasia," in *The Reticuloendothelial System,* International Academy of Pathology Monograph, Williams & Wilkins, Baltimore, 1975, p. 301.

86. Isaacs, R., *Ann. Intern. Med.* **11,** 657 (1937).

87. Schnitzer, B., Loesel, L. S., and Reed, R. E., *Cancer* **26,** 1082 (1970).

88. Braylan, R. C., Jaffe, E. S., Burbach, J. W., Frank, M. M., and Berard, C. W., *Cancer Res.,* **36,** 1619 (1976).

89. Pernis, B., Ferrarini, M., Forni, L., and Amante, L., "Immunoglobulins on Lymphocyte Membranes," in *Progress in Immunology,* First International Congress of Immunology (B. Amos, ed.), Academic Press, New York, 1971, p. 95.

90. Grey, H. M., Rabellino, E., and Pirofsky, B., *J. Clin. Invest.* **50,** 2368 (1971).

91. Wilson, J. D., and Nossal, G. J. V., *Lancet* **ii,** 788 (1971).

92. Aisenberg, A. C., and Bloch, K. J., *N. Engl. J. Med.* **287,** 273 (1972).

93. Aisenberg, A. C., Bloch, K. J., and Long, J. C., *Am. J. Med.* **55,** 184 (1973).

94. Ross, G. D., Rabellino, E. M., Polley, M. J., and Grey, H. M., *J. Clin. Invest,* **52,** 377 (1973).

95. Aisenberg, A. C., Long, J. C., and Wilkes, B., *J. Natl. Cancer Inst.* **52,** 13 (1974).

96. Frøland, S. S., Natvig, J. B., and Stavem, P., *Scand. J. Immunol.* **1,** 351 (1972).

97. Papamichail, M., Brown, J. C., and Holborow, E. J., *Lancet* **ii,** 850 (1971).

98. Piessens, W. F., Schur, P. H., Moloney, W. C., and Churchill, W. H., *N. Engl. J. Med.* **288,** 176 (1973).

99. Dickler, H. B., Siegal, F. P., Bentwich, Z. H., and Kunkel, H. G., *Clin. Exp. Immunol.* **14,** 97 (1973).

100. Fu, S. M., Winchester, R. J., Feizi, T., Walzer, P. D., and Kunkel, H. G., *Proc. Nat. Acad. Sci. USA* **71,** 4487–4490 (1974).

101. Preud'homme, J. L., Brouet, J. C., Clauvel, J. P., and Seligman, M., *Scand. J. Immunol.* **3,** 853–858 (1974).

102. Fu, S. M., Winchester, R. J., and Kunkel, H. G., *J. Immunol.* **114,** 250–252 (1975).

103. Pernis, B., Brouet, J. C., and Seligmann, M., *Eur. J. Immun.* **4,** 776 (1974).

104. Augener, W., Cohnen, G., and Brittinger, G., *Biomedicine* **21,** 6–8 (1974).

105. Shevach, E. M., Herberman, R., Frank, M. M., and Green, I., *J. Clin. Invest.* **51,** 1933 (1972).

106. Pincus, S., Bianco, C., and Nussenzweig, V., *Blood* **40,** 303 (1972).

107. MacKinney, A. A., Stohlman, F., and Brecher, G., *Blood* **19,** 349 (1962).

108. Theml, H., Trepel, F., Schick, P., Kaboth, W., and Begemann, H., *Blood* **42,** 623–636 (1973).

109. Salmon, S. E., and Seligmann, M., *Lancet* **ii,** 1230 (1974).

110. Marchalonis, J. J., Atwell, J. L., Haustein, D., *Biochimica et Biophysica Acta* **351,** 99–112 (1974).

111. Aisenberg, A. C., *N. Engl. J. Med.* **288,** 883 (1973).

112. Azar, H. A., Hill, W. T., and Osserman, E. F., *Am. J. Med.* **23,** 239 (1957).

113. Preud'homme, J. L., and Seligmann, M., *J. Clin. Invest.* **51,** 701 (1972).

114. Brown, G., Greaves, M. F., Lister, T. A., Rapson, N., and Papamichael, M., *Lancet* **ii,** 753–755 (1974).

115. Berard, C. W., O'Conor, G. T., Thomas, L. B., and Torloni, H., eds., *Bull. WHO* **40,** 601 (1969).

116. Arseneau, J. C., Canellos, G. P., Banks, P. M., Berard, C. W., Gralnick, H. R., and DeVita, V. T., *Am. J. Med.* **58,** 314 (1975).

117. Banks, P. M., Arseneau, J. C., Gralnick, H. R., Canellos, G. P., DeVita, V. T., and Berard, C. W., *Am. J. Med.* **58,** 322 (1975).

118. Mann, R. B., Jaffe, E. S., Braylan, R. C., Nanba, K., Frank, M. M., Ziegler, J. L., and Berard, C. W., *N. Engl. J. Med.* (in press).

119. Fialkow, P. J., Klein, E., Klein, G., Clifford, P., and Singh, S., *J. Exp. Med.* **138,** 89 (1973).

120. Kersey, J., Sabad, A., Gajl-Peczalska, K., Hallgren, H., Yunis, E. J., and Nesbit, M., *Am. J. Pathol.* **74,** 64A (1974) (abstract).

121. Binder, R. A., Jencks, J. A., Chun, B., Rath, C. E., *Cancer* **36,** 161 (1975).

122. Lukes, R. J., and Collins, R. D., *Br. J. Cancer* **31,** (Supp. II) 1 (1975).

123. Iversen, U., Iversen, O. H., Ziegler, J. L., Bluming, A. Z., and Kyalwazi, S. K., *Europ. J. Cancer* **8,** 305–310 (1972).

124. Kersey, J. H., Sabad, A., Gajl-Peczalska, K., Hallgren, H. M., Yunis, E. J., and Nesbit, M. E., *Science* **182,** 1355 (1973).

125. Smith, R. W., Terry, W. D., Buell, D. N., and Sell, R. W., *J. Immunol.* **110,** 884 (1973).

126. Chin, A. H., Saiki, J. H., Trujillo, J. M., and Williams, R. C., *Clin. Immunol. Immunopath.* **1,** 499 (1973).

127. Mokanakumar, T., Metzgar, R. S., and Miller, D. S., *Cell. Immunol.* **12,** 30 (1974).

128. Cotropia, J., *Proc. Am. Assoc. Cancer Res.* **15,** 29 (1974).

129. Jondal, M., Wigzell, H., and Aiuti, F., *Transplant. Rev.* **16,** 163 (1973).

130. Borella, L., and Sen, L., *J. Immunol.* **111,** 1257 (1973).

131. Davey, F. R., and Gottlieb, A. J., *Am. J. Clin. Path.* **62,** 818 (1974).

132. Sen, L., and Borella, L., *N. Engl. J. Med.* **292,** 828 (1975).

133. Catovsky, D., Goldman, J. M., Okos, A., Frisch, B., Galton, D. A. G., *Brit. Med. J.* **2,** 643 (1974).

134. Haegert, D. G., Stuart, J., Smith, J. L., *Brit. Med. J.* **1,** 312 (1975).

135. Flandrin, G., Brouet, J. C., Daniel, M. T., and Preud'homme, J. L., *Blood* **45,** 183 (1975).

136. Smith, J. L., Barker, C. W., Clein, G. P., and Collins, R. D., *Lancet* **i,** 74 (1973).

137. Castleberry, R. P., Toben, H. R., and Moreno, H., *Blood* **42,** 1025 (1973).

138. Kaplan, J., Mastrangelo, R., and Peterson, W. D., Jr., *Cancer Res.* **34,** 521 (1974).

139. Mann, R. B., Jaffe, E. S., Braylan, R. C., Eggleston, J. C., Ransom, L., Kaizer, H., and Berard, C. W., *Am. J. Med.* **58,** 307 (1975).

140. Jaffe, E. S., Braylan, R. C., Frank, M. M., Green, I., and Berard, C. W., *Blood* **48,** 213 (1976).

141. Shevach, E. M., Edelson, R., Frank, M. M., Lutzner, M., and Green, I., *Proc. Natl. Acad. Sci. USA* **71,** 863 (1974).

142. West, W., and Herberman, R. B., *Cell. Immunol.* **14,** 139 (1974).

143. Rappaport, H., and Thomas, L. B., *Cancer* **34,** 1198 (1974).

144. Brouet, J. C., Flandrin, G., and Seligmann, M., *N. Engl. J. Med.* **289,** 341 (1973).

145. Zucker-Franklin, D., Melton, J. W., III, and Quagliata, F., *Proc. Natl. Acad. Sci.* **71,** 1877 (1974).

146. Edelson, R. L., Kirkpatrick, C. H., Shevach, E. M., Schein, P. S., Smith, R. W., Green, I., and Lutzner, M. A., *Ann. Intern. Med.* **80,** 685 (1974).

147. Braylan, R., Variakojis, D., and Yachnin, S., *Blood* **42,** 1024 (1973).

148. Faguet, G. B., and Abele, D. C., *Clin. Res.* **22,** 388A (1974).

149. Flandrin, G., and Brouet, J. C., *Mayo Clin. Proc.* **49,** 575 (1974).

150. Thomas, L. B., and Rappaport, H., "Mycosis Fungoides and Its Relationship to Other Malignant Lymphomas," in *The Reticuloendothelial System,* IAP Monograph No. 16, Williams & Wilkins, Baltimore, 1975, pp. 243–261.

151. Jaffe, E. S., Shevach, E. M., Sussman, E. H., Frank, M. M., Green, I., and Berard, C. W., *Br. J. Cancer* **31** (Supp. II), 107–120 (1975).

152. Lennert, K., and Mestdagh, J., *Virchows Arch. Abt. A. Path. Anat.* **344,** 1 (1968).

153. Scheurlen, P. G., and Hellriegel, K. P., *Klin. Wsch.* **49,** 597 (1971).

154. Dameshek, W., *Blood* **21,** 243 (1963).

155. Brouet, J. C., Labaume, S., and Seligmann, M., *Br. J. Cancer* **31** (Supp. II), 121 (1975).

156. Stein, H., Lennert, K., and Parwaresch, M. R., *Lancet* **ii,** 855 (1972).

157. Brouet, J., Preud'homme, J., Seligmann, M., and Bernard, J., *Br. Med. J.* **4** (5883), 23–24 (1974).

158. Richter, M. N., *Am. J. Path.* **4,** 285 (1928).

159. Brouet, J. C., Preud'homme, J. L., Flandrin, G., Chelland, N., and Seligmann, M., *J. Natl. Cancer Inst.* **56,** 631 (1976).

160. Bouroncle, B. A., Wiseman, B. K., Dean, C. A., *Blood* **13,** 609 (1958).

161. Shrek, R., and Donnelly, W. J., *Blood* **27,** 199 (1966).

162. Burke, J. S., Byrne, G. E., Jr., and Rappaport, H., *Cancer* **33,** 1399 (1974).

163. Catovsky, D., Petitt, J. E., Galetto, J., Okos, A., and Galton, D. A. G., *Br. J. Haemat.* **26,** 29 (1974).

164. Burns, C. P., Maca, R. D., and Hoak, J. C., *Cancer Res.* **33,** 1615 (1973).

165. Rubin, A. D., Douglas, S. D., Chessin, L. N., Glade, P. R., and Dameshek, W., *Am. J. Med.* **47,** 149 (1969).

166. Rappaport, H., and Braylan, R. C., "Changing Concepts in the Classification of Malignant Neoplasms of the Hematopoietic System," in *The Reticuloendothelial System,* International Academy of Pathology Monograph, Williams & Wilkins, Baltimore, 1975, p. 1.

167. Fu, S. M., Winchester, R. J., Rai, K. R., and Kunkel, H. G., *Scand. J. Immunol.* **3,** 847 (1974).

168. Yam, L. T., Castold, G. L., Garvey, M. B., and Mitus, W. J., *Blood* **32,** 90 (1968).

169. Golomb, H. M., Braylan, R., and Polliack, A., *Brit. J. Haem.* **29,** 455 (1975).

170. Daniel, M. Th., and Flandrin, G., *Lab. Invest.* **30,** 1 (1974).

171. Scott, R. B., and Robb-Smith, A. H. T., *Lancet* **2,** 194 (1939).

172. Peckham, M. J., and Cooper, E. H., *Cancer* **24,** 135 (1969).

173. Leech, J., *Lancet* **ii,** 265 (1973).

174. Braylan, R. C., Jaffe, E. S., and Berard, C. W., *Lancet* **ii,** 1328 (1974).

175. Taylor, C. R., *Lancet* **ii,** 802 (1974).

176. Garvin, A. J., and Spicer, S. S., submitted for publication.

177. Green, I., Jaffe, E., Shevach, E., Frank, M., and Berard, C., *Fed. Proc.* **33,** 610 (1974).

178. Kaur, J., Catovsky, D., Spiers, A. S. D., and Galton, D. A. G., *Lancet* **ii,** 800 (1974).

179. Belpomme, D., Joseph, R., Navares, L., Gerard-Marchant, R., Huchet, R., Botto, I., Grandjon, D., and Mathe, G., *N. Engl. J. Med.* **291,** 1417 (1974).

180. Grifoni, V., Del Giacco, G. S., Manconi, P. E., Tognella, S., and Mantovani, G., *Lancet* **ii,** 332 (1975).

181. Pretlow, T. G., II, Luberoff, D. E., Hamilton, L. J., Weinberger, P. C., Maddox, W. A., and Durant, J. R., *Cancer.* **31,** 1120 (1973).

182. Kadin, M. E., Newcom, S. R., Gold, S. B., and Stites, D. P., *Lancet* **ii,** 167 (1974).

183. Longmire, R. L., McMillan, R., Yelonsky, R., Armstrong, S., Lang, J. E., and Craddock, G. G., *N. Engl. J. Med.* **289,** 763 (1973).

184. Lennert, K., Stein, H., and Kaiserling, E., *Br. J. Cancer* **31** (Supp. II), 29 (1975).

185. Dorfman, R. F., "The Non-Hodgkin's Lymphomas," in *The Reticuloendothelial System,* International Academy of Pathology Monograph, 1975, p. 262.

186. Frizzera, G., Moran, E., and Rappaport, H., *Lancet* **i**, 1070–1073 (1974).

187. Lukes, R. J., and Tindle, B. H., *N. Engl. J. Med.* **292,** 1 (1975).

188. Young, R. C., Corder, M. P., Haynes, H. A., and DeVita, V. T., *Am. J. Med.* **52,** 63 (1972).

189. Hersh, E. M., and Oppenheim, J. J., *New Engl. J. Med.* **273,** 1006 (1965).

190. Aisenberg, A. C., *New Engl. J. Med.* **270,** 508 (1966).

191. MacLennan, E. C. M., *Transpl. Rev.* **13,** 67 (1972).

192. Van Boxel, J. A., Stobo, J. D., Paul, W. E., and Green, I., *Science* **175,** 194 (1972).

193. O'Toole, C., Perlmann, P., Wigzell, H., Unsguard, B., and Zetterlind, C., *Lancet* **1,** 1085 (1973).

194. Paul, W. E., "Antigen Recognition and Cell Receptor Sites," in *Defence and Recognition* (R. R. Porter, ed., Butterworths, London, 1973, p. 329.

195. Han, T., Sokol, J. E., *Amer. J. Med.* **48,** 728 (1970).

196. Corder, M. P., Young, R. C., Brown, R. S., and DeVita, V., *Blood* **39,** 595 (1972).

197. Aisenberg, A. C., *J. Clin. Invest.* **41,** 1964 (1962).

198. Shier, W. W., Roth, A., Ostroff, G., and Schrift, M. H., *Amer. J. Med.* **20,** 94 (1956).

199. Levy, R., and Kaplan, H. S., *N.E.J.M.* **290,** 18 (1974).

200. DeVita, V. T., *N.E.J.M.* **289,** 801 (1973).

201. Schwartz, R. S., *N.E.J.M.* **290,** 397 (1974).

202. Kaplan, H. S., and Smithers, D. W., *Lancet* **2,** 1 (1959).

203. Green, I., Inkelas, M., and Allen, L. B., *Lancet* **1,** 30 (1960).

204. Muftuoglu, A., *N.E.J.M.* **277,** 125 (1967).

205. Scheurlen, P. G., Schneider, W., and Pappas, A., *Lancet* **11,** 1265 (1971).

206. Grifoni, V., Del Giacco, G. S., Parconi, P. E., and Montovani, G., *Italian J. Immun. Immunopath.* **1,** 21 (1970).

207. Matchett, K. M., Huang, A. T., and Kremer, W. B., *J. Clin. Invest.* **52,** 1908 (1973).

208. Ru;hl, H., Vogt, W., Bochert, G., Schmidt, S., Moelle, R., and Schaoua, H., *Clin. Exp. Immunol.* **19,** 55 (1975).

209. Twomey, J. J., Douglass, C. C., and Morris, S., *J. Nat. Cancer Inst.* **51,** 345 (1973).

210. Mintz, U., and Sachs, L., *Proc. Nat. Acad. Sci.* **72,** 2428 (1975).

211. Ru;hl, H., Vogt, W., Bochert, G., Schmidt, S., Moelle, R., and Schaoua, H., *Immunology* **26,** 989 (1974).

212. Ward, P. A., and Berneberg, J.-L., *N.E.J.M.* **290,** 76 (1974).

213. Cohen, S., Fisher, B., Yoshida, T., *N.E.J.M.* **290,** 882 (1974).

214. Yoshida, T., Edelson, R., Cohen, S., and Green, I., *J. Immunol.* **114,** 915 (1975).

215. Wybran, J., and Fudenberg, H. H., *J. Clin. Invest.* **52,** 1026 (1973).

216. Aiuti, F., and Wigzell, H., *Clin. Exp. Immunol.* **13,** 183 (1973).

217. Ramot, B., Many, A., Biniaminov, M., and Aghai, E., *Israel J. Med. Sci.* **9,** 657 (1973).

218. Peczalska, G. K. J., Hansen, J. A., Bloomfield, C. D., and Good, R. A., *J. Clin. Invest.* **52,** 3064 (1973).

219. Cohnen, G., Augener, W., Brittinger, G., and Douglas, S. D., *N.E.J.M.* **289,** 863 (1973).

220. Sullivan, J. L., Barry, D. W., Albrecht, P., and Lucas, S. J., *J. Immunol.* **114,** 1458 (1975).

221. Chase, M. W., *Cancer Res.* **26,** 109 (1966).

222. Oppenheim, J. J., Whang, J., and Frei, E., *Blood* **26,** 121 (1965).

223. Shaw, R. K., Swed, C., Boggs, D. R., Fahey, J. L., Frei, E., and Utz, J. P., *Arch. Int. Med.* **106,** 467 (1960).

224. Miller, D. G., *Ann. Int. Med.* **57,** 703 (1962).

225. Block, J. B., Haynes, H., Thompson, W. L., and Neiman, P., *J. Nat. Cancer Inst.* **42,** 973 (1969).

226. Cone, L., and Uhr, J. W., *J. Clin. Invest.* **43,** 2241 (1964).

227. Smith, M. J., Browne, E., and Slungaard, A., *Blood* **41,** 505 (1973).

228. Froland, S. S., and Stavem, P., *Lancet* **1,** 795 (1972).

229. Jones, L. H., and Hardisty, R. M., Wells, D. G., and Kay, H. M., *Brit. Med. J.* **2,** 329 (1971).

230. Robbins, J. H., and Levis, W. R., *Int. Arch. Allergy Appl. Immunol.* **30,** 580 (1970).

231. Robbins, J. H., and Levis, W. R., *Int. Arch. Allergy* **43,** 845 (1972).

232. Rubin, A. D., "In Vitro Evaluation of Lymphocyte Proliferation in Lymphoproliferative Disorders," in *Proceedings of the Fifth Leucocyte Culture Conference* (J. E. Harris, ed.), Academic Press, New York, p. 239.

233. Schweitzer, M., Melief, C. J. M., and Eijsvoogel, V. P., *Europ. J. Imm.* **3,** 121 (1973).

234. DaGuillard, F., "The Differing Responses of Lymphocytes to Mitogens," in *Proceedings of the Seventh Leukocyte Culture Conference* (F. Daguillard, ed.), Academic Press, New York, 1973, p. 571.

235. Chess, L., MacDermott, R. P., and Schlossman, S. F., *J. Immunol.* **113,** 113 (1974).

236. Lohrmann, H. P., Novikous, L., and Graw, R. G., *J. Exp. Med.* **139,** 1553 (1974).

237. Lohrman, H. P., Whand-Peng, J., *J. Exp. Med.* **140,** 54 (1974).

238. Kornfeld, S., *Biochem. Biophys. Acta* **192,** 542 (1969).

239. Novogrodsky, A., Biniaminov, M., Ramot, B., and Katchalski, E., *Blood* **40,** 311 (1972).

240. Glasgow, A. H., Nimberg, R. B., Menzoian, J. O., Saporoschetz, J., Cooperband, S. R., Schmid, K., and Mannick, J. A., *N.E.J.M.* 291, 1263 (1974).

241. Tavadia, H. B., Gandie, K. B., Nicoll, W. D., *Clin. Exp. Immun.* **16,** 177 (1974).

242. Perlmann, P., and Holm, G., *Adv. Immunol.* **11,** 117 (1969).

243. Flad, H. D., Huber, C., Bremer, K., Menne, H. D., and Huber, H., *Europ. J. Immun.* **3,** 688 (1973).

244. Harrison, M. R., Elfenbein, G. J., and Green, I., *J. Immunol.* **110,** 602 (1973).

245. Gall, P. R., Sighelboim, J., Ossorio, R. C., and Fahey, J. L., *Clin. Immunol. Immunopathol.* **3,** 377 (1975).

246. Moroz, C., Shalmon, L., and Hahn, J., *Europ. J. Immun.* **3,** 16 (1973).

247. Eijsvoogel, V. P., van Rood, J. J., duToit, E. D., and Schellekens, P., *Europ. J. Immun.* **2,** 413 (1972).

248. *In Vitro Methods of Cell-Mediated Immunity* (B. R. Bloom and P. R. Glade, eds.), Academic Press, New York, 1971, p. 333.

249. Ahmed, A., Edelson, R., Strong, D., Knudsen, A. C., Woody, J. N., Sell, K. W., and Green, I., Unpublished data.

250. Bennett, B., and Bloom, B. R., *Proc. Nat. Acad. Sci.* **59,** 756 (1968).

251. Salvin, J. B., Youngner, J. S., and Lederer, W. H., *Infect. and Immunity* **7,** 68 (1973).

252. Broder, S., Nelson, D., Durm, M., Blackman, M., and Waldman, T., *J. Clin. Invest.* (in press).

253. Waldman, T. A., Broder, S., Durm, M., Blaese, M., and Strober, W., *Lancet* **2,** 609 (1974).

254. Alter, B. J., and Bach, F. H., *Cell Immunol.* **1,** 207 (1970).

255. Schirrmacher, V., Martinez, J. D., Festenstein, H., *Nature* **255,** 155 (1975).

256. Levis, W. R., and Robbins, J. H., *Immunol.* **8,** 927 (1971).

257. Greineder, D., Rosenthal, A. S., *J. Immunol.* **114,** 1541 (1975).

258. Rode, H. N., Gordon, J., *J. Cell Immunol.* **13,** 87 (1974).

259. Levis, W. R., and Miller, A. E., *Lancet* **11,** 357 (1972).

260. Kennedy, J. C., and Mensah-Ekpaha, J. A., *J. Immunol.* **111,** 1639 (1973).

261. Harrison, M. R., and Paul, W. E., *J. Exp. Med.* **138,** 1602 (1973).

262. Greaves, M., and Janossy, G., *Trans. Rev.* **11,** 87 (1972).

263. Waxdal, M. J., and Basham, T. Y., *Nature* **251,** 153 (1974).

264. Jondal, M., and Klein, G., *J. Exp. Med.* **138,** 1365 (1973).

265. Greaves, M. F., Brown, G., and Rickinson, A. B., *Clin. Imm. and Immunopath.* **3,** 514 (1975).

266. Olding, L. B., Jensen, L. B., and Oldstone, M. B. A., *J. Exp. Med.* **141,** 561 (1975).

267. Woodruff, J. F., and Woodruff, J. J., *J. Immunol.* **112,** 2176 (1974).

268. Sullivan, J. L., Barry, D. W., Lucas, S. J., and Albrecht, P., *J. Exp. Med.* **142,** 773 (1975).

269. Benacerraf, B., and McDevitt, H. O., *Science* **175,** 273 (1972).

270. Green, I., *Immunogenetics* **1,** 4 (1974).

271. Gasser, D. L., and Silvero, W. K., *Adv. Immunol.* **18,** 1 (1974).

272. Klein, J., *Biology of the Mouse Histocompatibility Complex,* Springer Verlag, New York, 1975.

273. Geczy, A. F., DeWeck, A. L., and Shevach, E. M., *J. Immunol.* (in press).

274. Schreffler, D. C., and David, G., *Adv. Immunol.* **20,** 125 (1975).

275. *Histocompatibility Testing* (Jean Dausset and Jacque Colombani, eds.), Williams & Wilkins, Baltimore, 1972.

276. Wernet, P., and Kunkel, A. G., *J. Exp. Med.* **138,** 1021 (1973).

Chapter Eleven

Interactions of Lymphocytes with Oncogenic Viruses

MARTIN S. HIRSCH

Department of Medicine, Massachusetts General Hospital and Harvard Medical School, Boston, Massachusetts

Viruses with oncogenic properties are widely disseminated throughout the animal kingdom. Members of the herpes, adeno, papova, and oncornavirus groups may all be oncogenic in the appropriate host. Some of these oncogenic agents may be acquired exogenously, whereas others are activated from latent states within animal cells (1,2). In man, the relationships between viruses and cancer are much less clear. Several candidate human oncogenic viruses have been reported, including C- and B-type oncornaviruses (3–6), herpes simplex virus (7), Epstein-Barr virus (EBV) (8), cytomegalovirus (9), and papovaviruses (10). As of this writing, none of these agents has been firmly established as etiologically related to human cancer, although there is considerable circumstantial evidence implicating EBV as a causal agent in African Burkitt's lymphoma and/or nasopharyngeal carcinoma (8). Necessary and justified restraints on human experimentation make relationships between candidate viruses and cancer difficult to interpret, but it appears likely that several viruses may be oncogenic in man, as they are in experimental animals. There is no reason to suspect that man should differ from animals in his susceptibility to the oncogenic effects of viruses, either exogenous or endogenous.

Viruses may interact with lymphoid cells in a variety of ways, both beneficial and detrimental to the host (2,11–16). The relationships between potentially oncogenic viruses and lymphoid cells are particularly complex. In this chapter I will review several aspects of these relationships, concentrating on two well-

Research carried out in the author's laboratory was supported by PHS grant CA 12464–06 and by contract No. 1-CP 43222 within the Virus Cancer Program of the National Cancer Institute. The survey of the literature for this review was completed in January 1976.

studied systems, C-type oncornavirus infections of mice and EBV infections of man. When possible, I will extrapolate to certain other oncogenic virus model systems as well.

LYMPHOCYTES AND C-TYPE ONCORNAVIRUSES IN THE MOUSE

Several members of the C-type oncornavirus group can induce lymphoreticular or hematopoietic neoplasms when injected into mice. The mechanisms involved in the development of leukemias or lymphomas are not fully understood, but they may involve virus-induced immunosuppression and selective virus-induced autoimmunity, with consequent subversion of the host's antiviral and antitumor defense mechanisms.

Effects of Oncornaviruses on Immune Responses

Immunodepression.   Administration of murine leukemia viruses (MuLV) to appropriate hosts frequently results in the development of hyporesponsiveness to certain antigens. There appear to be marked differences between MuLV with short incubation periods from infection to neoplasia, e.g., Friend and Rauscher viruses, and MuLV with long incubation periods, e.g., Moloney and Gross viruses (14–16). Similarly, exogenous viruses behave differently from endogenous viruses (14).

The most widely studied immunosuppressive C-type virus is the Friend leukemia virus (MuLV-F), a complex of agents that can markedly affect both humoral and cell-mediated immune responses to a wide variety of antigens and mitogens (15,17–29). Infection of susceptible mice (e.g., BALB/c) leads to a rapid, profound, and prolonged depression of the ability to mount a humoral immune response; mice resistant to MuLV-F infection and leukemogenesis, e.g., C57BL/6 show only transient immunosuppression or none at all (18). F_1 hybrid mice have a susceptibility pattern of the more susceptible parent, in terms of both virus infection and immunosuppression (18). The degree of suppression is dependent on the dose of infectious virus administered; immunization with formalinized virus preparations protects against the immunosuppressive effects of subsequent MuLV-F infection (15). MuLV-F does not appear to act on fully differentiated, antibody-secreting effector cells (19) but does affect B lymphocytes in an earlier stage of differentiation (20). Partially differentiated memory B lymphocytes appear to become infected and subsequently inhibited from responding to a secondary challenge with *Vibrio cholerae* antigen (20). Since lymphocytes involved in the primary response to *V. cholerae* do not appear to be infected by MuLV-F, virus-infected mice are capable of responding to a primary challenge with this antigen (20). Thus, infection of lymphocytes by MuLV-F may be a prerequisite for the development of immunosuppression.

The mechanisms involved in depression of humoral responsiveness are not clear. The proliferative capacity of MuLV-F-infected lymphocytes is reduced as a consequence of infection (15), and both organ distribution and cell surface receptors on B-lymphocytes are altered (21,22). However, electron microscopic studies have indicated that individual virus-infected immunocytes may still be capable of forming antibody (23). Concomitant with development of immunosuppression are morphological changes in spleens of infected animals, particularly a diminution of villous cells and an increase of smooth cells having occasional holes in their surfaces (24); these changes are felt to represent a decrease in functional B lymphocytes. In addition to B cell abnormalities, recent studies suggest that MuLV-F or one of its component parts, the Rowson-Parr virus (RPV), can alter macrophage function, and that restoration of this function can reverse virus-induced immunosuppression (25,26). The presence of suppressor cells that release undefined immunosuppressive factors has also been described following MuLV-F infection (27).

Several cell-mediated immune responses are also reduced following murine infection with MuLV-F. These include skin graft rejection, macrophage migration inhibition, and lymphocyte-mediated cytotoxicity (15). Suppression is dependent on dose of infectious virus, temporal relationships of infection to challenge, and lymphoid organ tested (15,28,29). Although the mechanisms of this suppression are presently obscure, Ceglowski (15) has reported the presence of suppressor cells of cell-mediated immunity in the spleens of MuLV-F infected mice, analogous to similar suppressor cells observed in Moloney leukemia or sarcoma virus models (30,31). Unlike these other models, however, the MuLV-F infected splenic suppressor cells release an immunosuppressive factor that is trypsin-sensitive but resistant to nucleases, neuraminidase, anti-MuLV-F serum, and heating at 56°C for 30 minutes (15). The possibility of other contaminant viruses with immunosuppressive capacity, e.g., the minute virus of mice, in such preparations (32,33) must always be considered.

This brief review of the reported effects of just one murine C-type oncornavirus, MuLV-F, suggests the complexity of the interactions involved. It is clear that no single hypothesis can at present account for the diversity of findings described. It is also clear that generalizations cannot be extended from exogenously administered viruses to endogenous viruses (14) or from MuLV-F to other exogenous oncornaviruses (13,14,16). Divergent results obtained in different model systems may result from variations in strain or age of mouse, strain and dose of virus, target cell infected, route of virus administration, type of response observed, presence of contaminating virus, and timing of observations in relation to spread of infection and neoplasm. Mechanisms involved in virus-induced immunosuppression may include alterations in macrophage function, destruction of lymphocytes, inhibition of lymphocyte activation and proliferation, alteration of lymphocyte traffic, or stimulation of suppressor cells (13). The supposition that virus-induced immunosuppression contributes to virus-induced neoplasia is logical but as yet unproven; an alternative view that leukemia development may be a necessary step for the expression of virus-induced immunosuppression has also been proposed (14).

Autoimmunity.   In addition to producing immunosuppression, exogenous infection of certain lymphocyte subpopulations with C-type oncornaviruses can lead to the aberrant expression of lymphocyte-mediated autoimmunity (34–38). C3H/He mice, when infected as neonates with Moloney leukemia virus (MuLV-M), either vertically through maternal milk or exogenously by inoculation, become persistent virus carriers. These MuLV-M carriers develop thymic involution, characterized by pronounced intrathymic cell destruction, at approximately 3–4 months of age, and thereafter develop thymic lymphomas, resulting in death between 4–12 months. Prior to death, the malignant lymphoblasts present in the thymus appear to disseminate to peripheral lymphoid tissues and other organs. Using a microcytotoxicity assay, Proffitt et al. have found that during the course of lymphomagenesis in MuLV-M carriers, thymocytes become vigorously reactive against normal syngeneic fibroblast target cells, whereas they spare identically derived cells infected with MuLV-M (34–37). The autoaggressive cells may appear in the thymus as early as 1 month of age, but they are not detectable in peripheral lymphoid organs until the time lymphoma cells begin to disseminate (3–5 months of age). Transplantable lymphoma cells derived from MuLV-M carriers also exhibit the same pattern of selective autoaggressive behavior. Although some young (about 10-week-old) carrier lymphocytes also show reactivity against MuLV-associated antigens (39), this reactivity disappears as lymphoma development progresses.

The autoaggressive thymocytes from MuLV-M-carriers belong to a cortisone-resistant, nonadherent, light density, MuLV-M infected population of T cells (36). Although syngeneic target cells infected with Gross leukemia virus (MuLV-G) are also spared from cytolysis by MuLV-M-infected thymocytes, target cells infected with lymphocytic choriomeningitis (LCM) virus are not (37). Thus, the sparing appears to be specific for MuLV-related antigens. Thymocytes from LCM or lactic dehydrogenase (LDH) virus carrier mice show no cytotoxic activity against either uninfected or infected fibroblasts (37). Further specificity studies indicate that the thymocytes from MuLV-M-carriers react against cells from nearly all mouse strains so far tested; in contrast, no reactivity can be demonstrated against human, rat, or hamster cells (37).

MuLV-M induced thymocyte autoaggressiveness might, in part, account for viral persistence, thymic involution, subsequent immunosuppression and lymphomagenesis (39). Autoaggressive cells may help to destroy potentially reactive antiviral or antitumor cells, thereby allowing unrestricted proliferation of autoaggressive neoplastic cells, culminating in disseminated lymphoma. In addition to the activation of T cells having autoreactive potential, other cells having immunoregulatory activity, e.g., suppressor cells, may become activated by a similar mechanism during infection with MuLV-M (30), augmenting immunosuppression and subsequent oncogenesis.

Autoimmune phenomena may accompany other oncornavirus infections in mice or rats (40,41). Cell-mediated selective autoreactivity has also been noted in infections with Abelson leukemia virus (MuLV-A), an agent that induces predominantly B cell neoplasms (38).

Activation of Oncornaviruses from Lymphocytes

Most, if not all, murine strains carry DNA sequences in their genomes that code for the expression of C-type oncornavirus information (2,42,43). Expression of this information varies among strains, among mice within strains, and among anatomical sites and cell types within individual mice (42–45). It may vary from tight repression to production of fully infectious virus. Individual animals and probably individual cells may contain the necessary information to code for the production of several different types of C-type oncornaviruses, both ecotropic and xenotropic (46,47). Although it is well established that some of these endogenous viruses can be oncogenic when inoculated into other hosts, it is not clear whether they are oncogenic in the hosts from which they arise. Expression of C-type oncornaviruses can be accelerated or amplified in vivo by certain manipulations, e.g., X-irradiation or induction of graft-versus-host reactions (GVHR), which in turn can increase the incidence of lymphoreticular neoplasms (2,48–50). Infectious C-type oncornaviruses can be activated from lymphoid cells in vitro by stimulators of lymphocyte blastogenesis such as mixed lymphocyte reactions (51,52) and certain mitogens (53,54).

When young adult (BALB/c $\times$ A/J)F$_1$ mice are inoculated with splenocytes from similarly aged BALB/c mice, GVHR ensue, characterized by splenomegaly, depletion of small lymphocytes, hyperplasia of reticulum or histiocytic cells, and alterations of some immune functions. Subsequently, a significant percentage of these mice develop immunoblastic or reticulum cell sarcomas, predominantly of F$_1$ origin (55). After induction of GVHR but prior to lymphoma development, splenic C-type oncornaviruses, either ecotropic or xenotropic, are readily detectable in the majority of these animals; matched, uninjected F$_1$ or parental mice of comparable ages rarely have detectable virus (49,50,52). Treatment of parental cells with mitomycin-C or antitheta serum, or treatment of recipients with interferon, will diminish GVHR, inhibit virus activation, and reduce lymphomagenesis (51,56). GVHR-associated oncornaviruses may be oncogenic when inoculated into newborn mice of the same strain (50). Several recent studies indicate that normal mice can respond immunologically to endogenous C-type oncornaviruses (57–62). Although variable degrees of immunosuppression have been described following GVHR (63–65), it is unclear whether such animals are hyporesponsive to their own activated endogenous viruses or to virus-associated tumor antigens. A reasonable sequence of events is that during GVHR, oncornaviruses are activated from responsive lymphocytes, and that these viruses subsequently infect recipient immunoblasts; in the face of GVHR-induced immunosuppression both oncornaviruses and virus-altered immunoblasts proliferate, culminating in the development of malignant lymphoma.

Another murine model in which C-type oncornaviruses are immunologically activated involves the placement of murine skin grafts (DBA/2 or A/J) onto histoincompatible BALB/c recipients (66,66a). Recipients are subsequently treated with various immunosuppressive agents to prolong graft survival. Regimens that result in prolonged graft maintenance, e.g., high-dose antilymphocyte serum (ALS) or high-dose cyclophosphamide, lead to activation of both ecotropic and xenotropic C-type oncornaviruses (66a). Regimens that do not significantly prolong graft survival, e.g., low-dose cyclophosphamide or varying doses of cortisone, do not lead to virus activation. High-dose cyclophosphamide alone does not activate viruses, whereas high-dose ALS alone leads to a moderate incidence of virus activation. Kinetic studies indicate that viruses are first detected between 1–2 weeks following transplantation, in spleens and in regional nodes draining skin graft sites; thereafter, highest virus titers are detected in spleens (66a). The histological appearance of spleens in these mice is remarkably similar to that observed in mice undergoing GVHR, with depletion of small lymphocytes but hyperplasia of other elements. Viruses are not detected in thymuses, skin graft sites, or tails of graft recipients, nor are they found in donor grafts. These findings suggest that viruses are activated from recipient lymphoid cells reacting against donor antigens and that the replication of these viruses is facilitated by concomitant immunosuppression. The active viruses may be ecotropic or xenotropic, and at least some of the activated ecotropic viruses are oncogenic, inducing thymic lymphomas in neonatal NIH-Swiss mice (66a).

Mixed lymphocyte reactions in vitro between BALB/c and BALB/c × A/J)F$_1$ spleen cells may be associated with the activation of either ecotropic or xenotropic viruses (51,52). The activated viruses are seen budding exclusively from lymphoblasts (67), suggesting that the responding BALB/c cells, rather than the target F$_1$ cells, are the source of virus. Recently, certain nonspecific mitogens have also been shown to activate xenotropic viruses from murine lymphocytes (53,54). Bacterial lipopolysaccharide (LPS), a B-lymphocyte mitogen in mice, efficiently induces such viruses. Concanavalin A (Con A), a stimulator of both T and B cells, is a less effective virus-inducer than LPS, and phytohemagglutinin (PHA) does not induce C-type oncornaviruses at all. In one study the effects of LPS and Con A were enhanced by halogenated pyrimidines (53). These nucleoside derivatives can themselves, under certain conditions, activate C-type oncornaviruses from mouse lymphocytes (68). It appears that, although lymphocyte blastogenesis in vitro may be an important factor in virus activation, the selection of certain subpopulations of lymphocytes for stimulation may be more critical. Presently, it would seem that certain T lymphocytes may be stimulated during MLR to produce ecotropic or xenotropic viruses, whereas B lymphocytes may produce xenotropic viruses after appropriate mitogenic stimulation.

Culture of certain murine lymphocytes in vitro may also result in the spontaneous expression of some oncornavirus gene products (69) and occasionally in the production of infectious C-type oncornaviruses. This may reflect release from in vivo immunologic constraints on the production and expression of new antigens.

LYMPHOCYTES AND C-TYPE ONCORNAVIRUSES IN OTHER MAMMALS

Except for the mouse, lymphocyte-oncornavirus interactions have not been extensively studied in mammalian systems, despite the fact that oncornaviruses are widely found in nearly all mammalian species. Within the past few years reports have appeared of oncornavirus interactions with lymphoid cells in domestic cats. Cats may be infected with two distinct groups of oncornaviruses (70). One, the RD-114 group, is present in latent form in both healthy and tumor-bearing cats and can be readily induced from cat cells in vitro (71,72). This group of viruses is xenotropic and has not been reported to be oncogenic. The other group, composed of feline leukemia virus (FeLV) and feline sarcoma virus (FeSV), replicates well in cat cells, has not been induced from normal cat cells, and appears to be oncogenic for cats (70). Cats infected with FeLV, either spontaneously or experimentally, develop antibodies against feline oncornavirus-associated cell membrane antigen (FOCMA) (70,73). Prospective studies have indicated that low FOCMA antibody titers in the presence of FeLV are associated with a high incidence of leukemia, whereas high antibody titers are associated with resistance to leukemogenesis (73). FeLV itself can induce thymic atrophy and peripheral lymphocyte depletion (74–76), marked suppression of cell-mediated immunity (75), and an increased susceptibility to other infections (77). It is not yet known if virus-induced autoreactivity similar to that seen in MuLV-M carrier mice occurs in FeLV-infected cats, or if virus-induced immunosupression contributes directly to the development of leukemia.

Primate C-type oncornaviruses have recently been described in baboons (78), gibbon apes (79), woolly monkeys (80), and possibly in man (3–5). Lymphoreticular neoplasms have been associated with some of these isolates, and studies concerning interactions between lymphoid cells and primate oncornaviruses are in progress.

INTERACTIONS OF LYMPHOCYTES AND PRIMATE HERPESVIRUSES

Several mammalian herpesviruses have oncogenic properties when inoculated into secondary hosts in vivo. Transformation or "immortalization" of cells in vitro has also been accomplished with these agents. The interactions between host lymphocytes and potentially oncogenic herpesviruses have been most thoroughly studied in primate systems, including Epstein-Barr virus (EBV) and cytomegalovirus (CMV) in man and herpesviruses saimiri (HVS) and ateles (HVA) in subhuman primates.

Epstein-Barr Virus

The Epstein-Barr virus (EBV), first seen in cultures of Burkitt's lymphoma cells in 1964 (81), has been implicated as a cause of both infectious mononucleosis (82,83) and African Burkitt's lymphoma (8). The evidence that heterophile-positive mononucleosis is caused by EBV is overwhelming (83). The evidence suggesting that EBV is also an oncogenic virus includes the following:

1. The uniformly elevated antibody titers to EBV, but not to other viruses, in African patients with Burkitt's lymphoma, and the absence of similarly elevated titers in matched control populations (84).

2. The presence of EBV-associated antigens and EBV DNA in biopsies of Burkitt's lymphomas and in lymphoblastoid cell lines derived from these tumors (85–88).

3. The ability of EBV to "immortalize" neonatal human lymphocytes, permitting long-term cultures of these cells (89,90).

4. The oncogenic effect of cell-free EBV in subhuman primates (91–93). Although none of these points proves a causal relationship between EBV and African Burkitt's lymphoma, the circumstantial evidence suggests more than a fortuitous association.

Effects of EBV on Lymphocytes.   Human B lymphocytes appear to be the major target cells for EBV. Most, if not all, B lymphocytes have EBV receptors, and recent studies suggest that the complement receptors on these cells are closely related or identical to the EBV receptors (8). In contrast, T lymphocyte populations have not been shown to have EBV receptors (94). Although different strains of EBV may induce transformed cells with different biological and antigenic characteristics (95), infection of human umbilical cord lymphocytes generally results in stimulation of cellular DNA synthesis, development of Epstein-Barr nuclear antigen (EBNA), and lymphoblastoid transformation, all within the first week of culture (96–100). With longer time in culture, the number and percentage of cells positive for EBNA increases. The presence of EBNA, unlike the EBV-induced early antigen (EA) or viral capsid antigen (VCA), is compatible with cell proliferation (97). EA or VCA production, in contrast, signals entry into a productive lytic cycle and rarely occurs following exogenous EBV infection (96,97). The surface representation of nonviral antigens, e.g., histocompatibility (HLA) antigens, may also be altered by EBV infection and transformation (101). The addition of macrophages or fibroblasts to purified cultures of B lymphocytes facilitates immortalization, though neither macrophages nor fibroblasts themselves support EBV replication (102).

The sequence of events that follows in vivo infection with EBV is less clear. Infections frequently are subclinical, particularly in childhood. In adults, the incubation between exposure and clinical manifestations of infectious mononucleosis varies between 30–50 days. Among the abnormalities that may occur during the course of infectious mononucleosis are an atypical lymphocytosis in the peripheral blood, production of heterophile- and autoantibodies, and a diminution in cell-mediated responsiveness to certain antigens, despite an increase in spontaneous DNA synthesis among T cell populations (103,104). Most of the atypical lymphocytes present in peripheral blood are T lymphocytes, although a small proportion of early atypical cells appear to be B lymphocytes (103–107). During the acute phase of infectious mononucleosis, killer cells (probably T lymphocytes) specifically cytotoxic for B cell lines transformed by EBV can be found in peripheral blood (108–110). At this time intense lymphoproliferative changes are also found in thymus-dependent paracortical zones of lymph nodes (103). The intense T cell response against EBV-infected cells may result in a state of temporary anergy against other encountered antigens (103). It is not known whether EBV-infected B lymphocytes can also react in an autoimmune fashion against uninfected antiviral cells, in a way analogous to that suggested by murine leukemia virus models (34–37).

It is possible that the clinical syndrome of mononucleosis may represent a "civil war" between a vigorous T-lymphocyte-mediated rejection reaction against EBV-altered target B cells, which may themselves be autoreactive. A variety of humoral autoimmune responses may be observed during infectious mononucleosis (103), and when there is a deficiency in immunity against EBV-associated antigens, progressive fatal EBV-directed lymphoproliferation may ensue (111,112). Although infections EBV has not been found in blood during infectious mononucleosis (113), EBNA-positive cells have been found (114), and in vitro culture of such cells with umbilical cord lymphocytes readily results in the release of infectious virus (115,116). Following recovery from mononucleosis, both EBNA-positive B lymphoblasts and T lymphoblasts cytotoxic for EBNA-positive cells disappear from peripheral blood (114).

The succession of events that occurs during the pathogenesis of African Burkitt's lymphoma is far less clear, although it appears that EBV infection may antedate clinical lymphoma development by months to years (117,118). Burkitt's lymphoma biopsy cells contain EBV-DNA and EBNA, readily grow in culture, and may release infectious EBV shortly after in vitro propagation with umbilical cord leukocytes (8,116). Burkitt's lymphoma patients develop a variety of humoral antibody responses against EBV-associated antigens, some of which correlate with the clinical activity of the disease (83,119). Cell-mediated immunity against EBV-associated or unrelated antigens has not been thoroughly studied in Burkitt's lymphoma patients (83,124).

EBV-carrying lymphoblastoid lines derived from normal donors or patients with infectious mononucleosis differ in several respects from those derived from patients with Burkitt's lymphoma (121). These include growth characteristics, mobility, immunoglobulin production and secretion, surface antigen distribution, medium requirements, and clonality. In addition, lymphoblastoid cell lines derived from Burkitt's lymphomas regularly show a chromosomal abnormality (122–124), recently defined as an 8–14 translocation (124). Such a genetic alteration may influence the likelihood of EBV-induced transformations leading to lymphoma development, since lymphoid cell lines derived from patients with infectious mononucleosis have not contained this abnormality (123,124). However, the abnormality is neither present in all Burkitt's lymphoma lines containing EBV nor unique to lymphoma lines derived from Burkitt's tumors (124). Perhaps both chromosomal alteration and EBV infection are cofactors in the pathogenesis of Burkitt's lymphoma.

Activation of EBV from Lymphocytes.   EBV-infected lymphoid cells appear to retain viral DNA in two forms. Part exists in a covalently closed, free circular form and another part is integrated within the cell genome (125,126). As previously mentioned, many lymphoblastoid cell lines begin to produce EBV antigens and/or infectious virus after varying periods in culture. Some lymphoblastoid lines, e.g., most of those derived from cord leukocytes, are "non-producers" in that they are EA- and VCA-negative and do not produce infectious virus (116). Halogenated pyrimidines are effective inducers of EBV markers on some human lymphoblastoid lines (127–129). Activation of viral antigens by halogenated pyrimidines can be prevented by simultaneous treatment of cells with cytosine arabinoside or excess thymidine, indicating that the thymidine analogs must be incorporated into host cell DNA for viral activation to occur (128,129). In certain lymphoid lines, expression of EBV-associated antigens can also be increased by mitomycin C, actinomycin D, cytosine arabinoside, methotrexate, ultraviolet or X-irradiation, and arginine deprivation (129–133). Mixed leukocyte cultures between EBV genome-positive cells and EBV-negative umbilical cord cells may also result in activation of infectious virus with subsequent infection and immortalization of cord lymphocytes (115,116). It is not clear whether an allogeneic reaction is necessary for this sequence of events to occur, although it is likely that lymphocyte blastogenesis favors virus activation and subsequent infection of lymphocytes.

Cytomegalovirus

Human cytomegalovirus (CMV) resembles EBV in several respects. Both of these herpesviruses induce mononucleosis syndromes, and both have been implicated in oncogenic disorders (9,134). In addition, both remain latent within leukocytes for prolonged periods but can become activated during situations characterized by immunologic dysfunction (135,136), and following transfusion of fresh blood (137,138).

Although lymphocyte CMV interactions have not yet been well defined in man, a few preliminary observations have recently been made. Molecular-hybridization studies have indicated that CMV DNA sequences can be found associated with host DNA in peripheral leukocytes of normal blood donors (139). In addition, CMV has been reported to abortively infect B lymphoblastoid lines containing EBV genomes, but not T lymphoblastoid lines (140,141). It has not been shown whether latent CMV can be activated from human lymphoid cells. However, several observations suggest that human CMV can be activated in vivo following transfusion of fresh leukocyte-rich blood. Most studies have failed to demonstrate infectious CMV in donor blood (142–145) despite the presence of CMV DNA within leukocytes (139). Shortly after blood transfusion, a significant blastogenic response develops in the peripheral blood of recipients (146), perhaps representing an allogeneic reaction between donor and recipient leukocytes. Seroconversion to CMV frequently follows this type of response (138,147) and is occasionally associated with heterophile-negative mononucleosis. In such cases, CMV is isolatable from peripheral blood leukocytes or from urine, and a variety of serological abnormalities may occur, including antinuclear antibodies, cryoglobulins, and cold agglutinins (148). It appears that CMV may be activated from a latent state within donor leukocytes by a graft-versus-host or host-versus-graft reaction. In analogous murine model systems, mouse CMV has been activated or amplified in vivo by transfusion of leukocytes from latently infected mice into uninfected histoincompatible recipients (149) or by placement of histoincompatible skin grafts onto latently infected recipients (150). In vitro activation of latent murine CMV from splenic lymphocytes has also been described following allogeneic reactions or treatment with mitogens (151). Although immunosuppression following CMV infection in man has not yet been reported, murine infection with CMV results in both humoral and cellular hyporesponsiveness (152–154).

Simian Herpesviruses

Two herpesviruses of subhuman primates, *Herpesvirus saimiri* (HVS), a ubiquitous agent in squirrel monkeys, and *Herpesvirus ateles* (HVA), an agent common to spider monkeys, have been demonstrated to have oncogenic properties (155–157). These viruses have not been shown to be oncogenic in the species from which they originate, but they do induce lymphomas and leukemias when inoculated into a variety of other subhuman primates. Whereas the natural host excretes infectious virus and transmits the virus horizontally, experimentally inoculated species that develop lymphoproliferative disease do not express viral antigens or infectious virus. Both normal and neoplastic lymphoid cells carry herpesvirus genomes, however, and in vitro explantation results in rapid gene derepression and expression of viral antigens and infectious virus (157). Both HVS and HVA have a predilection for T lymphocytes, unlike the B cell tropism of EBV in man (158–160). T lymphoblastoid lines can be established from diseased animals or from marmoset lymphocytes transformed in vitro (158–160). A few cells from most lines contain antigens, and such cells may produce small amounts of infectious virus; upon prolonged culture, many lines become nonproducers with regard to both infectious virus and viral antigens (157). These nonproducer lines continue to carry viral genetic information but are not well induced by halogenated pyrimidines. No specific chromosomal aberrations have been demonstrated in HVS-carrying lymphoblastoid lines or in fresh leukocytes from diseased animals (161).

Inoculation of HVS or HVA into marmosets or owl monkeys results in the rapid induction of lymphoproliferative disease. Prior to overt lymphomagenesis, infected animals produce antibodies against various virus-associated antigens (162,163). Although cell-mediated responses against viral antigens have not been thoroughly evaluated, there is evidence of nonspecific depression of certain T lymphocyte functions, e.g., mitogen responsiveness, in infected animals (147). In general, mitogen reactivity is inversely proportional to the progression of disease, the degree of spontaneous lymphocyte blastogenesis, and the proportion of lymphocytes from which HVS can be recovered. It is possible that the lack of lymphoma development in natural hosts is a result of more efficient immune responsiveness against virus- or tumor-associated antigens. The nature of the defect of T lymphocyte responsiveness in lymphoma-susceptible owl monkeys is not clear. It has been proposed that either functional leukocytes may be "crowded out" by virus-infected cells that are not responsive to mitogens, or a subpopulation of suppressor cells may be activated by virus infection (164). The possible autoimmune elimination of normal cells by virus-infected T lymphocytes analogous to that proposed for Moloney leukemia virus (33–36) has not been explored.

Table 1   Lymphocyte Interactions with Herpesviruses and with C-type Oncornaviruses

Characteristic	Oncornaviruses	Herpesviruses
Virus genetic information	Acquired genetically or postnatally	Acquired by intrauterine or postnatal infection
Lymphocytes involved	T or B	T (e.g., HVS) or B (e.g., EBV)
Mechanism of virus induction	Spontaneous Chemical Radiation Immunological	Spontaneous Chemical Immunological (CMV)
Fate of induced cell	Lives	Dies
Infection in primary host:		
Antiviral immune response	Yes	Yes
Immunosuppression	Variable	Variable
Oncogenicity	?	?
Infection in secondary host:		
Antiviral immune response	Yes	Yes
Immunosuppression	Yes	Yes
Autoaggressiveness	Yes	?
Oncogenicity	Yes	Yes

CONCLUSIONS

It is instructive to compare the interactions of potentially oncogenic C-type oncornaviruses and host lymphocytes with the interactions of potentially oncogenic
herpesviruses and lymphocytes (Table 1). Whereas transmission of oncornavirus
genetic information may occur by either genetic or infectious routes, there is at
present no evidence that mammalian herpesviruses are genetically transmitted.
Nevertheless, in both situations virus genetic information may become incorporated into lymphocyte genomes. Varying degrees of genetic repression of virus
information may occur, but such repression may be at least partially overcome by
in vitro cell culture, treatment with certain nucleoside derivates or mitogens, or
allogeneic reactions in vivo or in vitro. Production of infectious oncornaviruses
by lymphoid cells is compatible with cell survival, whereas production of infectious herpesviruses uniformly leads to cell lysis. Within both groups are members
that may have tropisms for B lymphocytes or T lymphocytes and may even have
selective tropisms for subpopulations within these cell types. The functional
capacities of virus-infected cells may become disordered; oncornavirus infection
may direct lymphocytes to become autoaggressive and may interfere with their
ability to respond to antigens; herpesvirus infection may induce lymphocytes to
become autonomous or immortalized and may also interfere with their ability to
respond to mitogens or antigens. It is not known whether herpesviruses can
induce autoaggressiveness on the part of infected lymphocytes. Both groups of
viruses can induce antiviral immune responses in their hosts of origin, as well as
in subsequently infected hosts.

Although both herpesviruses and oncornaviruses can induce lymphoid neoplasms in secondarily infected hosts, it remains unclear whether they are oncogenic agents in their primary hosts. Secondarily infected hosts frequently develop diminished responsiveness to other antigens, and the hyporesponsiveness
generally worsens as the tumor burden increases. The mechanisms leading to
decreased responsiveness vary considerably and remain largely undefined. Similarly, the relationship between disordered immunity induced by exogenous oncogenic viruses and subsequent oncogenic events is unclear. Inhibition of antiviral immune mechanisms may lead to enhanced virus replication, with resultant
increased likelihood of a malignant transformation event. The proliferation of
virus-transformed cells or virus-induced autoaggressor cells may also be facilitated by virus-initiated immunosuppression of antitumor responses. Tumor cells
themselves may further augment immunosuppression by producing suppressor
factors or by acting autoaggressively. Thus, exogenous oncogenic viruses may
initiate a series of events in which immunosuppression is a fundamental intermediate step on the pathway to neoplasia.

The role of potentially oncogenic endogenous viruses in their natural hosts is
much less clear. Although certain immunologic events and radiation can induce the expression of latent agents, it is not clear whether these viruses are
necessary for the subsequent development of neoplasms. In some situations
expression of endogenous viruses can be related to the subsequent development
of neoplasia; in other situations viral expression may actually increase the immunogenicity and rejectability of tumors. Development of effective vaccines
and/or antiviral chemotherapeutic agents that can prevent activation of endogenous viruses or eliminate productive virus carrier states may be necessary to

answer questions regarding the role of endogenous viruses in the pathogenesis of lymphoreticular neoplasms.

ACKNOWLEDGMENTS

I wish to thank Drs. P. H. Black, M. R. Proffitt, C. R. Rinaldo, Jr., and H. B Simon for reviewing this manuscript.

REFERENCES

1. Gross, L., *Oncogenic Viruses,* 2nd Ed., Pergamon, Oxford, 1970.
2. Hirsch, M. S., and Black, P. H., *Adv. Virus Res.* **19,** 265 (1974).
3. Mak, T. W., Manaster, J., Howatson, A. F., McCulloch, E. A., and Till, J. E., *Proc. Nat. Acad. Sci.* **71,** 4336 (1974).
4. Teich, N. M., Weiss, R. A., Salahuddin, S. Z., Gallagher, R. E., Gillespie, D. H., and Gallo, R. C., *Nature* **256,** 551 (1975).
5. Nootor, K., Aarssen, A. M., Bentvelzen, P., DeGroot, F. G., and van Pelt, F. G., *Nature* **256,** 595 (1975).
6. McGrath, C. M., Grant, P. M., Soule, P. M., Glancy, T., and Rich, M. A., *Nature* **252,** 247 (1974).
7. Melnick, J. M., Adam, E., and Rawls, W. E., *Cancer* **34,** 1375 (1974).
8. Klein, G., *N. Eng. J. Med.* **293,** 1353 (1975).
9. Giraldo, G., Beth, E., Kourilsky, F. M., Henle, W., Henle, G., Miké, V., Huraux, J. M., Anderson, H. K., Gharbi, M. R., Kyalwazi, S. K., and Puissant, A., *Int. J. Cancer* **15,** 839 (1975).
10. Weiss, A. F., Portmann, R., Fischer, H., Simon, J., and Zang, K. D., *Proc. Nat. Acad. Sci.* **72,** 609 (1975).
11. Gressor, I., and Lang, D. F., *Prog. Med. Virol.* **8,** 62 (1966).
12. Wheelock, E. F., and Toy, S. T., *Adv. Immunol.* **16,** 123 (1973).
13. Woodruff, J. F., and Woodruff, J. J., in *Viral Immunology and Immunopathology* (A. Notkins, ed.), Academic Press, New York, 1975, p. 393.
14. Stutman, O., *Adv. Cancer Res.* **22,** 261 (1975).
15. Ceglowski, W., *Ann. N.Y. Acad. Sci.* (in press).
16. Dent. P. B., in *The Immune System and Infectious Diseases* (E. Neter and F. Milgrom, eds.), S. Karger, Basel, 1975, p. 95.
17. Ceglowski, W. S., Campbell, B., and Friedman, H., *J. Immunol.* **114,** 231 (1975).
18. Ceglowski, W. S., and Friedman, H., *Nature* **224,** 1318 (1969).
19. Ceglowski, W. S., and Friedman, H. *J. Immunol.* **103,** 460 (1969).
20. Cerny, J., and Warner, E. B., *J. Immunol.* **114,** 571 (1975).
21. Bainbridge, D. R., and Bendinelli, M., *J. Nat. Cancer Inst.* **49,** 773 (1972).
22. Kately, J. R., Holderbach, J., and Friedman, H., *J. Nat. Cancer Inst.* **53,** 1135 (1974).
23. Ceglowski, W. S., Koo, G. C., and Friedman, H., *Adv. Exp. Biol. Med.* **12,** 435 (1971).
24. Farber, P., Specter, S., and Friedman, H., *Science* **190,** 469 (1975).
25. Levy, M. H., and Wheelock, E. F., *J. Immunol.* **114,** 962 (1975).
26. Bendinelli, M., Kaplan, G. S., and Friedman, H., *J. Nat. Cancer Inst.* **55,** 1425 (1975).
27. Kately, J. R., Kamo, I., Kaplan, G., and Friedman, H., *J. Nat. Cancer Inst.* **53,** 1371 (1974).
28. Mortenson, R. F., Ceglowski, W. S., and Friedman, H., *J. Immunol.* **111,** 1810 (1973).
29. Mortenson, R. F., Ceglowski, W. S., and Friedman, H., *J. Immunol.* **112,** 2077 (1973).
30. Cerny, J., and Stiller, R. A., *J. Immunol.* **115,** 943 (1975).
31. Kirchner, H., Muchmore, A. V., Chused, T. M., Holden, H. T., and Herberman, R. B., *J. Immunol.* **114,** 206 (1975).

32. Bonnard, G. D., Manders, E. K., Campbell, D. A., Jr., Herberman, R. B., and Collins, M. J., Jr., *J. Exp. Med.* **143**, 187 (1976).

33. Herberman, R., unpublished observations.

34. Proffitt, M. R., Hirsch, M. S., and Black, P. H., *Science* **182**, 821 (1973).

35. Proffitt, M. R., Hirsch, M. S., Gheridian, B., McKenzie, I. F. C., and Black, P. H., *Int. J. Cancer* **15**, 221 (1975).

36. Proffitt, M. R., Hirsch, M. S., McKenzie, I. F. C., Gheridian, B., and Black, P. H., *Int. J. Cancer* **15**, 230 (1975).

37. Proffitt, M. R., Hirsch, M. S., Ellis, D. A., Gheridian, B., and Black, P. H., *J. Immunol.* **117**, 11 (1976).

38. Sklar, M., and Rowe, W., unpublished observations.

39. Proffitt, M. R., Hirsch, M. S., and Black, P. H., in *Autoimmunity* (N. Talal, ed.), Academic Press, New York (in press).

40. Cox, K. O., and Keast, D., *J. Nat. Cancer Inst.* **50**:941 (1973).

41. Kuzumaki, N., Kodama, T., Takeichi, N., and Kobayashi, H., *Int. J. Cancer* **14**:483 (1974).

42. Huebner, R. J., and Todaro, G. J., *Proc. Nat. Acad. Sci.* **64**:1087 (1969).

43. Todaro, G. J., and Huebner, R. J., *Proc. Nat. Acad. Sci.* **69**:1009 (1972).

44. Rowe, W. P., and Pincus, T., *J. Exp. Med.* **135**:429 (1972).

45. Lerner, R. A., Wilson, C. B., DelVillano, B. C., McConahey, P. J., and Dixon, F. J., *J. Exp. Med.* **143**:151 (1976).

46. Aoki, T., and Todaro, G. J., *Proc. Nat. Acad. Sci.* **70**:1598 (1973).

47. Aaronson, S. A., and Stephenson, J. R., *Proc. Nat. Acad. Sci.* **70**:2055 (1973).

48. Kaplan, H. S., *Cancer Res.* **27**:1325 (1967).

49. Hirsch, M. S., Black, P. H., Tracy, G. S., Leibowitz, S. G., and Schwartz, R. S., *Proc. Nat. Acad. Sci.* **67**:1914 (1970).

50. Armstrong, M. Y. K., Ruddle, N. H., Lipman, M. B., and Richards, F. F., *J. Exp. Med.* **137**:1163 (1973).

51. Hirsch, M. S., Phillips, S. M., Solnik, C., Black, P. H., Schwartz, R. S., and Carpenter, C. B., *Proc. Nat. Acad. Sci.* **69**:1069 (1972).

52. Sherr, C. J., Lieber, M. M., and Todaro, G. J., *Cell* **1**:55 (1974).

53. Moroni, C., Schumann, G., Robert-Guroff, M., Suter, E. R., and Martin, D., *Proc. Nat. Acad. Sci.* **72**:535 (1975).

54. Greenberger, J. S., Phillips, S. M., Stephenson, J. R., and Aaronson, S. A., *J. Immunol.* **115**:317 (1975).

55. Gleichmann, E., Gleichmann, H., Schwartz, R. S., Weinblatt, A., and Armstrong, M. Y. K., *J. Nat. Cancer Inst.* **54**:107 (1975).

56. Hirsch, M. S., Ellis, D. A., Proffitt, M. R., Black, P. H., and Chirigos, M. A., *Nature New Biol.* **244**:102 (1973).

57. Nowinski, R. C., and Kaehler, S. L., *Science* **185**:869 (1974).

58. Aaronson, S. A., and Stephenson, J. R., *Proc. Nat. Acad. Sci.* **71**:1957 (1974).

59. Ihle, J. N., Hanna, M. G., Jr., Roberson, L. E., and Kenney, F. T., *J. Exp. Med.* **139**, 1568 (1974).

60. Hirsch, M. S., Kelly, A. P., Proffitt, M. R., and Black, P. H., *Science* **187**, 959 (1975).

61. Herberman, R. B., Nunn, M. E., and Lavrin, D. H., *Int. J. Cancer* **16**, 216 (1975).

62. Zarling, J. M., Nowinski, R. C., and Bach, F. H., *Proc. Nat. Acad. Sci.* **72**, 2780 (1975).

63. Phillips, S. M., Gleichmann, H., Hirsch, M. S., Black, P., Merrill, J. P., Schwartz, R. S., and Carpenter, C. B., *Cell. Immunol.* **15**, 152 (1975).

64. Solnik, C., Gleichmann, H., Kavanah, M., and Schwartz, R. S., *Cancer Res.* **33**, 2068 (1973).

65. Grebe, S. C., and Streilein, J. W., *Adv. Immunol.* **22**, 120 (1976).

66. Hirsch, M. S., Ellis, D. A., Black, P. H., Monaco, A. P., and Wood, M. L., *Science* **180**, 500 (1973).

66a. Hirsch, M. S., Ellis, D. A., Kelly, A. P., Proffitt, M. R., Black, P. H., Monaco, A. P., and Wood, M. L., *Internl J. Cancer* **15**, 493 (1975).

67. André-Schwartz, J., Schwartz, R. S., Hirsch, M. S., Phillips, S. M., and Black, P. H., *J. Nat. Cancer Inst.* **51**, 507 (1973).

68. Phillips, S. M., Hirsch, M. S., André-Schwartz, J., Solnik, C., Black, P., Schwartz, R. S., Merrill, J. P., and Carpenter, C. B., *Cell. Immunol.* **15**, 169 (1975).

69. Lonai, P., Decléve, A., and Kaplan, H. S., *Proc. Nat. Acad. Sci.* **71**, 2008 (1974).

70. Essex, M., *Adv. Cancer Res.* **21**, 175 (1975).

71. Todaro, G. J., Benveniste, R. E., Lieber, M. M., and Livingston, D. M., *Virol.* **55**, 506 (1973).

72. Fischinger, P. J., Peebles, P. J., Nomura, S., and Haapala, D. K., *J. Virol.* **11**, 978 (1973).

73. Essex, M., Sliski, A., Cotter, S. M., Jakowski, R. M., and Hardy, W. D., Jr., *Science* **190**, 790 (1975).

74. Anderson, L. F., Jarrett, W. F. H., Jarrett, O., and Laird, H. M., *J. Nat. Cancer Inst.* **47**, 807 (1971).

75. Perryman, L. E., Hoover, E. A., and Yohn, D. S., *J. Nat. Cancer Inst.* **49**, 1357 (1972).

76. Hoover, E. A., Perryman, L. E., and Kociba, G. J., *Cancer Res.* **33**, 145 (1973).

77. Essex, M., Hardy, W. D., Jr., Cotter, S. M., Jakowski, R. M., and Sliski, A., *Inf. Imm.* **11**, 470 (1975).

78. Benveniste, R. E., Lieber, M. M., Livingston, D. M., Sherr, C. J., Todaro, G. J., and Kalter, S. S., *Nature* **248**, 17 (1974).

79. Kawakami, T. G., Huff, S. D., Buckeley, P. M., Dungworth, D. L., Synder, S. P., and Gilden, R. V., *Nature* **235**, 170 (1972).

80. Theilen, G. H., Gould, D., Fowler, M. E., and Dungworth, D. L., *J. Nat. Cancer Inst.* **47**, 881 (1971).

81. Epstein, M. A., Achong, B. G., and Barr, Y. M., *Lancet* **1**, 702 (1964).

82. Evans, A. S., Rothfield, N. F., and Niederman, J. C., *Lancet* **1**, 167 (1971).

83. Klein, G., *The Herpesviruses* (A. Kaplan, ed.), Academic Press, New York, 1973, p. 521.

84. Henle, G., Henle, W., Clifford, P., Diehl, V., Kafuko, G. W., Kirya, B. G., Klein, G., Morrow, R. H., Munube, G., Pike, P., Tukei, P., and Ziegler, J., *J. Nat. Cancer Inst.* **43**, 1147 (1969).

85. Lindahl, T., Klein, G., Reedman, B. M., Johansson, B., and Singh, S., *Intern. J. Cancer* **13**, 764 (1974).

86. Reedman, B. M., and Klein, G., *Intern. J. Cancer* **11**, 499 (1973).

87. Nonoyama, M., Huang, C. H., Pagano, J. S., Klein, G., and Singh, S., *Proc. Nat. Acad. Sci.* **70**, 3265 (1973).

88. zurHausen, H., Schulte-Holthausen, H., Klein, G., Henle, W., Henle, G., Clifford, P., and Santesson, L., *Nature* **228**, 1056 (1970).

89. Pope, J. H., Horne, M. K., and Scott, W., *Int. J. Cancer* **4**, 255 (1969).

90. Miller, G., *Yale J. Biol. Med.* **43**, 358 (1971).

91. Shope, T., Dechairo, D., and Miller, G., *Proc. Nat. Acad. Sci.* **70**, 2487 (1973).

92. Werner, J., Wolf, H., Apodacca, J., and zurHausen, H., *Intern. J. Cancer* **15**, 1000 (1975).

93. Epstein, M. A., zurHausen, H., Ball, G., and Rabin, H., *Intern. J. Cancer* **15**, 17 (1975).

94. Greaves, F. M., Brown, G., and Rickinson, A. B., *Clin. Immunol. Immunopathol.* **3**, 514 (1975).

95. Katsuki, T., and Hinuma, Y., *Intern, J. Cancer* **15** 203 (1975).

96. Robinson, J., and Miller, G., *J. Virol.* **15**, 1065 (1975).

97. Leibold, W., Flanagan, T. D., Menezes, J., and Klein, G., *J. Nat. Cancer Inst.* **54**, 65 (1975).

98. Yata, J., Desgranges, C., Nakagawa, T., Faure, M. C., and De Thé, G., *Intern, J. Cancer* **15**, 377 (1975).

99. Moss, D. J., and Pope, J. H., *Intern. J. Cancer* **15**, 503 (1975).

100. Menezes, J., Jondal, M., Leibold, W., and Dorval, G., *Inf. Immun.* **13**, 303 (1976).

101. McCune, J. M., Humphreys, R. E., Yocum, R. R., and Strominger, J. L., *Proc. Nat. Acad. Sci.* **72**, 3206 (1975).

102. Schneider, U., and zurHausen, H., *Intern, J. Cancer* **15**, 59 (1975).

103. Carter, R. L., *Lancet* **1**, 824 (1975).

104. Mangi, R., Niederman, J. C., Kelleher, J. E., Dwyer, J. M., Evans, A. S., and Kantor, F. S., *N. Eng. J. Med.* **291,** 1149 (1974).

105. Papamichail, M., Sheldon, P. J., and Holborow, E. J., *Clin. Exp. Immunol.* **18,** 1 (1974).

106. Denman, A. M., and Pelton, B. K., *Clin. Exp. Immunol.* **18,** 13 (1974).

107. Pattengale, P. K., Smith, R. W., and Perlin, E., *N. Eng. J. Med.* **291,** 1145 (1974).

108. Svedmyr, E., and Jondal, M., *Proc. Nat. Acad. Sci.* **72,** 1622 (1975).

109. Royston, I., Sullivan, J. L., Periman, P. O., and Perlin, E., *N. Eng. J. Med.* **293,** 1159 (1975).

110. Hutt, L. M., Huang, Y. T., Dascomb, H. E., and Pagano, J. S., *J. Immunol.* **115,** 243 (1975).

111. Bar, R. S., DeLor, C. J., Clausen, K. P., Hurtubise, P., Henle, W., and Hewetson, J., *N. Eng. J. Med.* **290,** 363 (1974).

112. Purtilo, D. T., Cassel, C. K., Yang, J. P., Harper, R., Stephenson, S. R., Landing, B. H., and Vawter, G. F., *Lancet* **1,** 935 (1975).

113. Rickinson, A. B., Epstein, M. A., and Crawford, D. H., *Nature,* **258,** 236 (1975).

114. Klein, G., Svedmyr, E., Jondal, M., and Persson, P. O., *Intern. J. Cancer* **17,** 21 (1976).

115. Rickinson, A. B., Jarvis, J. E., Crawford, D. H., and Epstein, M. A., *Int. J. Cancer* **14,** 704 (1974).

116. Dalens, M., Zech, L., and Klein, G., *Int. J. Cancer* **16,** 1008 (1975).

117. Cohen, M. H., Hirshaut, Y., Stevens, D., Hull, E. W., Davis, J. H., and Carbone, P. P., *Ann. Intern. Med.* **73,** 591 (1970).

118. Magrath, I., Henle, W., Owor, R., and Olweny, C., *N. Eng. J. Med.* **292,** 261 (1975).

119. Henle, G., Henle, W., and Klein, G., *Intern. J. Cancer* **8,** 272 (1971).

120. Fass, L., Herberman, R. B., Ziegler, J., and Morrow, R. H., *J. Nat. Cancer Inst.* **44,** 145 (1970).

121. Nilsson, K., and Pontén, J., *Int. J. Cancer* **15,** 321 (1975).

122. Manolov, G., and Manolova, Y., *Nature* **237,** 33 (1972).

123. Jarvis, J. E., Ball, G., Rickinson, A. B., and Epstein, M. A., *Intern. J. Cancer* **14,** 716 (1974).

124. Zech, L., Haglund, U., Nilsson, K., and Klein, G., *Int. J. Cancer* **17,** 47 (1976).

125. Nonoyama, M., and Tanaka, A., *Cold Spring Harbor Symp. Quantit. Biol.* **39,** 807 (1974).

126. Adams, A., and Lindahl, T., *Proc. Nat. Acad. Sci.* **72,** 1477 (1975).

127. Gerber, P., *Proc. Nat. Acad. Sci.* **69,** 83 (1972).

128. Hampar, B., Derge, J. G., Martos, L. M., and Walker, J. L., *Proc. Nat. Acad. Sci.* **69,** 78 (1972).

129. Klein, G., and Dombos, L., *Int. J. Cancer* **11,** 327 (1973).

130. Yata, J., Klein, G., Hewetson, J., and Gergely, L., *Int. J. Cancer* **5,** 394 (1970).

131. Gergely, L., Klein, G., and Ernberg, I., *Int. J. Cancer* **7,** 293 (1971).

132. Henle, W., and Henle, G., *J. Virol.* **2,** 182 (1968).

133. Lai. P. K., MacKay-Scollay, E. M., and Alpers, M. P., *J. Gen. Virol.* **21,** 135 (1973).

134. Rapp, F., *Adv. Cancer Res.* **19,** 265 (1974).

135. Strauch, B., Andrews, L., Siegel, N., and Miller, G., *Lancet* **1,** 234 (1974).

136. Fiala, M., Payne, J. E., Berne, T. V., Moore, T. C., Henle, W., Montgomerie, J. Z., Chatterjee, S. N., and Guze, L. B., *J. Inf. Dis.* **132,** 421 (1975).

137. Solem, J., and Jorgenson, W., *Acta Med. Scandinav.* **186,** 433 (1969).

138. Caúl, E. O., Clarke, S. K. R., Mott, M. G., Perham, T. G. M., and Wilson, R. S. E., **1,** 777 (1971).

139. Pagano, J. S., *J. Inf. Dis.* **132,** 209 (1975).

140. Huang, E. S., and Pagano, J. S., in *Proceedings of the Second International Symposium on Oncogenesis and Herpes Viruses,* Nuremberg, Germany, 1975 (in press).

141. Joncas, J. H., Menezes, J., and Huang, E. S., *Nature* **258,** 432 (1975).

142. Mirkovic, R., Werch, J., South, M. A., and Benyesh-Melnick, M., *Inf. Imm.* **3,** 45 (1971).

143. Wentworth, B. B., and Alexander, E. R., *Amer. J. Epidem.* **94,** 496 (1971).

144. Perham, T. G. M., Caul, E. O., Conway, P. J., and Mott, M. G., *Brit. J. Hematol.* **20,** 307 (1971).

145. Kane, R. C., Rousseau, W. E., Noble, G. R., Tegtmeier, G. E., Wulff, H., Herndon, H. B., Chin, T. D. Y., and Bayer, W. C., *Inf. Imm.* **11,** 719 (1975).

146. Schechter, G. P., Soehnlen, F., and McFarland, W., *N. Eng. J. Med.* **287,** 1169 (1972).

147. Prince, A. M., Szmuness, W., Millian, S. J., and David, D. S., *N. Eng. J. Med.* **284**, 1125 (1971).

148. Kantor, G. L., Goldberg, L. S., Johnson, B. L., Jr., Derechin, M. M., and Barnett, E. V., *Ann. Int. Med.* **73**, 553 (1970).

149. Lang, D. J., unpublished observations.

150. Wu, B. C., Dowling, J. N., Armstrong, J. A., and Ho, M., *Science* **190**, 56 (1975).

151. Olding, L. B., Jensen, F. C., and Oldstone, M. B. A., *J. Exp. Med.* **141**, 561 (1975).

152. Osburn, J. E., Blazkovec, A. A., and Walker, D. L., *J. Immunol.* **100**, 835 (1968).

153. Howard, R. J., and Najarian, J. S., *Clin. Exp. Immunol.* **18**, 109 (1974).

154. Howard, R. J., Miller, J., and Najarian, J. S., *Clin. Exp. Immunol.* **18**, 119 (1974).

155. Meléndez, L. V., Hunt, R. D., Daniel, M. D., Fraser, C. E. O., Barahona, H. H., King, N. W., and Garcia, F. G., *Fed. Proc.* **31**, 1643 (1972).

156. Deinhardt, F., Falk, L. A., and Wolfe, L. G., *Cancer Res.* **33**, 1424 (1973).

157. Deinhardt, F. W., Falk, L. A., and Wolfe, L. G., *Adv. Cancer Res.* **19**, 167 (1974).

158. Wallen, W. C., Neubauer, R. H., Rabin, H., and Cicmanec, J. L., *J. Nat. Cancer Inst.* **51**, 967 (1973).

159. Deinhardt, F., Falk, L. A., and Wolfe, L. G., *Cancer Res.* **34**, 1241 (1974).

160. Falk, L., Wright, J., Wolfe, L., and Deinhardt, F., *Int. J. Cancer* **14**, 244 (1974).

161. Marczynska, B., Falk, L. A., Wolfe, L. G., and Deinhardt, F., *J. Nat. Cancer Inst.* **50**, 331 (1973).

162. Pearson, G., Ablashi, D., Orr, T., Rabin, H., and Armstrong, G., *J. Nat. Cancer Inst.* **49**, 1417 (1972).

163. Falk, L. A., Wolfe, L. G., and Deinhardt, F., *J. Nat. Cancer Inst.* **51**, 165 (1973).

164. Wallen, W. C., Rabin, H., Neubauer, R. H., and Cicmanec, J. L., *J. Nat. Cancer Inst.* **54**, 679 (1975).

Chapter Twelve

Regulation of Inflammatory Responses in Neoplastic Disease

PETER A. WARD AND STANLEY COHEN

Department of Pathology, University of Connecticut Health Center, Farmington, Connecticut

The concept of "immune surveillance" has led to the belief that the immune response may represent a major defense mechanism against neoplastic disease. Evidence for and against this hypothesis has been presented in Chapter 2. Regardless of the degree to which immune surveillance is operative in the natural state, it now seems clear that it is possible to modulate immune responses in tumor-bearing animals and in human patients with neoplasms. Great progress has been made in the separation, purification, and detection of tumor-specific antigens, and immunologic mechanisms of tumor cell destruction have been elucidated. These studies have prompted a variety of experimental approaches to immunotherapy. Much of this volume is devoted to these approaches.

To date, only limited success has been achieved. There is a great disparity between the relative ease with which one can kill tumor cells in vitro and curing a host of a neoplasm in vivo. This difficulty can only in part be ascribed to such factors as tumor mass or the presence of tumor in "protected" sites. It seems reasonable to postulate that there are specific mechanisms operating in vivo to limit the capacity of the immune response to control malignant growth. Some of the possible factors involved have been touched upon throughout this book. One of the best studied and understood involves a process known as immunologic enhancement, which is discussed in detail in Chapter 6. There is a great deal of evidence that blocking factors are present in animals and human patients with tumors, and that such factors are responsible for enhancement. These have been associated with antibody, antigen, or immune complexes.

As discussed in Chapters 3 and 4, many of the immunologic mechanisms of tumor cell destruction actually involve the inflammatory response. Immunologic reactions, mainly of the cell-mediated variety, lead to the accumulation and activation of inflammatory cells. The macrophage appears to be the major participant in such reactions, but other cells with phagocytic potential such as neutrophils, basophils, and eosinophils have also been implicated in this mechanism, both in infections and in neoplastic disease. It is reasonable to assume that anything which interferes with recruitment or activation of inflammatory cells at the sites where they are needed will serve to frustrate the process of host defense. In this chapter we will briefly describe two mechanisms by which this can occur in neoplastic disease. The first involves the elaboration of specific inhibitory factors which block the activity of inflammatory mediators such as complement-derived and lymphokine chemotactic factors. The second involves regulation of the expression of cell-mediated immunity by lymphokines themselves. Both these mechanisms, which at present are incompletely understood, may prove to play an important role in vivo.

REGULATION BY INHIBITORY FACTORS

It is now well established that animals as well as humans with malignant tumors fail to demonstrate delayed-type dermal inflammatory reactions after the injection of a variety of antigens, including fungal extracts and bacterial products (1,2). This inability to accumulate inflammatory cells has been associated with a more serious prognosis. The defect has disappeared with successful surgical treatment of the tumor; the failure of the defect to disappear after treatment of the tumor has been associated with the recurrence of the tumor and/or metastatic spread. With the current interest in immunotherapy and the widely held belief that immunologic defenses against malignant tumors involve a role for lymphocytes and monocytes, any defect that impairs the ability of the host to mobilize these cells in response to local stimuli could logically compromise host defenses against cancer.

The fact that contact-type skin reactions (usually incited by dinitrochlorobenzene) and delayed-type hypersensitivity reactions (induced by extracts or products of microorganisms or by histocompatibility differences) are T lymphocyte dependent, and the occasional demonstration that T cells from cancer patients are hyporesponsive to antigenic stimuli in various in vitro tests, had led to the assumption that an acquired T cell defect accounts for these observations in malignant states. However, there are bits of information that do not fit in with this explanation. For example, many cancer patients have lymphocytes in the circulation that are normally reactive to antigenic stimuli. Furthermore, there is now evidence that cancer patients fail to respond with a cellular inflammatory reaction to nonspecific stimuli or irritants, such as croton oil (3). Thus, it would appear that a generalized defect in the mobilization (accumulation) of inflammatory cells may occur in the cancer-bearing state.

Several sets of observations relate to possible mechanisms of defective inflammation in the cancer state. The studies of Fauvre et al. suggest that inflammatory cells do indeed fail to accumulate in and around tumors and that malignant cells seem to "repel" macrophages (4). These studies have been carried out in vitro as well as in vivo, and the authors postulate that a product of the malignant cell causes macrophages to "keep their distance" when near cancer cells in vitro. A similar or identical product has been postulated in vivo, preventing mice from responding with a cellular inflammatory response when tumor cells are injected intracutaneously. These studies thus direct attention towards a tumor cell product with antimacrophage properties.

A second series of observations has focused on acquired chemotactic defects in cancer patients. Baum has published results from assays of chemotactic responsiveness using neutrophils from humans (5). A large percentage of these patients show significant impairment in the chemotactic response of neutrophils; it has been concluded that the basis for this defect is an acquired leukocyte abnormality which cannot be ascribed to a serum-associated inhibitor. Directing attention to the blood monocyte, similar observations have been reported by Snyderman et al. in man and, recently, also in mice (6). Human monocytes from many cancer patients are significantly defective in chemotaxis, and the defect cannot be corrected by washing the cells and resuspending them in fresh normal serum. The defect involves chemotactic response of blood monocytes to the complement-derived (C5) leukotactic factor as well as the lymphocyte-derived chemotactic factor. The monocyte chemotactic defect is reported to occur in patients with malignant tumors, disappearing with successful surgical removal of the tumor, and is diminished with immunotherapy (BCG). Some recent preliminary observations have suggested that the chemotactic defect involving monocytes may be due, at least in part, to the presence of an inhibitor in the serum (see below).

In very recent studies Pike and Snyderman report that extracts of fibosarcoma, lymphosarcoma, hepatoma, and teratosarcoma cells contain a heat-stable (resistant to boiling) factor, of low molecular weight (circa 10,000), that will impair the in vitro chemotactic responses of monocytes, but not neutrophils, to lymphocyte and complement-derived chemotactic factors (7). A similar material was not found in extracts of fibroblasts and hepatic cells. This inhibition reduced the numbers of monocytes that ordinarily appear following intraperitoneal injection of phytohemagglutin. It is also reported that, when injected along with the synegenic tumor cells, the extract leads to enhancement of tumor cell growth. The assumption, based on these results, is that the presence of monocytes in or around malignant tumor cells leads to suppression in proliferation of tumor cells and that substances, such as the extract from tumor cells, will preclude the accumulation of monocytes via suppression of chemotaxis. Whether the inhibitor can be demonstrated in vivo, and to what extent the inhibitor can explain the earlier observations of Snyderman et al., remain to be determined. Nevertheless, if those studies can be confirmed, they will provide evidence that the inflammatory response can be directly blocked by a product from tumor cells.

In the past few years two naturally occurring inhibitors, which seem to regulate the leukotactic system, have been discovered, and there is evidence that each inhibitor may play a role in suppression of leukotaxis in certain cancer-bearing states. These inhibitors are known as the chemotactic factor inactivator (CFI) and the cell-directed inhibitor of chemotaxis. When possible, data will be cited that emphasize the possible role of each inhibitor in causing suppression of the leukotactic system.

Somewhat surprisingly, CFI was first discovered when leukocytes from patients with Hodgkin's disease were being assessed for their leukotactic responsiveness (8,9). It has been known for several years that some patients with Hodgkin's disease do not develop tuberculin-type reactions to intradermally injected antigens, that these patients fail to reject skin homografts in the usual manner, and that accumulation of inflammatory cells (both neutrophils as well as mononuclear cells) in these patients is defective (10). The assessment of in vitro lymphocyte function (blastogenesis after contact with antigen) in Hodgkin's patients has failed to provide a coherent and consistent picture to explain the inflammatory defect. The in vitro leukotactic studies indicated that nearly half of all Hodgkin's patients are leukotactically defective, and that this defect is due to the presence of a serum-associated inhibitor. In the course of these studies it became apparent that Hodgkin's patients do not have a unique inhibitor; rather, they have abnormally large amounts of a naturally occurring CFI. When contrasted with serum from normal donors, serum samples from Hodgkin's patients contained CFI in blood nearly fivefold above the normal, low level.

CFI is an irreversible inhibitor of leukotactic factors (complement-derived, lymphocyte-generated, and bacterial-associated). The inhibition is both time-, temperature-, and concentration-dependent. It was originally postulated that CFI acted as an enzyme, since irreversible binding between the inhibitor and the chemotactic factors could not be demonstrated. Careful fractionation of human serum revealed CFI to be present in a biphasic pattern, as an α-globulin CFI (molecular weight, circa 50,000) and a β-globulin (molecular weight, circa 150,000) (11). Both CFI's have recently been demonstrated to have an aminopeptidase activity, and, while there is no formal proof that this is the mechanism by which inactivation of the naturally occurring chemotactic factors occurs, there is direct proof that the aminopeptidase activity accounts for the ability of CFI to inactivate synthetic di- and tri-peptides that are highly active (at nanomolar concentrations) as chemotactic factors (12). Substrate specificity for the two CFI's has been revealed by the fact that the α-globulin CFI specifically inactivates the C5 chemotactic peptide, while the β-globulin CFI specifically inactivates the C3 chemotactic peptide. These findings have helped to explain the early observation that Hodgkin patients had selective elevations in the C5, but not the C3 chemotactic factor inactivator. The features of CFI are summarized in Table 1.

The biological significance of CFI has been underscored by the diversity of chemotactic factors that can be inhibited by CFI (see above) as well as by the recent observation that CFI can inhibit not only the lymphocyte-derived monocyte chemotactic factor but also the migration inhibitory factor (MIF) produced by stimulated lymphoid cells (13). Depending on one's view about the relevance of lymphokines to mediate a wide variety of inflammatory reactions, CFI begins to assume an increasingly interesting role in the regulation of inflammatory responses. Besides Hodgkin's disease, CFI has also been found to be present in association with malignant tumor cells (14). The ascitic fluids associated with Walker carcinosarcoma or Novikoff hepatoma cells in rats and malignant mastocytoma in mice have been found to contain a CFI activity, as have homogenates of the tumor cells (15). No evidence of "spillover" of CFI into the serum of tumor-bearing animals has been found. While it is also possible to find a CFI activity in homogenates of most normal tissues, the origin of the CFI present in the tumor-induced ascitic fluids has not been determined. Nevertheless, the CFI present in these fluids would seem to preclude leukocyte accumulation that depends upon chemotactic mediators. These observations may explain why so

Table 1   Chemotactic Factor Inactivators

Tumor association:	Hodgkin's disease, transplantable tumors of rats and mice (carcinosarcoma cells, Novikoff hepatoma cells, malignant mastocytoma cells).
Nontumor association:	Hepatic cirrhosis, sarcoid, lepromatous leprosy.
Specificity of action:	Inactivates chemotactic factors of complement, lymphocytes, and bacterial origin, as well as synthetic leukotactic peptides.
Basis of action:	Degradation of chemotactic factors through aminopeptidase activity.
Physical-chemical features:	Heat labile, two forms in human serum: an α-globulin (estimated molecular weight of 50,000) specifically inactivates the C5 chemotactic factor; a β-globulin (estimated molecular weight of 150,000) specifically inactivates the C3 chemotactic peptide.

few inflammatory cells find their way to intermingle with the malignant cells. The data would also provide an explanation for the observations of Fauvre et al.

The tumor-associated CFI inactivates the bacterial as well as the complement-derived chemotactic factors and has been also demonstrated in homogenates of tumor cells. Subcellular fractionation has revealed CFI to be present in the microsomal fraction. Concern has also focused on the presence of tumor cells of CFI in non-tumor-associated inflammatory exudates. Peritoneal exudates which have been induced by glycogen and are rich in neutrophilic granulocytes do not contain a CFI activity. Thus, the presence of a CFI activity in the peritoneal cavity of rats or mice bearing malignant cells may serve as a barrier to the influx of inflammatory cells in response to the tumor. This would be in keeping with the observations that few inflammatory cells are found in the peritoneal cavities when the malignant cells are present.

The association of CFI with malignant tumors is not an exclusive one. In fact, it appears in the human that, except for Hodgkin's disease, elevations in serum levels of CFI are usually associated with nonmalignant diseases which have, as a feature, the inability of the individual to mount a delayed-type hypersensitivity response. Patients whose serum contains elevated levels of CFI are anergic. Patients with hepatic cirrhosis, sarcoid, lepromatous leprosy, and many patients with no apparent systemic disease have a significant incidence (75% of all cases) of elevated levels of CFI. In lepromatous leprosy there is a striking correlation between high levels of CFI in the serum and depressed or absent delayed hypersensitivity responses to intradermally injected antigens. In lepromatous leprosy it has also been shown (not unexpectedly in view of the CFI levels) that the ability to accumulate in skin inflammatory sites both neutrophils as well as monocytes is markedly depressed. Thus, there is a good correlation between elevations in levels of CFI and a defect in the ability to accumulate leukocytes at sites of inflammatory stimuli.

Table 2   Cell-Directed Inhibitor of Chemotaxis

Tumor association:	Present in serum of human patients with a variety of carcinomas and sarcomas.
Nontumor association:	Listeria meningitis (case finding) and in hepatic cirrhosis.
Specificity of action:	Reversibly impairs chemotactic responsiveness of neutrophils and monocytes to a variety of chemotactic stimuli (complement, bacterial, and lymphocyte-derived chemotactic factors). Also, the phagocytic function of neutrophils is impaired.
Basis of action:	Unknown.
Physical-chemical features:	Heat stable, present in human serum as a β-globulin with an estimated molecular weight of 200,000.

Another inhibitor that may play an important role in suppression of the inflammatory response in the cancer-bearing state is the cell-directed inhibitor (CDI) of leukotaxis. CDI was first discovered in the serum of a patient with Listeria meningitis. Subsequently, it was realized that a similar, or identical, inhibitor could be found in normal human serum, but in lower concentration. CDI reversibly inhibits chemotactic responses of neutrophils as well as monocytes by a direct effect on the leukocytes. The leukocytes are rendered nonresponsive to a variety of chemotactic stimuli, including the C3 and C5 chemotactic factors, the bacterial chemotactic factors, and the lymphokine-associated monocyte chemotactic factor. In addition to chemotactic responses, phagocytic responses of the neutrophil are also suppressed, as assessed quantitatively by impaired uptake of radiolabeled immune precipitates (containing antigen-antibody complexes). Nearly two-thirds of humans with cancer have elevated levels (ranging up to tenfold above the normal levels) of CDI. Elevated blood levels of CDI are associated with carcinomas as well as sarcomas. No obvious association of CDI with the organ or tissue origin of the tumor, or with the histologic pattern of the tumor, has been found. Nor is it known if CDI is being produced by the tumor, in a manner analogous to the well-known phenomenon of ectopic hormone production by carcinomas of the lung. The general features of CDI are described in Table 2. The observations of CDI associated with malignancies in the human could explain the recent observations of leukotactic defects involving neutrophils and monocytes. Whether the presence of high levels of CDI correlate with depressed inflammatory reactions in the skin (see above) of cancer patients cannot be determined at the present time.

These observations suggest that the well-accepted reports of defective inflammatory responses in humans and animals with malignant tumors may be explicable on the basis of imbalances in control of the leukotactic systems. If there are to be successful immunologic defenses against tumors, these leukotactic defects will have to be circumvented.

ROLE OF ENDOGENOUS LYMPHOKINES IN REGULATION

The previous section discussed the role of endogenous inhibitors of inflammatory mediators. These substances may be detected in normal animals and also are produced by various tumor cells. They can, as part of their spectrum of activity, suppress or interfere with the activity of lymphokine mediators and thus in theory can suppress inflammatory manifestations of cell-mediated immunity.

Recent work has suggested another regulatory mechanism for the control of cell-mediated immune reactions in vivo at the effector or efferent level. Surprisingly, this mechanism involves the lymphokines themselves. The observations leading to this conclusion will be presented in detail.

Studies in several laboratories (16–18) have demonstrated that migration inhibition factor (MIF) is dectectable in the circulation of mice and guinea pigs with delayed hypersensitivity. In the latter study (18), the kinetics of appearance of serum MIF were investigated. It was found that serum MIF reached a peak 6 to 12 hours after the intravenous challenge of actively immunized animals with specific antigen. This timing correlated with, but was slightly later than, the reduction in peripheral blood monocyte levels which was also seen in the experimental animals.

This association of the systemic appearance of MIF and an alteration in a cell population which is known to play a major role in manifestations of cell-mediated immunity suggested the possibility of modifying these reactions by administration of exogenous mediators. Since no attempt has been made to explore the whole range of possible serum lymphokines in the previous experiments, and since few monospecific lymphokine preparations exist, we chose to administer whole supernatants, rich in MIF activity, that also contained multiple other lymphokines. It was found (18) that the intravenous injection of such supernatants, but not control preparations, resulted in a marked suppression of delayed hypersensitivity skin reactions in animals that had been previously immunized. It should be noted that these recipient animals were immunized to antigens unrelated to those used to immunize the animals that served as lymphocyte donors for the culture supernatants.

The ability of exogenous lymphokines to suppress cutaneous delayed hypersensitivity suggests that endogenous lymphokine, when present systemically, might play a similar role. Experimental desensitization in the guinea pig may be a model for this effect, since the conditions of antigen administration here are precisely those used to induce serum MIF (19), and preliminary experiments have demonstrated that desensitization can be passively transferred with serum.

The above results prompted an exploration of serum MIF in man. To date, such activity has been found consistently in the group of lymphoproliferative diseases. Cohen et al. (20) reported the presence of MIF in serum of 14 to 16 patients with non-Hodgkin's lymphoma, 10 of 13 with Hodgkin's disease, and 4 of 5 with chronic lymphocytic leukemia. In addition 1 of 3 patients with multiple myeloma had low but detectable serum activity. In contrast, less than 3% of controls, including normals and patients with a wide variety of other diseases, had detectable serum MIF. Of great interest in terms of the present discussion is the fact that many patients with these disorders have complete or partial anergy, as was discussed for Hodgkin's disease in the previous section. The animal experiments described above suggest that the lymphokine in the circulation may contribute to this anergy. As yet no large-scale correlative study of degree of anergy, serum lymphokine activity, and presence of other serum factors, etc., has been done. However, preliminary results suggest that the same subset of Hodgkin's patients may have both serum CFI and MIF activity.

In the above study the cellular source of the serum MIF was not determined, although the pathologic cells themselves are the most likely candidates. The fact that some cases involve T cells and others involve B cells is not surprising, in view of recent reports by ourselves (21) and others (22,23) that B as well as T cells can produce MIF. In a subsequent study involving the Sezary syndrome (24) more direct evidence was obtained that the neoplastic lymphoid cells were the source of the MIF.

The extension of these findings to nonlymphoid tumors has not yet been made. The best candidates for study are those clinical situations where there is an association of cutaneous anergy, a large tumor mass, and demonstrated immune response against tumor antigens in vitro. This latter could be secondary to active immunotherapy. A further extension of these studies must involve the demonstration that systemic lymphokines can suppress other manifestations of cell-mediated immunity, in addition to cutaneous delayed hypersensitivity. Some candidates include the macrophage disappearance reaction, grafts, and possible local tumor rejection itself.

Regardless of the outcome of such studies, it is clear that lymphokines can act in a paradoxical manner, i.e., as suppressive agents. The mechanism of this reaction is not yet well understood. It appears likely that the cellular targets of the lymphokines (such as macrophages) that are effectors of cell-mediated immunity may be immobilized, activated, or otherwise preempted systemically and thus be relatively unavailable for reaction at the specific site of an evolving immunologic reaction.

SUMMARY AND CONCLUSIONS

Regulation of the immune response to tumors can occur at either the afferent or efferent limbs of that response. Mechanisms involving both have been described in a variety of experimental settings. One aspect relating to the terminal part of the efferent limb has received little attention. This relates to the induction of inflammatory reactions by the immune system. In this chapter we have discussed two ways in which this immunologically induced inflammatory response can be modulated, one involving inhibitors of leukotaxis and the other involving excess lymphokines. These represent prototypes for two kinds of regulatory activity. Regulation, in theory, can occur either via the participation of a variety of endogenous inhibitory factors, of which CFI is an example, or by the "spillover" of various excess mediators themselves into the general circulation. This latter affects local inflammatory reactions by preventing the establishment of local gradients and preempting and/or activating cells at inappropriate sites. These kinds of mechanisms are probably operative normally as sources of feedback control for inflammation. In addition, under pathological conditions, such as neoplastic disease, they may inadvertently limit host defense.

REFERENCES

1. Eilber, F. R., and Morton, D. L., *Cancer* **25,** 362 (1970).

2. Hughes, L. E., and Mackay, W. D., *Brit. Med. J.* **2,** 1346 (1965).

3. Johnson, M. W., Maibach, H. I., and Salmon, S. E., *N. Engl. J. Med.* **284,** 1255 (1971).

4. Fauvre, R. M., Kevin, B., Jacob, H., Gaillard, J. A., and Jacob, F., *Proc. Natl. Acad. Sci. USA,* **71** 4052 (1974).

5. Baum, J., in *The Phagocytic Cell in Host Resistance* (J. A. Bellanti and D. H. Dayton, eds.), Raven Press, New York, 1975, pp. 283–290.

6. Snyderman, R., and Stahl, C., in *The Phagocytic Cell in Host Resistance* (J. A. Bellanti and D. H. Dayton, eds.), Raven Press, New York, 1975, pp. 267–277.

7. Pike, M. C., and Snyderman, R., *Fed. Proc.* **35,** 388 (abstract) (1976).

8. Berenberg, J. L., and Ward, P. A., *J. Clin. Invest.* **52,** 1200 (1973).

9. Ward, P. A., and Berenberg, J. L., *N. Engl. J. Med.* **290,** 76 (1974).

10. Laneb, D., Pilney, F., Kelly, W. D., and Good, R. A., *J. Immunol.* **89,** 555 (1962).

11. Till, G., and Ward, P. A., *J. Immunol.* **114,** 843 (1975).

12. Ward, P. A., and Ozols, J., *J. Clin. Invest.* 1976 (in press)

13. Ward, P. A., and Rocklin, R. E., *J. Immunol.* **115,** 309 (1975).

14. Brozna, J. P., and Ward, P. A., *J. Clin. Invest.* **56,** 616 (1975).

15. Cohen, M. C., Brozna, J., Ward, P. A., and Cohen, S., *Fed. Proc.* **35,** 388 (abstract), (1976).

16. Yamamoto, K., and Takahashi, Y., *Nature* **233,** 261 (1971).

17. Salvin, S. B., Youngner, J. S., and Lederer, W. H., *Infect. Immun.* **7,** 68 (1973).

18. Yoshida, T., and Cohen, S., *J. Immunol.* **112,** 1540 (1974).

19. Sonozaki, H., Papermaster, V., Yoshida, T., and Cohen, S., *J. Immunol.* **115,** 1657 (1975).

20. Cohen, S., Fisher, B., Yoshida, T., and Bettigole, R. E., *N. Engl. J. Med.,* **290,** 882 (1974).

21. Yoshida, T., Sonozaki, H., and Cohen, S., *J. Exp. Med.* **138,** 784 (1973).

22. Rocklin, R. E., MacDermott, R. P., Chess, L., Schlossman, S. F., and David, J. R., *J. Exp. Med.* **140,** 1303 (1974).

23. Bloom, B. R., and Shevach, E., *J. Exp. Med.* **142,** 1306 (1975).

24. Yoshida, T., Edelson, R., Cohen, S., and Green, I., *J. Immunol.* **114,** 915 (1975).

Index